Applied Epidemiologic Principles and Concepts

This book provides practical knowledge to clinicians and biomedical researchers using biological and biochemical specimen/samples in order to understand
health and disease processes at cellular, clinical, and population levels. The
concepts and techniques provided will help researchers design and conduct
studies, then translate data from bench to clinics in an attempt to improve the
health of patients and populations. This book presents the extreme complexity of epidemiologic research in a concise manner that will address the issue
of confounders, thus allowing for more valid inferences and yielding results
that are more reliable and accurate.

Laurens Holmes Jr. was trained in internal medicine, specializing in immu-
nology and infectious diseases prior to his expertise in epidemiology-with-
biostatistics. Over the past two decades, Dr. Holmes had been working in
cancer epidemiology, control, and prevention. His involvement in chronic
disease epidemiology, control, and prevention includes signal amplification
and stratification in risk modeling and health disparities in hypertension, and
diabetes mellitus with large legacy (preexisting U.S. National Health Statistics
Center) data.

T0179042

Applied Epidemiologic Principles and Concepts

Clinicians' Guide to Study Design and Conduct

Laurens Holmes Jr., MD, DrPH

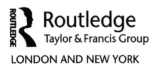

Routledge
Taylor & Francis Group

LONDON AND NEW YORK

First published 2018 by Routledge

2 Park Square, Milton Park, Abingdon, Oxon OX14 4RN
605 Third Avenue, New York, NY 10017

Routledge is an imprint of the Taylor & Francis Group, an informa business

First issued in paperback 2021

Library of Congress Cataloging-in-Publication Data

Names: Holmes, Larry, Jr., 1960- author.
Title: Applied epidemiologic principles and concepts : clinicians' guide to study design and conduct / Laurens Holmes Jr.
Description: Abingdon, Oxon ; New York, NY : Routledge, 2018. | Includes bibliographical references and index.
Identifiers: LCCN 2017018332| ISBN 9781498733786 (hardback) | ISBN 9781315369761 (ebook)
Subjects: | MESH: Epidemiologic Research Design
Classification: LCC RA651 | NLM WA 950 | DDC 614.4072--dc23
LC record available at https://lccn.loc.gov/2017018332

ISBN: 978-1-4987-3378-6 (hbk)
ISBN: 978-0-367-56008-9 (pbk)

*Dedicated to **Palmer Beasly, MD, MPH** (Dean Emeritus, UTSPH), and **James Steele, DVM, MPH** (Retired Assistant US Surgeon General and Professor Emeritus, UTSPH), both in memoriam!*

Contents

Foreword

Clinical medicine and surgery had evolved from the observation of individual patients to a group of patients and currently the examination of "big data" for clinical decision-making in improving care of our current and prospective patients. With this dynamic evolution comes challenges in design and appropriate interpretation of information generated from these large legacy data assessments. Specifically, for clinical research to benefit from the evolving technology in big data approach, clinicians and those working with patients to improve their care need to be properly informed on design, conduct, analysis, and interpretation of information from big data assessment.

Medicine and surgery continue to make advances by means of evidence judged to be objectively drawn from the care of individual patients. The natural observation of individuals remains the basis for our researchable questions' formulation and the subsequent hypothesis testing. The effectiveness of evidence-based medicine or surgery is dependent on how critical we are in evaluating evidence in order to inform our practice. However, these evaluations, no matter how objective, are never absolute; rather, they are probabilistic, as we will never know with absolute certainty how to treat a future patient who was not a part of our study. Despite the obstacles facing us today in attempting to provide an objective evaluation of our patients, since all of our decisions are based on judgment of some evidence, we have progressed from relying on expert opinion to the body of evidence accumulated from randomized, controlled clinical trials, as well as cohort investigations, prospective and retrospective.

Conducting a clinical trial yields more reliable and valid evidence from the data relative to nonexperimental or observational designs; however, although termed the *gold standard*, its validity depends on how well it is designed and conducted prior to outcome data collection, analysis, results, interpretation, and dissemination. The designs and techniques used to draw statistical inferences are often beyond the average clinician's understanding. A text that brings study conceptualization, hypothesis formulation, design, conduct, and analysis and interpretation of the results is long overdue and highly anticipated. Epidemiology is involved with design process, which is essential, since no amount of statistical modeling, no matter how sophisticated, can remove the error of design.

The text *Applied Epidemiologic Principles and Concepts* has filled this gap, not only in the way complex designs are explained but in the simplification of statistical concepts that had rarely been explained in such a way before. This text has been prepared intentionally to include rudimentary level information, so as to benefit clinicians who lack a sophisticated mathematical background or previous advanced knowledge of epidemiology, as well as other research-ers who may want to conduct clinical research and consumers of research products, who may benefit from the design process explained in this book. It is with this expectation and enthusiasm that we recommend this text to clini-cians in all fields of clinical, biomedical, and population-based research. The examples provided by the author to simplify designs and research methods are familiar to surgeons, as well as to clinicians in other specialties of medicine.

Although statistical inference is essential in our application of the research findings to clinical decision-making regarding the care of our patients, it alone, without clinical relevance or importance, can be very misleading or even meaningless. The author has attempted to deemphasize p value in the interpretation of epidemiologic or clinical research findings by stressing the importance of effect size and confidence intervals, which allow for the quan-tification of evidence and precision, respectively. For example, a large study, due to a large sample size as big data that minimizes variability, may show a statistically significant difference which, in reality, the effect size is too insig-nificant to warrant any clinical importance. In contrast, the results of a small study, such as is frequently seen in clinical trials or surgical research, may have a large effect on clinical relevance but not be statistically significant at ($p > 0.05$). Thus, without considering the magnitude of the effect size with the confidence interval, we tend to regard these studies as negative findings, which is erroneous, since absence of evidence, based simply on an arbitrary significance level of 5%, does not necessarily mean evidence of absence.[1] In effect, clinical research results cannot be adequately interpreted without con-sidering the biologic and clinical significance of the data before the statistical stability of the findings (p value and 95% confidence interval), since p value, as observed by the authors, merely reflects the size of the study and not the measure of evidence.

In recommending this text, it is our hope that this book will benefit cli-nicians, research fellows, clinical fellows, graduate interns, doctoral, post-doctoral students in medical and clinical settings, nurses, clinical research coordinators, physical therapists, and all those involved in designing and conducting clinical research and analyzing research data for statistical and clinical relevance. Convincingly, knowledge gained from this text will lead to improvement of patient care through well-conceptualized research. Therefore, with the knowledge that no book is complete, no matter its content or volume, especially a book of this nature, which is prepared to guide clinicians and others involved in clinical and medical research on design, conduct, analysis, and interpretation of findings, we contend that this book will benefit clinicians and others who are interested in applying appropriate design to research conduct, analysis, and interpretation of findings.

Finally, we are optimistic that this book will bridge the gap between knowledge and practice of clinical research, especially for clinicians in a busy practice who are passionate about making a difference in their patients' care through research and education.

Kirk Dabney, MD, MHCDS
Associate Director
Cerebral Palsy Program
and Clinical Director
Health Equity & Inclusion Office
Nemours/A.I. duPont Hospital for Children
Wilmington, Delaware

Richard Bowen, MD
Former Chairman
Orthopedic Department
A.I. duPont Hospital for Children
Wilmington, Delaware

1. D. G. Altman and J. M. Bland, "Absence of Evidence Is Not Evidence of Absence," *BMJ* 311 (1995): 485.

Preface

We often conceive of epidemiology in either simplistic or complex terms, and neither of these is accurate. To illustrate this, complexities in epidemiology could be achieved by considering a study to determine the correlation between serum lipid profile as total cholesterol, high-density lipoprotein, low-density lipoprotein, triglycerides, and total body fatness or obesity measured by body mass index (BMI) in children. Two laboratories measured serum lipid profile and one observed a correlation with BMI while the other did not. Which is the reliable finding? Could these differences reflect interlaboratory variability or sampling error? To address this question, one needs to examine the context of blood drawing since fasting blood levels may provide a better indicator of serum lipid. Epidemiologic studies could be easily derailed given the inability to identify and address possible confounding. Therefore, understanding the principles and concepts used in epidemiologic studies' design and conduct to answer clinical research questions facilitates accurate and reliable findings in these areas. Another similar example in a health fair setting involved geography and health, termed *healthography*. The risk of dying in one zip code, A, was 59.5 per 100,000 and the other zip code, B, was 35.4 per 100,000. There is a common sense and nonepidemiologic tendency to conclude that there is increased risk of dying in zip code A. To arrive at such inference, one must first find out the age distribution of these two zip codes since advancing age is associated with increased mortality. Indeed, zip code A is comparable to the US population while zip code B is the Mexican population. These two examples are indicative of the need to understand epidemiologic concepts such as confounding by age or effect measure modification prior to undertaking a clinical or translational research.

This textbook describes the basics of research in medical and clinical settings as well as the concepts and application of epidemiologic designs in research conduct. Design transcends statistical techniques, and no matter how sophisticated a statistical modeling, errors of design/sampling cannot be corrected. The author of this textbook has presented a complex field in a very simplified and reader-friendly manner with the intent that such presentation will facilitate the understanding of design process and epidemiologic thinking in clinical research. Additionally, this book provides a very basic explanation of how to examine the data collected from research conduct, the possibility of confounders, and how to address such confounders, thus disentangling such effects for reliable and valid inference on the association between exposure and the outcome of interest.

Research is presented as an exercise around measurement, with measurement error inevitable in its conduct, hence the inherent uncertainties of all findings in clinical and medical research. *Applied Epidemiologic Principles and Concepts* covers research conceptualization, namely, research objectives, questions, hypothesis, design, sampling, implementation, data collection, analysis, results, and interpretation. While the primary focus of epidemiology is to assess the relationship between exposure (risk or predisposing factor) and outcome (disease or health-related event), causal association is presented in a simplified manner, including the role of quantitative evidence synthesis (QES) in causal inference. Epidemiology has evolved over the past three decades, resulting in several fields being developed. This text presents in brief the perspectives and future of epidemiology in the era of the molecular basis of medicine, big data, "3 Ts," and systems science. Epidemiologic evidence is more reliable if conceptualized and conducted within the context of translational, transdisciplinary, and team science. With molecular epidemiology, we are better equipped with tools to identify molecular, genetic, and cellular indicators of risk as well as biologic alterations in the early stages of disease, and with 3 Ts and systems science, we are more capable of providing more accurate and reliable inference on causality and outcomes research. Further, the author argues that unless sampling error and confounding are identified and addressed, clinical and translational research findings will remain largely inconsistent, implying inconsequential epidemiology. Epidemiology is further challenged in creating a meaningful collegiality in the process of evidence discovery with the intent to improve population and patient health. Despite all the efforts of traditional epidemiologic methods and approach today, risk factors for many diseases and health outcomes are not fully understood. As a basic science of public health and clinical medicine, and with the ongoing emphasis on social determinants of health, advanced epidemiologic methods require team science and translational approach to embrace socio-epigenomics and genomics in risk identification and risk adapted intervention mapping.

Appropriate knowledge of research conceptualization, design, and statistical inference is essential for conducting clinical and biomedical research. This knowledge is acquired through the understanding of nonexperimental and experimental epidemiologic designs and the choice of the appropriate test statistic for statistical inference. However, regardless of how sophisticated the statistical technique employed for statistical inference is, study conceptualization and design mainly adequate sampling process are the building blocks of valid and reliable scientific evidence. Since clinical research is performed to improve patients' care, it remains relevant to assess not only the statistical significance but also the clinical and biologic importance of the findings, for clinical decision-making in the care of an individual patient. Therefore, the aim of this book is to provide clinicians, biomedical researchers, graduate students in research methodology, students of public health, and all those involved in clinical/translational research with a simplified but concise overview of the principles and practice of epidemiology. In addition, the author stresses common flaws in the conduct, analysis, and interpretation of epidemiologic study.

Valid and reliable scientific research is that which considers the following elements in arriving at the truth from the data, namely, biological relevance, clinical importance, and statistical stability and precision (statistical inference based on the *p* value and the 90%, 95%, and 99% confidence interval).

The interpretation of results of new research must rely on factual association or effect and the alternative explanation, namely, systematic error, random error (precision), confounding, and effect measure modifier. Therefore, unless these perspectives are disentangled, the results from any given research cannot be considered valid and reliable. However, even with this disentanglement, all study findings remain inconclusive with some degree of uncertainty, hence the random error quantification (*p* value).

This book presents a comprehensive guide on how to conduct clinical and medical research—mainly, research question formulation, study implementation, hypothesis testing using appropriate test statistics to analyze the data, and results interpretation. In so doing, it attempts to illustrate the basic concepts used in study conceptualization, epidemiologic design, and appropriate test statistics for statistical inference from the data. Therefore, although statistical inference is emphasized throughout the presentation in this text, equal emphasis is placed on clinical relevance or importance and biological relevance in the interpretation of the study results.

Specifically, this book describes in basic terms and concepts how to conduct clinical and medical research using epidemiologic designs. The author presents epidemiology as the main profession in the transdisciplinary and team science approaches to the understanding of complex ecologic model of disease and health. Clinicians, even those without preliminary or infantile knowledge of epidemiologic designs, could benefit immensely on what, when, where, who, and how studies are conceptualized, data collected as planned with the scale of measurement of the outcome and independent variables, data edited, cleaned and processed prior to analysis, appropriate analysis based on statistical assumptions and rationale, results tabulation for scientific appraisal, and results interpretation and inference. Unlike most epidemiologic texts, this is one of the few books that attempts to simplify complex epidemiologic methods for users of epidemiologic research namely clinicians. Additionally, it is rare to find an epidemiology textbook with integration of basic research methodology into epidemiologic designs. Finally, research innovation and the current challenges of epidemiology are presented in this book to reflect the currency of the materials and the approach.

A study could be statistically significant but biologically and clinically irrelevant, since the statistical stability of a study does not rule out bias and confounding. The *p* value is deemphasized, while the use of effect size or magnitude and confidence intervals in the interpretation of results for application in clinical decision-making is recommended. The use of *p* value as the measure of evidence could lead to an erroneous interpretation of the effectiveness of a treatment. For example, studies with large sample sizes and very little or insignificant effects of no clinical importance may be statistically significant, while studies with small samples though a large magnitude of effects are labeled "negative result."[1] Such results are due to low statistical power and increasing variability, hence the inability to pass the arbitrary litmus test of the 5% significance level.

Epidemiology Conceptualized

Epidemiologic investigation and practice, as old as the history of modern medicine, date back to Hippocrates (circa 2,400 years ago). In recommending the appropriate practice of medicine, Hippocrates appealed to the physicians' ability to understand the role of environmental factors in predisposition to disease and health in the community. During the Middle Ages and the Renaissance, epidemiologic principles continued to influence the practice of medicine, as demonstrated in *De Morbis Artificum* (1713) by Ramazinni and the works on scrotal cancer in relation to chimney sweeps by Percival Pott in 1775.

With the works of John Snow, a British physician (1854), on cholera mortality in London, the era of scientific epidemiology began. By examining the distribution/pattern of mortality and cholera in London, Snow postulated that cholera was caused by contaminated water.

Epidemiology Today

There are several definitions of epidemiology, but a practical definition is necessary for the understanding of this human science. Epidemiology is the basic science of public health. The objective of this discipline is to assess the distribution and determinants of disease, disabilities, injuries, natural disasters (tsunamis, hurricanes, tornados, and earthquakes) and health-related events at the population level. Epidemiologic investigation or research focuses on a specific population. The basic issue is to assess the groups of people at higher risk: women, children, men, pregnant women, teenagers, whites, African Americans, Hispanics, Asians, poor, affluent, gay, lesbians, transgender, married, single, older individuals, obese/overweight etc. Epidemiology also examines the frequency of the disease or the event of interest changes over time. In addition, epidemiology examines the variation of the disease of interest from place to place. Simply, descriptive epidemiology attempts to address the distribution of disease with respect to "who," "when," and "where." For example, cancer epidemiologists attempt to describe the occurrence of prostate cancer by observing the differences in populations due to age, socioeconomic status, occupation, geographic locale, race/ethnicity, etc. Epidemiology also attempts to address the association between the disease (outcome) and exposure (risk factor). For example, why are some men at high risk for prostate cancer? Does race/ethnicity increase the risk for prostate cancer? Simply, is the association causal or spurious? This process involves the effort to determine whether a factor (exposure) is associated with the disease (outcome). In the example with prostate cancer, such exposure includes a high-fat diet, race/ethnicity, advancing age, pesticides, family history of prostate cancer, and so on. Whether or not the association is factual or a result of chance remains the focus of epidemiologic research. The questions to be raised are as follows: Is prostate cancer associated with pesticides? Does pesticide cause prostate cancer?

Epidemiology often goes beyond disease-exposure association or relationship to establish causal association (association to causation). In this process of causal inference, it depends on certain criteria, one of which is the strength or magnitude of association, leading to the recommendation of preventive measures. However, complete knowledge of the causal mechanism is not necessary prior to preventive measures for disease control. Further, findings from epidemiologic research facilitate the prioritization of health issues and the development and implementation of intervention programs for disease control and health promotion.

This book is conceptually organized in three sections. Section I deals with research methods and epidemiologic complexities in terms of design and analysis, Section II deals with epidemiologic designs, as well as causal inference, while Section III delves into perspectives, epidemiologic challenges, and special topics in epidemiology, namely, epidemiologic tree, challenges, emerging fields, consequentialist perspective of epidemiology and epidemiologic role in health and healthcare policy formulation. Throughout this book, attempts are made to describe the research methods and nonexperimental as well as experimental designs. Section I comprises research methods and design complexities with an attempt to describe the following:

- Research objectives and purposes
- Research questions
- Hypothesis statements: null and alternative
- Rationales for research, clinical reasoning, and diagnostic tests
- Study conceptualization and conduct—research question, data collection, data management, hypothesis testing, data analysis
- Confounding
- Effect measure modification
- Diagnostic and screening test

Section II comprises the epidemiologic study designs with an attempt to describe the basic notion of epidemiology and the designs used in clinical research:

- The notion of epidemiology and the measures of disease occurrence/ frequency and the measure of disease association/effect
- Ecologic studies
- Cross-sectional designs
- Case-control studies
- Cohort studies: prospective, retrospective, and ambidirectional
- Clinical trials or experimental designs
- QES, meta-analysis, scientific study appraisal, and causal inference

Section III consists of perspectives, challenges, future, and special topics in epidemiology in illustrating the purposive role of epidemiology in facilitating the goal of public health, mainly disease control and health promotion. Additionally, this section presents the integrative dimension of epidemiology.

- Epidemiologic perspectives: advances, challenges, emerging fields, and the future
- Consequentialist epidemiology
- Role of epidemiology in health and healthcare policy formulation

Section I has five chapters. The first two chapters deal with the basic descriptions of scientific research at the clinical and population levels and how the knowledge gained from the population could be applied to the understanding of individual patients in the future. The attempt is made in these chapters to discuss clinical reasoning and the use of diagnostic tests (sensitivity and specificity) in clinical decision-making. The notions, numbers needed to treat, and numbers needed to harm are discussed later in the chapter on causal inference. These chapters delve into clinical research conceptualization, design involving subject recruitment, variable ascertainment, data collection, data management, data analysis, and the outline of the research proposal.

In Section II, epidemiologic principles and methods are presented with the intent to stress the importance of a careful design in conducting clinical research. Epidemiology remains the basic science of clinical medicine and public health that deals with disease, disabilities, injury, and health-related event distributions and determinants and the application of this knowledge to the control and prevention of disease, disabilities, injuries, and related health events at the population level. Depending on the research question and whether or not the outcome (disease or event of interest) has occurred prior to the commencement of the study or the investigator assigns subjects to treatment or control, an appropriate design is selected for the clinical research. The measures of effects or point estimates are discussed with concrete examples to illustrate the application of epidemiologic principles in arriving at a reliable and valid result. Designs are illustrated with flow charts, figures, and boxes for distinctions and similarities. The hierarchy of study design is demonstrated with randomized clinical trial (RCT) and the associated meta-analysis and QES as the design that yields the most reliable and valid evidence from data. Although RCTs are considered the "gold standard" of clinical research, it is sometimes not feasible to use this design because of ethical considerations, hence the alternative need for prospective cohort design.

Interpreting research findings is equally as essential as conducting the study itself. Interpretation of research findings must be informative and constructive in order to identify future research needs. A research result cannot be considered valid unless we disentangle the role of bias and confounding from a statistically significant finding, as a result can be statistically significant and yet driven by measurement, selection, and information bias as well as confounding. While my background in basic medical sciences and clinical medicine (internal medicine) allows me to appreciate the importance of biologic and clinical relevance in the interpretation of research findings, biostatisticians without similar training must look beyond random variation (p value and confidence interval) in the interpretation and utilization of clinical and translational research findings. Therefore, quantifying the random error with p value (a meaningful null hypothesis with a strong case against the null hypothesis requires the use of significance level) without a confidence interval deprives the reader of the ability to assess the clinical importance of the range of values in the interval. Using Fisher's arbitrary p value cutoff point for type I error (alpha level) tolerance, a p value of 0.05 need not provide strong evidence against the null hypothesis, but p less than 0.0001 does.[2] The precise p value should be presented, without reference to arbitrary thresholds. Therefore, results of clinical and translational research should not be presented as "significant" or "nonsignificant" but should be interpreted in the context of the type of study and other available evidence. Second, systematic error and confounding should always be considered for findings with low p values, as well as the potentials for effect measure modifier (if any) in the explanation of the results. Neyman and Pearson describe their accurate observation:

> No test based upon a theory of probability can by itself provide any valuable evidence of the truth or falsehood of a hypothesis. But we may look at the puvrpose of tests from another viewpoint. Without hoping to know whether each separate hypothesis is true or false, we may search for rules to govern our behavior with regard to them, in following which we insure that, in the long run of experience, we shall not often be wrong.[3]

This text is expected to provide practical knowledge to clinicians and translationists, implying all researchers using biological and biochemical specimen or samples in an attempt to understand health and diseases processes at cellular (preclinical and laboratory), clinical, and population levels, additionally all those who translate such data from bench to clinics in an attempt to improve the health and well-being of the patients they see.

Specifically, this book describes in basic terms and concepts how to conduct clinical research using epidemiologic designs. The author presents epidemiology as the main discipline so to speak in the transdisciplinary and translational approaches to the understanding of complex ecologic model of disease and health. Clinicians, even those without preliminary or those with infantile knowledge of epidemiologic designs, could benefit immensely from this text, namely, on what, when, where, who, and how studies are conceptualized; data collected as planned with the scale of measurement of the outcome and independent variables; data edited, cleaned, and processed prior to analysis; appropriate analysis based on statistical assumptions and rationale; results tabulation for scientific appraisal; and result interpretation and inference. Unlike most epidemiologic texts, this is one of the few books that attempt to simplify complex epidemiologic methods for users of epidemiologic research namely clinicians. Additionally, it is extremely rare to access a book with integration of basic research methodology into epidemiologic designs. Finally, research innovation and the current challenges of epidemiology are presented in this book to reflect the currency of the materials and the approach.

Epidemiology is an ever-changing discipline. The author has consulted with data judged to be accurate at the moment of the presentation of these materials for publication. However, due to rapid changes in risk factor identification and biomarkers of disease, the limitations of human knowledge, and the possibility of errors, the author wishes to be insulated from any responsibility due to error arising from the use of this text. Since epidemiology is an inexact science and scientific knowledge is cumulative, indicative of the need for replication science in our continuous effort to improve health, caution must be applied in the use and application of the information in this text. Therefore, readers are advised to consult with other sources of similar data for the confirmation of the information therein.

1. D. G. Altman and J. M. Bland, "Absence of Evidence Is Not Evidence of Absence," *BMJ* 311 (1995): 485.
2. R. A. Fisher, *Statistical Methods and Scientific Inference* (London: Collins Macmillan, 1973).
3. J. Neyman and E. Pearson, "On the Problem of the Most Efficient Tests of Statistical Hypotheses," *Philos Trans Roy Soc A* 231 (1933): 289–337.

Acknowledgments

In preparing this book, so many people contributed directly or indirectly to the materials provided here. In order to make this book practical, data collected from different studies were used. I wish to express sincere gratitude to those who permitted the use of their data to illustrate the design techniques used in this book.

The attempt to create a simplified book in epidemiology remains challenging because of variability in the epidemiologic reasoning of those who require such materials. The simplification, so to speak, of the design process in evidence in clinical research came from my interaction with research and clinical fellows at the Nemours Orthopedic Department, who worked with me and gave me the reason to write this book. They are Drs. K. Durga, M. Ali, S. Joo, T. Palocaren, T. Haumont, M.J. Cornes, A. Tahbet, A. Atanda, J. Connor, M. Oto, M. Kadhim, and A. Karatas. The clinical research fellows and surgical residents in the orthopedic department also motivated the preparation of this text. Thank you for your interest in the evidence-based journal club.

My colleagues at the Nemours Orthopedic Department, Nemours Center for Childhood Cancer Research, and the University of Delaware, College of Health Sciences, also inspired this preparation via questions on study design, sample size, and power estimations, p value and confidence interval (CI) interpretation, and the preference of 95% CI to p value in terms of statistical stability. They are Drs. Richard Bowen, Kirk Dabney, Suken Shah, Tariq Rahman, George Dodge, Pete Gabos, Freeman Miller, Richard Kruse, Nahir Thacker, Kenneth Rogers, William Mackenzie, Sigrid Rajaskaren, Raj Rajasekaren, Paul Pitel, Jim Richards, and Stephen Stanhope.

I am indebted in a special way to peers in epidemiology and translational science, namely, Professor Bradley Pollock (UCDavis), Professor Reza Shaker (MCW), Professor Barry Borman (Massey University, NZ), and Professor Kenneth Rothman (Boston University), and for those not mentioned here, for the encouragement to present this material in a special setting, clinical and translational science environment.

I am unable to express adequately my gratitude to my kids (Maddy, Mackenzie, Landon, Aiden, and Devin) for their understanding and acceptance of the time I spent away from them to work on this book. To my siblings (Brian, Victor, Paul, Anne, and Julie), cousins (Victor, Charles, and Eka), nephews, aunts, uncles, and colleagues (Drs. Doriel Ward and Orysla Garrison, among others), I sincerely acknowledge what you all mean to me and will continue to mean to me in my aggressive intellectual search to make sense out of data by dedicating time and effort to educating and informing those in clinical research on how to draw inference and combine it with clinical importance in decision-making to improve patients' care.

Laurens Holmes, Jr.

Author

Laurens (Larry) Holmes, Jr., educated at the Catholic University of Rome, Italy; the University of the Health Sciences, Antigua; School of Medicine, University of Amsterdam, Faculty of Medicine; and the University of Texas, Texas Medical Center, School of Public Health, is a former chief epidemiologist (Orthopedic Department), head of the Epidemiology Laboratory at the Nemours Center for Childhood Cancer Research, and principal research scientist at the Nemours/A.I. DuPont Children's Hospital, Office of Health Equity & Inclusion. He is also an adjunct professor of clinical trials and molecular epidemiology in the Department of Biological Sciences, University of Delaware, Newark, Delaware.
He is recognized for his work on epidemiology and control of prostate cancer but has also published papers on other aspects of hormone-related malignancies and cardiovascular and chronic disease epidemiology utilizing various statistical methods, including the log binomial family, exact logistic model, and probability estimation from the logistic model by margin. Dr. Holmes is a strong proponent of reality in the statistical modeling of cancer and nonexperimental research data, where he presents on the rationale for tabular analysis in most nonexperimental research data, which are often not randomly sampled (probability sampling), rendering statistical inference application meaningless to such data. Since controlling for known confounders of variabilities in subgroup health and healthcare outcomes often fails to remove or explain these imbalances, a feasible alternative is to consider subgroup biologic/cellular events/molecular level variances or differences. Molecular epidemiology needs to focus on validation and characterization of biomarkers of risk/predisposition, severity, and progression as well as prognosis by race/ethnicity and sex. Professor Holmes's ongoing research is on the assessment of molecular determinants of racial/ethnic as well as sex disparities in disease incidence, prevalence, severity, progression, prognosis, and mortality. One of the biostatistical approaches to addressing valid inference in biomedical and clinical research is a model that amplifies signals in the data before risk stratification, implying the role of biostatistics as a tool in scientific evidence discovery—*"data signal amplification and risk stratification"*—was proposed by Dr. Holmes.

Section I

Basic research design principles and study inference

We often conceive epidemiology in either simplistic or complex terms, and neither of these is accurate. To illustrate these complexities in epidemiology, consider a study to determine the correlation between serum lipid and total body fatness or obesity in children. If two laboratories measured serum lipid and one observed a correlation while the other did not, which is the reliable finding? To address this question, one needs to examine the context of blood drawing since fasting blood level (FBL) may provide a better indicator of serum lipid as well as the size of the sample (patients or participants). Epidemiologic studies could be easily derailed given the inability to identify and address possible confounding such as FBL and non-FBL sample as well as sampling error (representative sample). Therefore, understanding the principles and concepts used in epidemiologic studies design and conduct to answer clinical research questions facilitate accurate and reliable evidence discovery in clinical medicine and public health. Another similar example in a health care setting involves geography or place and health, termed "healthography." The risk of dying in one zip code, A, was 59.5 per 100,000 and in the other zip code, B, was 35.4 per 100,000. There is a common sense and nonepidemiologic tendency to conclude that there is increased risk of dying in zip code A. To arrive at such inference, one must first find out the age distribution of these two zip codes since advancing age is associated with increased risk or dying or mortality. Indeed, zip code A is comparable to the US population, while zip code B is the Mexican population. These two examples are indicative of the need to understand epidemiologic concepts prior to undertaking a clinical or translational research.

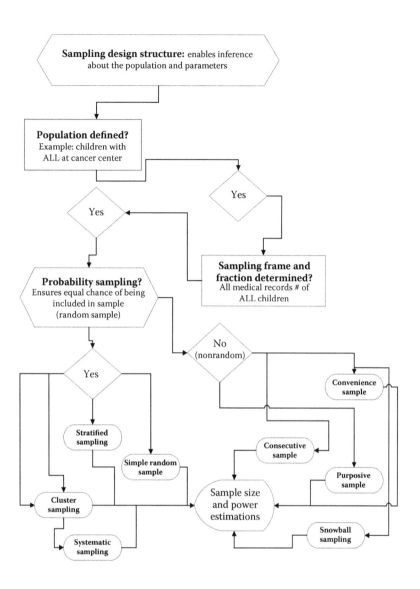

1 Epidemiologic research conceptualization and rationale

1.1 Introduction

Research remains an exercise around measurement, with measurement error inevitable in its conduct, hence the inherent uncertainties of all findings in clinical and translational research. Research conceptualization, namely, research objectives, questions, hypothesis, design, implementation, data collection, analysis, results, and interpretation, requires careful planning and execution. While the primary focus of epidemiology is to assess the relationship between exposure (risk or predisposing factor) and outcome (disease or health-related event), causal association depends on the ability to design, conduct, and replicate studies for patterns and direction of evidence.

Scientific research is a systematic, controlled, empirical, and critical investigation of natural phenomena guided by theories and hypotheses about the presumed relations among them.[1-3] Consequently, research implies an organized and systematic way of finding solutions to questions.[4] This attempt requires that solutions to the postulated questions be approached when it is feasible, interesting, novel, ethical, and relevant.[2] Clinical research thus involves three basic elements:

1 Conceptualization
2 Design process
3 Statistical inference

As will be discussed further in this text, fundamental thinking in clinical research involves these elements:

a Biologic relevance
b Clinical importance
c Statistical stability

The statistical inference allows conclusions to be drawn from data because the entire population is never studied. The combination of this tripartite approach to evidence discovery from the data remains the cornerstone of valid and reliable results from clinical studies and their cautious interpretation in the attempt to improve patient care.

Conducting research involves planning, and that requires the measurement and quantification of the variables in the study, careful administration of well-designed instruments, data collection, appropriate analysis, and the interpretation of results. Depending on the research question and the type of design, this process could be very time-consuming and complex. For example, in clinical trials, an elaborate protocol for participants' enrollment, randomization, and treatment administration is used to ensure appropriate documentation of events during the trial.

The materials in this chapter will enable readers to understand research conceptualization and the distinction between clinical population medicine and epidemiology as well as their implications in epidemiologic/population-based clinical and biomedical research. This chapter, as a brief overview of research processes, focuses on the description of terms applied in research conceptualization and provides practical examples—process of research conduct, research objectives, purpose of research, research questions, hypotheses, and the description of clinical and population medicine within a research context (Figure 1.1).

1.2   Structure and function of research

Conducting research involves several processes (Figure 1.2):

a   *A well-defined problem statement, research questions, purposes, and potential benefits of the study to science, society, and humanity*

For example, one may formulate a research question around the effectiveness of treatment in improving some pathologic conditions—does cervical spine surgery stabilize the spine in children with skeletal dysplasia (SKD)? Clinicians and biomedical researchers should realize that research questions are not study topics, since such topics are generally broad and research questions must be very specific. Specifically, research questions should be formulated in such a way that they can be answered by observable evidence. Therefore, unless the research question is feasible, it cannot answer the question posed in a measurable manner.

b   *Identification of the theory and assumptions and a search of background literature to address the magnitude of the problem*

Such a literature review is aimed at identifying what has been done in terms of previous research, the gap in literature, and what the proposed study intends to add or contribute to the existing body of knowledge in the field. It is a common mistake made by novice researchers to avoid the intensive literature review of the subject of their interest until the research question and study designs are formulated. We caution against such an approach since there is a possibility

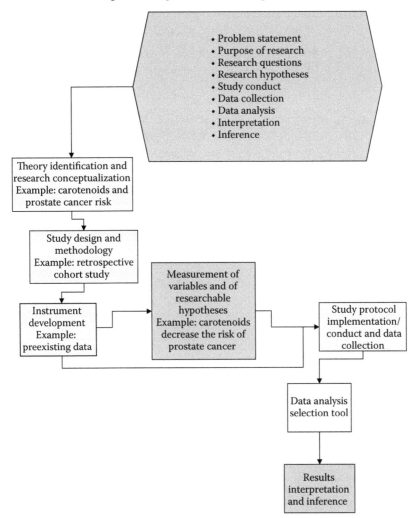

Figure 1.1 Design process and function.

that such questions have already been answered. It may lead to a study that is not novel and hence will have very little to offer to science in medicine.

c *Measurement of variables and statement of researchable hypotheses*

Research is basically an exercise with measurement, which is always subject to errors. Good research aims, therefore, at minimizing measurement error, thus reducing variability in what is being measured.

d *Identification of the appropriate study design and methodology to fit the research question or hypothesis*

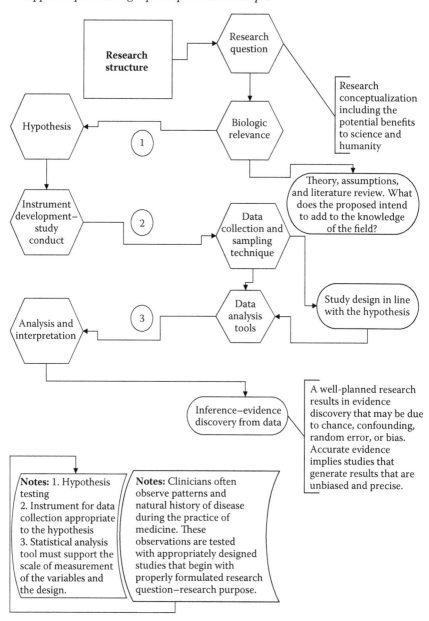

Figure 1.2 Research structure.

For example, in the previously mentioned illustration with cervical spine surgery and SKD, the selected design may be the one that involves the administration of surgery to all patients with SKD, which makes it a single sample design with repeated measure. The design could be prospective or retrospective (these terms will be defined and clarified later in the text).

e *Development of an instrument for data gathering and identifying an appropriate sampling technique*

Since the generalization of findings requires probability sampling of study subjects prior to baseline or preoperative data collection, the sample must be drawn from the population of patients with the same condition. Practically, every sample in the study must have a nonzero probability of being selected for the study.

f *Selection of data analysis tools or statistical techniques to test the hypothesis or answer the research question and presentation of results and interpretation*

For example, in the illustration with SKD, the null hypothesis may be that cervical spine surgery does not stabilize the spine in children with SKD. In testing this hypothesis, one can use a paired *t*-test or repeated-measure analysis of variance (ANOVA) if two or more than two measurement times were used and the outcome was measured on a continuous scale. These tests will be explained later in the text.

g *Offering conclusions that are based on the data as well as what the data suggests and recommendations*[5-7]

1.3   Objective of study/research purpose

Research conceptualization begins with the purpose of the study, which is a statement that describes the intent and the direction of the study.[2,5] The purpose statement or purpose of a study is the rationale behind the study.[5,8] Although the purpose of the study is often used interchangeably with the research question or the problem statement, they are distinct entities and should be very clearly differentiated in the proposal development and manuscript preparation phases of the study. Simply, the purpose of the study describes the objectives, intent,[5] and aims of the study. The research question therefore remains a specific statement that needs to be answered, following the hypothesis testing in quantitative research.

In clinical, epidemiologic, or biomedical research, the purpose of a study is the statement of the overall objective of the study. This statement identifies the independent and response variables as well as how the variables will be measured and the design to be used to achieve the expected relationship, correlation, or association. In published articles, we often use words and phrases such as *relationship, mean comparison, effectiveness, efficacy*, and *association* to express the nexus or link between the response, outcome, or dependent variable and the independent, predictor, explanatory, or antecedent variable. For example, in the previous illustration, the purpose of the study may be stated as, "To examine the effectiveness of cervical spine surgery in stabilizing the spine in children with SKD."

The *objective* of a study is a concise statement describing the intent of the research. Such objectives can be evaluated from several standpoints or dimensions. For example, if the objective of a study is to assess the role of electrocautery in the development of deep wound infection in pediatric patients with neuromuscular scoliosis and electrocautery cannot be measured directly but is dependent on an "indirect measure termed proxy," then it is not a good study objective. Therefore, in clinical, experimental, and nonexperimental studies, a good study objective is that which is measurable.[8] For example, if the objective of a study was to examine the effectiveness and safety of posterior spine fusion in correcting curve deformities and maintaining correction in children with leukodystrophy (degenerative disease of the white matter of the brain), the measurement of the effectiveness would be the postoperative reduction in the major curve angles (thoracic and thoracolumbar curves), while safety will be measured by less complications (psuedoathrosis, instrument failure, and screw pull out) following surgery.

In practice, while the purpose of the study may not be easily differentiated from the objective, the research question remains a concise statement about the study objective. A research question's purpose is to imply what issue the research will address. Similarly, the purpose of the study is a broad scope of what the study intends to accomplish in terms of benefits to society, medicine, and science (Figure 1.3).

BOX 1.1   STUDY OBJECTIVE/RESEARCH PURPOSE

- Purpose of study—why the study was conducted (completed study) or will be conducted (proposal).
- Intent of the study—the motivation for the study
- Expression of the main idea or concept behind the study
- Identification of independent and dependent variables in biomedical and epidemiologic studies
- Hypothetical example: The purpose of the study was to determine the risk of deep wound infection (outcome/response/dependent variable) associated with the intraoperative cell server (independent/predictor/explanatory variable) following spine fusion in children with cerebral palsy, using retrospective cohort design (case-only).
- Often stated in the last paragraph of the introduction section of original articles in published manuscripts.

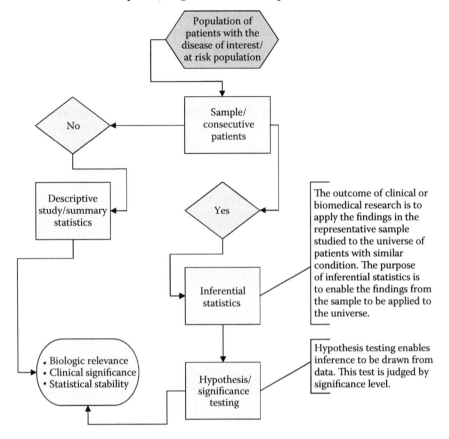

Figure 1.3 Research evidence discovery.

1.4   Research questions and study hypotheses

1.4.1   *Research questions*

Fundamental to clinical research is a clear statement of the question proposed to be answered. This question should be carefully selected and clearly defined prior to beginning to conduct research.[9] For example, a research question may be framed in the context of trying to determine whether a new treatment, compared with the current or standard treatment, reduces the risk of coronary heart disease (CHD). Research questions could be primary or secondary. The primary question refers to the main outcome of the study.[9] For example, "Does angiotensin converting enzyme (ACE) inhibitor reduce the incidence of CHD?" A secondary research question aimed at a secondary outcome may assess physical activities or look at racial/ethnic variation in the response to ACE inhibitor. For example, the secondary research question may be stated as, "Are there racial/ethnic differences in CHD incidence reduction following ACE inhibitor use?" Yet another example of a primary research question may be, "Does ADT prolong the survival of elderly men diagnosed with prostate cancer (CaP)?" and the secondary question may be, "Is there a difference in CaP survival in elderly men diagnosed with loco-regional versus metastatic disease?" (Figure 1.4).

Depending on the research question, participants may be randomly assigned to different treatments or procedures. This approach, which is called a human experiment or clinical trial, will be discussed at some length in the upcoming section on design. If a clinical trial is not feasible (ethical considerations), the researcher may collect data on participants (independent, dependent, or response variables and confounding) and conduct a nonexperimental study.

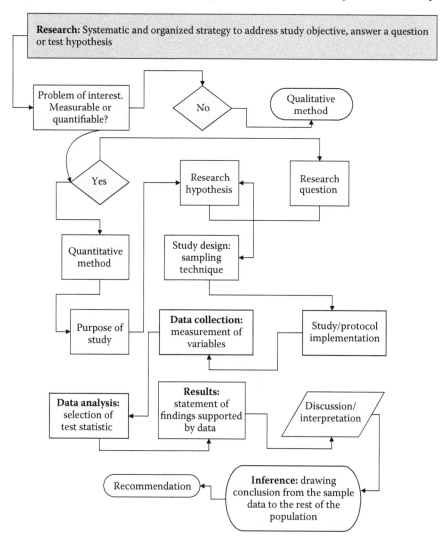

Figure 1.4 Basic elements of research.

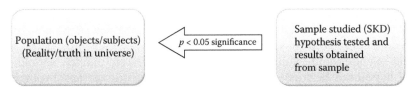

Figure 1.5 Generalizability of study finding to the targeted population.

The information on confounding variables is collected in order to statistically control for the influence of the confounding on the response, dependent, or outcome variable (nonexperimental studies' results may be influenced by selection biases and confounding if not minimized and controlled for respectively). If the intent is to generalize from the research participants to a larger population, as is often the case in epidemiologic (nonexperimental) and experimental studies, the investigator will utilize probability sampling to select participants (sampling technique). This approach allows every study subject the same probability of being selected from the general population for inclusion in the study sample and the variables to be studied to be termed "random variables" (suitable for hypothesis testing).[10,11] In such a situation, statistical inference can then be applied to the study, implying the generalization of the findings beyond the sample studied to the larger population (Figure 1.5).

1.4.2   Study hypothesis

Hypothesis testing is essential in quantitative study designs.[7] The hypothesis of a study is a statement that provides the basis for the examination of the significance of the findings.[2] Whenever an investigator wishes to make a statement beyond the sample data (descriptive statistics) or simply draw an inference from the data, hypothesis testing is required. A hypothesis is a statement about the population or simply the universe/world that is testable. An example of a hypothesis statement could be, "Selenium in combination with vitamin D decreases the risk of CaP." To assess this association, the investigator needs to examine the data for evidence against the null hypothesis. If the data provide evidence against the null hypothesis (no association), the null hypothesis is rejected; in contrast, if data fail to provide evidence against the null hypothesis, the null hypothesis is not rejected, thus negating any inclination to the alternative hypothesis of association between the response and independent variable.[12] While hypotheses will be described more in this text's companion, the biostatistics, it serves to note here that hypothesis testing includes the following:

a   Generation of the study hypothesis and the definition of the null hypothesis
b   Determination of the level below which results are considered statistically significant, implying α level 0.05
c   Identification and selection of the appropriate statistical test for determining whether to accept or reject the null hypothesis

In determining whether or not an association exists, the investigator must first assume that the null hypothesis is true and then determine how likely the data collected from selenium with vitamin D are. Generally, if the data from selenium and vitamin D and CaP are extremely unlikely should the null hypothesis be true, then there is evidence against the null hypothesis; in contrast, if the data in question are not unlikely if the null hypothesis were true, then there is no evidence against the null hypothesis.[12,13] While hypotheses in medical and clinical sciences are often stated as alternative hypotheses, the testing of a hypothesis assumes the null—no difference. For example, there is no difference in CaP risk among men who take selenium combined with vitamin D compared to those who do not. In clinical sciences, hypothesis testing involves single-group as well as two- and multiple-group comparison. Examples of such tests are single-group means using a single or one-sample t-test, population proportion using z statistics (tests difference between the sample proportion and hypostasized population proportion), differences between population proportions, and differences between population means.[14,15] The appropriate statistics and their assumptions are an essential part of these materials and are presented in detail in subsequent chapters.

1.5 Primary versus secondary outcomes

The primary outcomes represent what the investigators intend to measure to answer their questions.[6,8,9] This outcome is measured by the primary response variable. A primary response variable may be the incidence of a disease, disease severity, a biochemical end point (such as prostate-specific antigen [PSA] level), or a biomarker (such as for CaP diagnosis). As an example, in a diabetes mellitus (DM) study, if the primary outcome is disease incidence, the response variable may be the blood glucose ascertainment in a follow-up study of overweight and normal-weight adults until the diagnosis of DM by well-defined clinical and laboratory measures. If the outcome is DM severity, the response variable may be measured by retinopathy, the need for lower extremity amputation, erectile dysfunction in men, vascular stenosis, and/or the occurrence of comorbidities during the study period. With mortality as the primary outcome, death from all causes or from a given disease remains a clear, feasible, and reliable measure of the outcome. For example, the effectiveness of androgen-deprivation therapy in the treatment of locoregional CaP may be measured by the number of deaths due to CaP or cause-nonspecific mortality occurring in the treatment arm (ADT) versus control arm (non-ADT). These variables (response and independent) may be measured on a continuous, nominal, or discrete scale, as will be illustrated in detail in the upcoming chapters. A study may also be conducted to assess other outcomes, which are not primary to the research question, termed *secondary outcomes* and measured by secondary variables. In this case, care should be taken to consider secondary outcomes that are

more relevant to the primary research questions, since the more secondary outcome measures selected, the more likelihood for one to encounter
a nonsignificant result, as well as inconsistent and conflicting findings.[9] A
secondary response variable may be a biochemical failure, in which the primary response is death from the tumor. For example, if a study is conducted
to examine the effectiveness of tamoxifen in prolonging survival of older
women with nonoperable breast cancer, tumor grade/size may represent a
secondary outcome measure, while mortality remains the measure of survival as the primary outcome.

1.5.1 Scales of measurement

A continuous scale for the outcome measure (granted that it is clinically relevant, such as PSA level, blood glucose level) carries an advantage of utilizing
a reduced sample size to show a difference between the treatment and control
groups, should such an effect really exist,[9] and facilitates the use of a more
powerful test statistic, termed *parametric* (normality assumed). In contrast,
if the primary outcome measure is not death and the study population represents senior or older old adults with higher mortality risk, then there may be
a sample size issue that may underpower the study, leading to type II error.
These concepts are clearly described in upcoming chapters and in the companion volume of this text (biostatistics).

1.5.2 Clinical versus population-based research

Clinical medicine focuses on individual patients. It is not evidenced based
unless it is population based. Population medicine, which may be used
interchangeably with population or public health, remains the collective effort of the society to remain healthy.[16,17] To fulfill this task, public
health utilizes sound research principles to conduct research into disease control and prevention at the population level.[18] The management
of individual patients in clinical medicine is based on the best available
research data, which are derived from well-defined and measured evidence.[19,20] Whereas population medicine or public health may represent
the notion of preventive health practices at the population level, implying what the population does to remain healthy, clinical medicine is diagnostic and therapeutic.[18]

In practice, there is an interrelationship between population and clinical
medicine. The practice of clinical medicine or patient care is dependent on
population-based data.[18,20] For example, the use of antihistamines (H2 block-
ers) in gastric hyperacidity or antihypertensive drugs, such as beta-blockers,
to control hypertension in individual patients is based on data from clinical trials on the efficacy and community-based routine use of such agents
and the effectiveness in the population. Consequently, the decision to place a
patient on a chemoprophylactic agent for the prevention of cerebrovascular

accident is based on what is known about the agent at the population level and the probability that the individual patient may represent the population and therefore be responsive to the agent if administered in a comparable manner as in the clinical trial or nonexperimental prospective studies (this is the basis of routine patient treatment).

1.5.3   Epidemiologic / population-based research

The notion of epidemiologic research reflects scientific enquiry at a specific population level. Epidemiologic research therefore tends to be characterized as population based and is not as simple as clinicians and researchers might assume. In the physical sciences, results hold the same in similar physical circumstances; however, epidemiologic investigation involves humans in specific populations, and since humans are genetically and psychosocially heterogeneous, the results could be paralyzed by confounding, rendering the finding nonfactual. Epidemiology is considered the basic and core science of public health and is simply defined as the study of the distribution and determinants of disease, disabilities, injuries, and health-related events at the population level. With this definition, epidemiologic methods are not simple in terms of application, requiring basic education and training in some concepts like incidence rate involving person-time, incidence density, confounding, effect measure modifiers, causation and causal inference, association, random error quantification, and p value function. It is because of this need to inform clinicians and biomedical researchers on the appropriate application of these concepts in design and inference process in research, that this book was conceived. To illustrate the complexities of epidemiologic principles, let us consider two groups of patients. The average age of death of patients with infantile scoliosis (A) is 1.5 years, while the average age at death of patients with adolescent scoliosis (B) is 14 years. Does this mean that those in group A have a greater risk of dying? The age at death in this comparison does not reflect the risk of death but merely characterizes those who die. Thus, to maintain that one group is at a higher risk relative to the other without controlling for the age distribution of these two groups prior to comparison is epidemiologically fallacious. Second, the age at onset of death does not account for the proportion of those who died. The materials in subsequent chapters will allow us to avoid such errors or fallacies in the interpretation of our results and to draw appropriate inference.

Epidemiologic designs are generally used to estimate risk and measure incidence rate/density as well as prevalence. More complex designs are used to compare measures of disease occurrence, leading to causal prediction as well as impact of disease in a defined human population.[21] Epidemiologic designs or methods include ecologic, cross-sectional (prevalence studies), case control, cohort, and hybrids (Figure 1.6).[18]

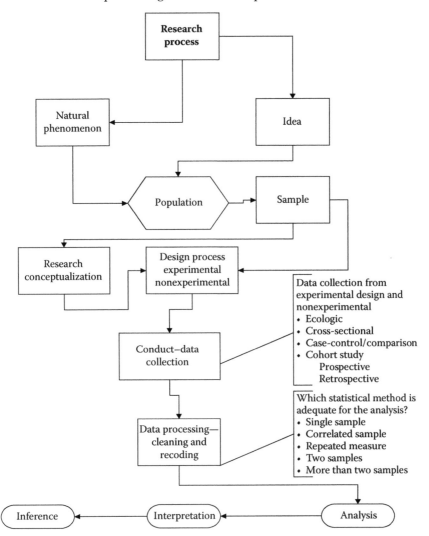

Figure 1.6 Research process and design.

1.5.4   *Research rationale*

The purpose of research as the intent or the rationale behind the study was presented earlier in this chapter. Clinical research is conducted primarily to enhance therapeutics, implying the intent to improve patients' care. The application of this concept in biomedical sciences, public health, and clinical medicine signaled a departure from nihilism, which claimed that disease improved without therapy. The scientific medical discoveries on pellagra, DM, penicillin, and sulfonamide provide reliable data on medicinal benefits in therapeutics. Today, with biomedical and clinical research, clinical investigators applying reliable and valid research methodologies can show the efficacy and effectiveness of agents and devices, competing therapies, combination treatments, comparative effectiveness, and diagnostic and screening criteria for most diseases.

In claiming the advantage of therapeutics in medicine (complementary versus traditional), there is a need for clinical investigators, who may be expert physicians and who are indeed researchers, to understand the biological theories and the complexities of disease. Though the biological and clinical importance of a disease is essential in formulating the research question, the clinician is also expected to acquire statistical reasoning. The combination of these two models enhances the analysis and the interpretation of the data from clinical research. Therefore, in clinical research, there is an investigator (clinical) who examines the formal hypothesis or established biology based on the work in the clinical settings (experience, observation, and data), as well as another investigator (biostatistician/epidemiologist) whose contribution is to generalize observations from the sample to the target population, as well as combine empirical (observation and data) and theory-based knowledge (probability and determinism) to the understanding of the results of the study. Despite these distinctions, an effective clinical research involves the understanding of these two models of thinking or reasoning by the investigators, clinicians, and epidemiologists/biostatisticians. Without this integration, our effort toward design and interpretation of research findings is limited, since making reasonable, accurate, and reliable inferences from data in the presence of uncertainty remains the cornerstone of clinical research results, utilized in improving the health care of future patients. In stressing the essence of this integration, one is not claiming the relevance of statistical reasoning over biological and clinical importance, since clinical research thinking is fundamentally biologic, clinical, and statistical.

The approach to biomedical and clinical research, as mentioned earlier, involves the following:

1   Research conceptualization
2   Design process
3   Statistical inference

In clinical medicine, the research conceptualization may involve outcome of partial intracapsular tonsillectomy (PITA) in children with obstructive sleep apnea syndrome (OSAS). The design process may involve repeated measure implying the baseline data of sleep study parameters before and after PITA, with a follow-up time to determine the effect of PITA in improving sleep architecture. The statistical inference, given that adequate numbers (sample size and power estimations) of children studied, involves the use of repeated measures ANOVA (RANOVA). Finally, statistical stability is examined in ruling out random variation using the p value (significance level) and 95% confidence interval (precision). The research conceptualization may require a clinical investigator or clinician utilizing his or her experience in the management of patients with malignancy (leukemia, for example), observation, and data to formulate a hypothesis regarding therapeutics. A case-comparison/control design could be applied here in which the treated group, termed *cases*, are placed on the new drug X, while the comparison group, also termed *control*, are placed on a standard care drug Y and followed for the assessment of outcome (death or biochemical failure). The statistical inference and the interpretation of the results are similar to the previous example with the outcome of OSAS following PITA.

Historically, central to clinical research and therapeutics is the concept of disease screening and diagnostic testing. We can view disease diagnosis and the diagnostic test as key elements in the ascertainment of subjects for clinical research. Inappropriate patient ascertainment may result in selection, information, and misclassification bias (discussed in subsequent chapters). This historical concept remains valid in research conduct and is the main material elaborated upon in this chapter. The sensitivity, specificity, predictive values, and likelihood ratio are described with examples. Thus, the validity of the results obtained in clinical research depends on how adequately the subjects were identified and assigned to treatment (experimental design or clinical trial) or followed after exposure (observational design).

1.5.5   Why conduct clinical research?

Research in biomedical science, clinical medicine and public health is a response to a health or health-related issue. Thus, research conducted commences with question formulation, followed by the design plans to answer the question, data collection and analysis, drawing conclusions from the results or findings, and information sharing through publication or dissemination. For example, a reason to conduct research may be to understand the natural history of a disease, such as a unicameral bone cyst, which is a benign tumor of the bone. Another example of the natural history of a disease is the data from the Swedish prospective cohort study of men diagnosed with CaP and followed for 10 years without specific treatment (watchful waiting or observational management) for CaP. In the latter example, with the primary end point being cause-specific mortality (CaP dead), the experience of this group was compared, and a 10-year relative survival of 87.0% was reported.[22] The natural history of disease refers loosely to the collectivity of the actual sequence of events since this phenomenon (actual sequence of events) can vary widely among patients.[23] In more concrete terms, we normally refer to the natural history of a disease as the assessment of the actual sequence of events for many patients in order to obtain some estimates of these events. In this respect, the natural history of disease can be characterized using measures of disease occurrence, such as case fatality, mortality rate, median survival time, etc. Research may also be conducted to relate laboratory data or information with screening, diagnosis, treatment, and prognosis. For example, a researcher/

investigator may wish to use the laboratory value for blood glucose level to screen, diagnose, and determine the prognosis of DM patients. Finally, a natural history of a disease may be studied in a randomized, placebo-controlled clinical trial, where treatment is allocated to one group, while the other group (control) is given the placebo. The result in the control group without the treatment represents the natural history of the disease studied (Figure 1.7).

Primary to research in clinical medicine is to address questions pertaining to screening, diagnosis, treatment, and outcome of care (prognosis), with the ultimate goal being the improvement of patients' care. This effort involves these tasks:

1   Protocol development and management/coordination
2   Recruitment and data collection/entry
3   Data management and analysis
4   Making sense of the data through interpretation and inference

The clinical researcher should have a clear idea of the concept to be measured. This step allows the investigator to clearly address the research questions. The statement of such question must reflect the scale of measurement of the variable, such as nominal, ordinal, interval, or ratio (to be discussed in Chapter 3). The reliability of the variables to be measured (if questionnaires are used to collect information) has to be examined on the basis of the stability of the response to the question over time—a sort of test and retest reliability. As is often seen in clinical research involving radiographic measure, reliability could be measured by examining the agreement between two observers or surgeons (interrater reliability). Very important is the validity or accuracy of the measure, which is simply the extent to which the empirically observed association between measures of the concepts agree with the testable hypothesis about the association between variables assessed.

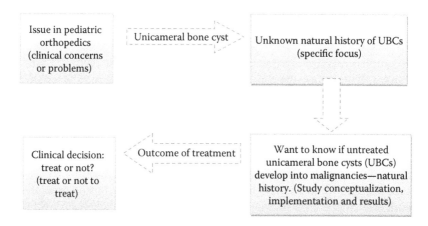

Figure 1.7 Rationale for research.

1.6 Study subjects

Clinical research may involve human subjects. For example, clinical 1 researchers may be interested in finding out if a certain drug (n34) enhances programmed cell death (apoptosis) in children with neuroblastoma. A case-control nonexperimental epidemiologic design may be proposed for this investigation. The issues to be addressed include study subject selection, since the control—children not administered n34—must be comparable to those administered the active treatment mice (n34 neuroblastoma). If randomization process was used, such selection is feasible, minimizing selection bias, sampling, and generalization errors.

1.6.1 Subject selection

Investigators must select samples that are representative of the patient population, implying the performance of the investigation on a number of patients large enough to minimize random error (increased sample representativeness) in order to generalize the study findings to the targeted population of patients. An example of a study sample would be children with adolescent idiopathic scoliosis who underwent posterior spinal fusion for curve deformities correction between 2000 and 2011. Another example is the sample of asthmatic children for cromolyn sodium as an adjunct therapeutic agent in the treatment of uncontrolled asthma in this population. Well-structured inclusion and exclusion criteria are essential in appropriate subject selection to ensure that the study findings are reasonably generalized. Therefore, criteria should be selected in such a manner that the generalization of the study findings to the targeted population is feasible. However, contrary to scientific community such as the National Institutes of Health (NIH) requirement of "total or comprehensive inclusion" (women, children, racial/ethnic minorities), any sample could be studied such as estrogen and osteoporosis in postmenopausal women, provided the study findings are not overgeneralized.

1.7 Sampling

Clinical researchers must determine a priori who should be in the sample. Part of the rationale behind sampling, among other considerations (research complexity and efficiency, limited resources), is to increase precision (minimize sampling variability) and ensure accuracy of the estimates, such as the mean or proportion. Commonly used probability sampling techniques include a simple random sample, a systematic random sample, and a stratified sample as well as a cluster sample. It is, however, important to note that while the appropriate probability sampling technique is essential in limiting sampling variability, eliminating random error is impossible and there remains the possibility of random variability, hence the need to quantify such errors (random) by probability value (p).

The utility of findings from an inferential study depends on appropriate sampling. Sampling as a desirable approach in research is based on the rationale of an appropriate sample representing the target population. While study size may be influenced by the available resources, the study sample must reflect the characteristics of the targeted population. A sample is described as a subset of the targeted population, which is always desirable, given the impossibility of studying the entire population. In clinical research, the study sample rarely meets the requirement for probability sampling. In this context, convenient (subjects who meet criteria and are accessible to investigators) and consecutive (entire patient population over a long period of time) samples are often used.

Inferential studies that quantify random error require probability sampling. This approach ensures that the study sample represents the targeted population and that data derived from such a sampling technique reflect the true experience in the population from which the study sample was drawn. These techniques, which include the simple random sample, stratified sample, systematic sample, and the cluster sample, will be discussed in detail in the next chapter. Despite this recommendation, there are exceptions to the application of inference to the target population namely disease registry such as SEER data and consecutive sample. In effect, random error is quantifiable in these two situations despite the nonprobability sample used (Figure 1.8).

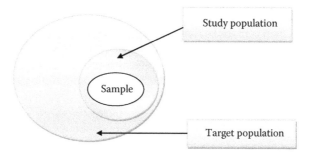

Figure 1.8 **Sample as a representative unit of the target population.** The design of the study involves the selection of sample from the source or referenced population that produced the study population (sampling frame). For example, if a study is proposed to examine the effect of DNA methylation on brain/CNS tumors development using a case-control design, the sample may be a unit or portion from the children diagnosed with brain/CNS tumors and children without the outcome of interest. With a predetermined sample based on the sample size estimation, the cases are sampled from the sampling frame (list of all patients with brain/CNS tumor), and the sampling fraction is obtained based on the sample size, and using systematic random sampling, the sampling fraction determines which patient to choose with known and equal probability until the sample size is obtained for the case (one group). The same process is applied to the control from the source population.

1.8   Generalization

When studying physical phenomena, we can apply the findings easily without determining how to reasonably apply the findings to a geographic location in which the phenomenon was not observed. However, biologic or biomedical studies differ because of the heterogeneity of the species and the changing environmental conditions. Can we generalize the findings of a study based on a consecutive sample? This question requires the investigators to determine whether the sample is comparable to a probability sample to justify generalization. For example, if the investigator estimates that the consecutive sample was large enough to minimize random error (representative sample), then such a study finding could be generalized to a target population with the assumption that the sampling technique used is similar to the probability sampling technique. In contrast, if the consecutive sample is judged not to minimize random error, such a finding should not be generalized. Consequently, such studies' results should be presented with descriptive statistics, without any attempt to quantify random error.

1.8.1 Sample size estimation

The exact sample needed to conduct a study in order to determine the difference between the groups studied or the effect of treatment on patients treated remains unknown and, hence, the notion of estimation. The information needed to estimate the required sample for a study includes the effect size. For example, if a clinician is interested in observing the benefit of drug A compared to the standard of care in reducing asthma symptoms among overweight/obsess children, she/he may utilize an effect size of 10% as a clinically acceptable minimum difference between standard care and new drug for such an agent to inform and change clinical practice. Since two independent samples are involved, the measure of effect may be relative odds or odds ratio, relative risk, hazard ratio, risk difference, etc. The statistical power $(1 - \beta)$ is required with the minimum power of 80% as the ability to detect the minimum difference of 10% (RR, 1.10) based on the predetermined effect size (Figure 1.9). The type I error tolerance is required in quantifying the

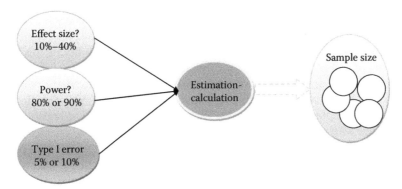

Figure 1.9 Process and factors influencing sample estimation.

random error from the representative sample, with the known and equal probability of being included in the study. This error tolerance is conventionally set at 5% ($p = 0.05$), implying the rejection of the null hypothesis should the point estimate obtained from the sample is due to chance and hence violates the representative sample notion in justifying the generalization of the findings to the targeted population (N) (Figure 1.9).

1.9   Sample size and power estimations

While this issue will be discussed in detail, the importance of understanding the essence of the study size needed for the research project needs to be mentioned early. Sample size estimation is important at the beginning of the design of a research project. In inferential or analytic study, the findings require generalization. This process involves a clear statement of the null and alternative hypotheses, indicating the direction of the test, selecting the test statistic based on the scale of measurement of the outcome and independent or predictor variables, clinically reasonable effect size, variability, and the statement of type I error tolerance and type II errors. Given the importance of power, an adequate sample size is necessary in order to avoid missing a real difference and concluding that there is no difference. Subsequent chapters will provide details on specific statistical test settings (t-test, chi-square, correlation coefficient, logistic regression, survival analysis, structural equation, ANOVA, and analysis of covariance [ANCOVA]) and on how to estimate the study size. However, researchers must plan to address loss to follow-up by compensating for the attrition rate, as well as to increase the study size while utilizing multivariable statistical modeling to adjust for confounding at the analysis phase of the research.

Sample size estimation reflects the feasibility of study and remains one of the elements that could result in a decision not to approve a study for funding. If indeed the researchers are unable to illustrate that there is an adequate sample size and power for the proposed study, invariably, the future contribution of the proposed project to science, public health, and medicine is questionable. Supposing a study is proposed to examine the survival advantage of children with rhabdomyosarcoma placed on immunotherapy plus chemotherapy relative to patients with chemotherapy alone, the feasibility of this study in terms of sample size and power estimations could be stated as: the sample size estimation for the benefit of immunotherapy in pediatric rhabdomyosarcoma was based on 36 months event-free survival rate of 50% for those on chemotherapy plus immunotherapy. We aimed to detect a hazard ratio of 0.80 associated with chemotherapy plus immunotherapy relative to chemotherapy alone. In effect 264 children per arm was required ($n = 528$), with 85% power, two-tailed test, 5% type I error tolerance and Cox proportional hazard test. To compensate for 15% dropout or attrition rate, the total number of patients recruited was $n = 608$.

1.10 Summary

The goal of clinical research in general is to provide useful data or information on the observed phenomenon, usually achieved through a methodic approach to answering the research question/s and test the hypothesis. This goal is expressed in the attempt to draw inference from the study results regarding the truth in the universe or targeted population. With this as the goal of research, investigators begin with research questions, formulate hypotheses (null and alternative), perform the test, and answer the research questions. Clinical research is a systematic, empirical, critical, and sometimes controlled investigation of phenomena in patients' settings (diagnostic, therapeutic, and preventive). The approach could be divided into these categories:

1 Research conceptualization
2 Design process
3 Statistical inference

This process involves a well-defined problem statement, research questions, purposes, and potential benefits of the study to science and humanity; identification of the theory and assumptions; a search of background literature; measurement of variables; statement of researchable hypotheses; presentation of operational definitions and measurement; and selection of the appropriate study design. In addition, it requires determination of the methodology to fit the research question or hypothesis, development of an instrument or tools for data gathering, identification of an appropriate sampling technique, selection of a data analysis tool or statistical technique to test the hypothesis or answer the research question, and presentation of the results and interpretation and conclusions that are based on the data as well as what the data suggests and recommendations for clinical research.

The *purpose* of a study is the statement of the overall objective of the study and identifies the independent (predictor or explanatory) and response (outcome or dependent) variables as well as how the variables will be measured and the design is to be used to achieve the expected relationship or association. The *objective* of the study describes the intent. Research questions and hypotheses are two basic ways of assessing the relationship or association between study variables. In quantitative studies, hypothesis testing is essential in drawing an inference or in making a statement beyond the sample data. Simply, *hypothesis* refers to a statement about the population or simply the universe/world that is testable.

The evidence from clinical research is dependent on how well the data has been interpreted regarding these elements:

1 Biologic relevance of the findings
2 Clinical importance of the observed data, implying the effect size

3 Statistical stability, which is the measure of how representative the sample is relative to the population; it is measured by the confidence intervals (90,95,99), as well as the *p* value

Questions for discussion

1 Suppose that drug X is an established antimicrobial agent against ulcerative colitis. Investigators wish to study drug Y, a newly manufactured steriodal.
   a What are the research question and the purpose of the study?
   b State the hypothesis to be tested.
   c What is the outcome variable, and what is an appropriate scale of measurement?
   d Which design or designs will be feasible in this study?
   e Would it be a good idea to have a placebo group in this study and compare three groups instead of two?
2 Suppose we wish to examine the relationship between low birth weight and cerebral palsies (CPs) incidence.
   a What would the hypothesis be?
   b How will the study population be selected?
   c Suppose you wish to compare the incidence rate of CP between the exposed and the unexposed subjects, what would be an appropriate study design?
   d How should we assess the relationship between the outcome and independent variable in this example?
   e What could serve as a threat to validity in the selected design?
3 Consider a group of children ages 2 to 14 years with a low hemoglobin level; you wish to see if there is familial aggregation of low hemoglobin level.
   a Which study design would be adequate in examining the hypothesis in this context?
   b What is the hypothesis?
   c What other factors would you consider in assessing this relationship?

References

1. R. B. Kerlinger, *Behavioral Research: A Conceptual Approach* (New York: Rinehart and Winston, 1979).
2. S. B. Hulley, S. R. Cummings, W. S. Browner et al. *Designing Clinical Research*, 2nd ed. (Philadelphia, PA: Lippincott, Williams & Wilkins, 2001).
3. M. Angell, "Caring for Women's Health—What Is the Problem?" *N Engl J Med* 329 (1993): 271–272.
4. E. Babbie, *The Practice of Social Research,* 9th ed. (Belmont, CA: Wadsworth/ Thomson Learning, 2001).

5. J. W. Creswell, *Research Design: Qualitative, Quantitative and Mixed Methods Approaches*, 2nd ed. (Thousand Oaks, CA: Sage Publication, 2003).
6. G. Keppel, *Design and Analysis: A Researcher's Handbook*, 3rd ed. (New York: Guilford, 1998).
7. L. F. Locke, W. W. Spiruso, and S. J. Silverman, *Proposals that Work: A Guide for Planning Dissertations and Grant Proposals*, 4th ed. (Thousand Oaks, CA: Sage Publication, 2000).
8. B. G. Leventhal and R. E. Wittes, *Research Methods in Clinical Oncology* (New York: Raven Press, 1988).
9. L. M. Friedman, C. D. Furberg, and D. L. DeMets, *Fundamentals of Clinical Trials*, 3rd ed. (New York: Springer, 1988).
10. W. D. DuPont, *Statistical Modeling for Biomedical Researchers* (Cambridge, UK: Cambridge University Press, 2003).
11. L. E. Braitman, "Statistical Estimates and Clinical Trials," *J Biopharm Stat* 3 (1993): 249–256.
12. T. D. V. Swinscow and M. J. Campbell, *Statistics at Square One*, 9th ed. (London, UK: BMJ Books, 2002).
13. D. G. Altman, "Statistics in Medical Journals," *Stat Med* 1 (1982): 59–71.
14. J. L. Garb, *Understanding Medical Research: A Practitioner's Guide* (Boston: Little, Brown, and Company, 2000).
15. B. Rosner, *Fundamentals of Biostatistics*, 5th ed. (Belmont, CA: Duxbury Press, 2000).
16. Institute of Medicine, *Healthy Communities* (Washington, DC: National Academy Press, 1996).
17. Institute of Medicine, *The Future of Public Health* (Washington, DC: National Academy Press, 1988).
18. L. Holmes, *Basics of Public Health Core Competencies* (Sudbury, MA: Jones and Bartlett Publishers, 2009).
19. D. L. Sackett, W. S. Richardson, W. Rosenberg, and R. B. Haynes, *Evidence-Based Medicine: How to Practice and Teach Evidence-Based Medicine*, 2nd ed. (Edinburg: Churchill Livingstone, 2000)
20. D. L. Katz, *Clinical Epidemiology & Evidence-Based Medicine: Fundamental Principles of Clinical Reasoning & Research* (Thousand Oaks, CA: Sage, 2001).
21. K. Rothman, *Epidemiology: An Introduction* (New York: Oxford University Press, 2002).
22. J. E. Johansson, H. O. Adami, S. O. Anderson et al. "High 10-year Survival Rate in Patients with Early, Untreated Prostatic Cancer," *JAMA* 267 (1992): 216–219.
23. R. S. Greenberg et al. *Medical Epidemiology*, 4th ed. (New York: Lange, 2005).

2 Clinical research proposal development and protocol

2.1 Introduction

Clinical research is an attempt to advance efficient, objective, and reliable knowledge regarding therapeutics as well as diagnostics and prevention. In contrast with patient care, which is derived from chance occurrence and experience, clinical research is more efficient, since it applies theory and data to the improvement of care. Defining clinical research is not a simple task. But operationally, clinical research is the application of research methodology in a clinical setting to study conceptualization, design process, conduct, analysis, and statistical inference. Conducting clinical research is interdisciplinary in approach including clinical, epidemiologic, statistical, ethical, and managerial considerations.

Clinical research involves clinicians in the study conceptualization. However, since fairly large investigations in this field involve the biology of the disease or outcome as well as the clinical implications of the data to improve care, epidemiologic and statistical considerations are essential in designing and conducting clinical research. Depending on the design, some disciplines may weigh more than others in design and conduct. For example, a clinical trial involves trial methodologists, who are very highly quantitative and who may be clinicians, epidemiologists, and statisticians. With this, conducting clinical research involves collaboration between these disciplines with the involvement of epidemiologists and biostatisticians at the conceptualization or planning stages of the study. The rationale for this recommendation of team science is to prevent design and methodological issues, avoid measurement and design errors, and streamline the study prior to conducting it and doing analyses.

In presenting a chapter on designing and conducting research, the primary challenge is the inclusion of all the aspects of clinical research. The emphasis in this chapter is on the science of clinical research, given the author's background. Therefore, there are important aspects of clinical research that are not covered here in detail, namely, administration, funding, and infrastructure. The purpose of clinical research is to provide the basis for clinical-care decision making, diagnosis, treatment, prognosis, and prevention of disease.

This chapter attempts to show how a good design may lead to reliable answers to the research question or hypothesis.

An adequate analysis of clinical research data is as necessary as the design used to generate the data. A well-designed clinical research study should minimize bias by employing reliable and valid measurements and random sampling (unbiased estimates) and minimize variability from simple random sampling by utilizing large samples of patients or participants in the study. This process has become feasible recently but allows for fatal errors unless used properly. Whereas this chapter and other chapters on statistical inference present how to make sense out of data, data analysis requires the analyst to understand the design and the assumptions of the test statistic and understand the methods and limitations of the statistical techniques. Therefore, clinical researchers should merge analytic strategy into clinicians' understanding of the rationale and limitations of the analysis and the statisticians' understanding of the biology and clinical implications, if applicable, of the data. Since one cannot overemphasize this marriage, the design and conduct of clinical research should involve these two players from research conceptualization.

2.2   Study conceptualization

Research conceptualization refers to the specification of terms used in the research as well as the planning of the operation of the study or research project. This term could also apply to the design and planning required for implementing or conducting the study. However, as used in this presentation, it refers to the first phase of clinical research study, which focuses on the biology as well as the clinical implications of the research question, the hypothesis, and how these could be addressed with an appropriate design. Specifically, we refer to conceptualization when attempting to measure as precisely as we possibly can the variables used in our research, implying the precise definition of variables as concepts for the research.

2.2.1   Study conceptualization requires variable ascertainment

Conceptualization in terms of variable ascertainment is the process of identifying and clarifying the concept, leading to the specification of variable measures. For example, an investigator intends to examine the etiologic role of maternal steroid used during pregnancy in a group of children with cerebral palsy (CP) (cases) and without CP (control). Maternal use of steroids may be conceptualized by dosage, frequency, trimester of gestation at time of use, type of steroid, route of administration, and duration of use. The specification of this variable also involves the scale of measurement: binary, continuous, or categorical. Maternal steroid use may be measured on a continuous scale involving the dosage of the steroid in milligrams, which may allow the investigator to examine the severity of CP with the dosage of steroid used during pregnancy. Further, steroid use could be measured on a binary scale, with "ever used steroid during the pregnancy of the CP child/non-CP control child" and "never used steroid during the pregnancy of the CP child/non-CP control child." A categorical scale could be used as well, which allows the mild, moderate, and severe (based on the dosage) use of steroids during pregnancy to assess the dose response severity of CP. Therefore, the closer the measure is to the biologic hypothesis proposed to be tested by steroid use, the more likely it is to measure the association between the response or outcome (CP) and the independent variable (maternal steroid use).

Besides variable ascertainment, study conceptualization requires the description of operational definitions of terms used in the study. For example, in a study conducted to examine the factors associated with deep wound infection following spine fusion to correct curve deformities in adolescents with neuromuscular scoliosis, investigators may measure parental socioeconomic status by education, income, and poverty. These measures serve to define socioeconomic status in this study operationally.

2.2.2   Conceptualization and confounding

2.2.2.1   Confounding: Distortion or bias?

Conceptualization requires identification of confounding variables (third extraneous variables that influence the measure of effect between the exposure and outcome). Since patients and research participants live in a noncontrolled environment, there are extraneous factors that if not evenly distributed may affect the relationship between exposure and outcome. For example, investigators wanted to assess the outcome of surgery plus radiation or surgery alone on the survival of children with nephroblastoma. If a parental history of nephroblastoma, stage at diagnosis, or age at diagnosis is associated with the outcome (survival), then these variables may possibly influence survival and require adjustment in a multivariable model (simultaneous adjustment) or stratification to control for a single confounding variable. Also, matching at the design phase could be used to balance some of these confounders. Confounding will be discussed later in this presentation, as a threat to the internal validity of studies. Further, it is important to note that confounding, though not a bias, may lead to a biased estimate of an outcome, given a risk variable.

BOX 2.1   ELEMENTS AND CHARACTERISTICS OF CONFOUNDERS

A confounder is an agent or extraneous factor that accounts for differences in disease occurrence or frequency or measures of the effect between the exposed and unexposed.
- It predicts disease frequency in the unexposed or referent population. For example, in the association between oral cancer and

---

alcohol consumption, smoking is considered confounding if it is associated with both oral cancer and alcohol consumption.

- A confounder is not qualified by this association only.
- To qualify as a confounder, smoking must be associated with the occurrence of oral cancer in the unexposed or referent group, apart from its association with alcohol consumption.
- Also, smoking must be associated with oral cancer among non-alcohol consumers.
- If the effect of alcohol consumption is mediated through the effect of smoking, then it is not a confounder, regardless of whether there is an effect of exposure (alcohol consumption) on oral cancer (outcome or disease).
- Any variate that represents a step or in the pathway between the exposure and disease does not represent a confounder but could be termed an intermediate variate.
    - **Alcohol consumption → Smoking → Oral cancer**
- Surrogate confounders are factors associated with confounders. For example, in chronologic age and aging, chronologic age is a surrogate confounder.
- **Features of confounder—it** must be:
    - An extraneous risk factor for disease
    - Associated with the exposure in the source population or the population at risk from which the case is derived
    - Must not be affected by the exposure or disease, implying that it cannot be an intermediate in the causal pathway between the disease and exposure

2.2.3   Validity and reliability

A good study design enhances the scientific validity of the clinical research, and measurement criteria serve to enhance study conceptualization. Therefore, a predefined measure to address the reliability and validity of measurement is required in the study conceptualization phase of a sound research project. There are several types of validity to assess in research; *validity* refers to the extent, magnitude, or degree to which an empirical measure adequately reflects the meaning of the proposed study variable. The degree to which a scale or an instrument measures what it is supposed to measure represents validity. For example, an investigator wishes to examine the lung capacity of asthmatic children before and after albuterol inhalation via a pocket nebulizer; he or she uses two measures with different calibrations for before and after the measurement of lung capacity. Since the instrument is different, the measure is invalid, thus compromising the internal validity of the study and introducing measurement error into the result. *Reliability* or *reproducibility* refers to the power or ability of an instrument to provide or reproduce the measure. For example, if an instrument is used to measure the systolic blood pressure (BP), this measure is reliable if it produces the same result when there is no change in an individual's systolic BP. Another example is the use of a scale to measure

---

BOX 2.2   STUDY ACCURACY: VALIDITY—SYSTEMATIC ERROR (BIAS) AND RANDOM ERROR

ACCURACY

The objective of a study, which is an exercise in measurement, is to obtain a valid and precise estimate of the effect size or measure of disease occurrence.

- The value of a parameter is estimated with little error.
- It is related to the handling of *systematic errors* or biases and *random error*.
- It involves the generalization of findings from the study to the relevant target or source population.
- It comprises *validity* and *precision*.
  - Validity refers to the estimate or effect size that has little systematic error (biases).
  - There are two components of validity: internal and external.
- *Internal validity* refers to the accuracy of the effect measure of the inferences drawn in relation to the source population.
  - Inference of the source population
  - A prerequisite for external validity
  - Measures of internal validity are (a) confounding, (b) selection bias, and (c) information bias (measurement error).
- *External validity* refers to the accuracy of the effect measure of the inferences in relation to individuals outside the source population.
  - It involves representation of the study population to the general population.
  - Do factors that differentiate the larger or general population from the study population modify the effect or the measure of the effect in the study?
  - It involves a combination of epidemiologic and other sources, for example pathophysiology.
  - It is related to criteria for causal inference.
- *Precision* refers to estimate or measure of effect or disease occurrence with little random error.

weight in kilograms. If the mean weight of all children with achondroplasia in a study of 246 children is 31.7 kg today and the measure is repeated the next day, a scale would be unreliable if the mean score of the same children the next day is 51.7 kg, provided the data were entered accurately. It is therefore important to note that reliability is not accuracy but the scale's ability to provide the same measures, as illustrated in the mean body weight example. Consequently, reliability and validity are essential attributes of design and must be determined at the conceptualization of a study prior to data collection.

2.3   Research question

A good research design is one in which study participants contribute answers to the biological or clinical questions. What is a research question and when is it applied in proposal development, conducting a study, and report preparations are questions that must be contemplated prior to beginning research.

A research question is simply a statement that identifies the object, phenomenon, or issue to be studied. In clinical medicine, as well as in biomedical sciences that involve animal experiment, the initial approach to conducting research is the formulation of a research question, which will be transformed into a hypothesis in a quantitative study or objective in a qualitative design. The research question is formulated in such a way that it defines the nature of intervention (independent variable) and the primary end point or outcome (response variable). Here is an example of a feasible research question: does cervical fusion with instrumentation increase cervical stability in children with skeletal dysplasia? This formulation identifies the following:

a   The study or patient population is stated as children with skeletal dysplasia.
b   The independent variable is identified as cervical fusion (surgery).
c   The outcome or response, also called the *dependent variable*, is stated as cervical spine stability.

Here is another example of a feasible research question: does autograft compared with allograft achieve more solid fusion in pediatric patients with spondyloepiphyseal dysplasia?

a   The study or patient population is stated as pediatric patients with spondyloepiphyseal dysplasia.
b   The independent variable is identified as cervical fusion with autograft compared with allograft.
c   The outcome or response (dependent variable) is stated as solid fusion.

Several examples could be stated to enable one to formulate a feasible research question. However, regardless of the area of clinical research, it is essential to note that a good research question must involve the following components:

a   Knowledge of the area or subject of research, which is possible to obtain through a critical review of literature on the topic of interest. For example, to examine in the pediatric population, the benefit of autograft compared with allograft in achieving solid fusion compared with athrodesis fusion, the researcher must review literature on the proportion of solid fusion achieved with autograft relative to allograft, assess the different instrumentation used in these studies, examine the heterogeneity of the disorders, and determine the statistical power of these studies as well as the design used to answer the research questions.

b   Determining whether or not a research question could be formulated to fill the gap in knowledge and clinical practice based on his or her critical review of literature.

c   Determining whether or not a similar study as proposed has been performed before in a similar population.

d   Examining the relevance of the question to increasing knowledge and understanding in the specific clinical area among clinicians, researchers, and students.

e   Determining the feasibility of translating the proposed research question into a study (for example, if a study is designed to determine whether or not electrocautery increases the risk of deep wound infection in children with neuromuscular scoliosis and electrocautery cannot be appropriately measured, it might introduce a significant amount of measurement, information, and selection biases and, hence, misclassification bias into the result of the study; such a research question is not considered to be feasible). However, the research question must be interesting, ethical, relevant (there is a current need to address this issue given the cost of hospitalization and the morbidity associated with deep wound infection in children with neuromuscular scoliosis), and novel.

2.3.1   *Research question in planning and conducting study*

Whether biomedical, observational, or social/behavioral sciences research, the first step in formulating a testable hypothesis in quantitative research design is to determine the measures of the primary end point and secondary end points (if any); the independent variable, such as the treatment (medication, surgery, radiation, etc.); and the specific population to be studied. Therefore, research question consideration is required during the planning phase of the study, when developing the study proposal, during the preparation of the scientific report for the sponsors (in a funded project), and during manuscript preparation for a scientific journal (Figure 2.1).

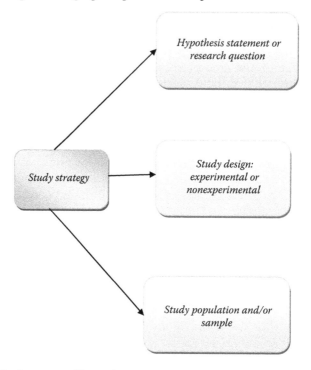

Figure 2.1 **Study strategy illustrating the design method, hypothesis or research question (mainly qualitative studies), and study population and sample.** The strategy requires the identification of primary and secondary objectives. Additionally, the type of design and the subjects must be clearly described. The study must describe the measurement clearly in terms of what should be measured from the samples or subjects. Further, the sample size and how it was derived as well as the statistical analysis plan should be clearly described.

2.4   Study background

A literature review is performed to provide an introduction to or background for the specific area of interest or research question to be answered. Whereas published literature that is critically appraised provides scholarship in the field or area to be researched, useful information can also be obtained on current breakthroughs in the area by investigators using summary proceedings from recent meetings as well as contact with senior investigators still active in the field.[1] The introduction of an original article or quantitative research project, whether in a proposal or completed study form (manuscript or report), is structured around the following:

a   An overview or scope of the clinical or health problem to be researched or studied—this information may embrace the prevalence, incidence, etiology, survival, cure rate, and comorbidity associated with the condition to be studied. Simply, it demonstrates the magnitude of the problem and its clinical relevance, establishing the rationale behind the study of this issue. For example, a retrospective cohort study designed to examine intraoperative factors associated with deep wound infection in pediatric patients following spine fusion to correct curve deformities may present the magnitude of the deep wound infection, known and possible etiologies, and the rationale for further studies to examine further risk variables as well as the specific overall objective in its introduction. Consider a hypothetical introduction:

I   Hypothetical introduction (magnitude or scope of clinical issue): The prevalence of deep wound infection following spine fusion in neuromuscular scoliosis varies with patient population, ranging from 9.3% to 34.6%, and is associated with multiple etiologic factors, some of which remain to be established, including intraoperative predisposing factors. The known etiologic factors include skin abrasion and breakdown due to instrumentation, while postulated risk variables include estimated blood loss, cell saver and packed red blood cells, and electrocautery. There are no studies to our knowledge that have examined the intraoperative factors, namely, packed red blood cells, cell saver, and estimated blood loss following posterior spine fusion in pediatric patients with neuromuscular scoliosis as risk factors for deep wound infection.

b A summary of studies including meta-analysis performed with respect to the research question. For example, the research question may ask if the intraoperative factors, namely, cell saver, packed red blood cells, and estimated blood loss risk factors for deep wound infection following spine fusion in pediatric patients with neuromuscular scoliosis.

I   Hypothetical introduction (critical summary of previous studies): Studies X, Y, and Z observed the prevalence of deep wound infection to be 23.6%, 12.3%, and 9.3%, respectively. These studies all observed rod instrumentation to be associated with deep wound infection following spine fusion for neuromuscular scoliosis. Study A assessed the risk of deep wound infection in patients with neuromuscular scoliosis and found deep wound infection to inversely correlate with cell saver. A recent retrospective cohort study (B) reported 30% prevalence of deep wound infection in patients with neuromuscular and adolescent idiopathic scoliosis and a significant increased risk of 23% deep wound infection among those who did not receive packed red blood cells compared to those who did. These studies, although demonstrating risks associated with deep wound infection, present with a heterogeneous patient population and small samples, limiting their statistical power.

c A statement on the current study filling in the gap—this paragraph is prepared to address the need for the current study to fill the gap in knowledge and clinical practice. It also states the approach to be utilized in filling this gap.

I   Hypothetical introduction (current study): This current study was proposed to determine the role of intraoperative factors in the development of deep wound infection following posterior spine fusion in pediatric patients with neuromuscular scoliosis. We postulated that cell saver and blood loss may increase the risk of deep would infection while packed red blood cells may decrease such risk in our sample. A retrospective cohort design with an unconditional logistic regression model was used to test these hypotheses.

2.5   Protocol implementation

Clinical study implementation involves performing the study as described in the protocol. This responsibility is described in detail in books in this field and will be mentioned in brief in the chapter on clinical trials as experimental design involving humans. It includes but is not limited to finalizing the study materials, site selection, staffing and training, strategies for communicating with sites, regulators, cost management, site initiation, enrollment options, data management setup and testing, monitoring procedures and training, auditing, safety monitoring, reports, and the Data and Safety Monitoring Board.

Good scientific practices are presented by organizations and agencies that protect human subjects in research as well as organizations that are concerned with scientific research integrity. Here are the recommendations:

a   Obtain an informed consent prior to the enrollment of eligible subjects in research. For example, a prospective study to examine the outcome of spine fusion tricalcium phosphate as a substitute to a bone graft in adolescent idiopathic scoliosis will require parental informed consent and permission as well as child assent prior to the enrolment of patients in this study.
b   Compliance to the study plan by following the research protocol guidelines.
c   Accurate data collection.
d   Appropriate reporting—accurate management of data and inference from the analysis.
e   Maintaining complete and accurate study files—data administration is also a component of data management, and
f   Recording and reporting unanticipated problems.

Further information about bias, conflict of interest, data gathering, and confidentiality regarding information sharing has been described and clearly recommended by the Institute of Medicine. This information is available at http://www.iom.edu/?id=5759.

BOX 2.3   ELEMENTS OF STUDY PROPOSAL

- *Title*—reflects the content and design and must be descriptive and concise
- *Abstract*—a concise summary of the protocol and contains the specific aims and hypothesis (quantitative designs), purpose or objective of the study, materials and methods, and the significance (clinical, public health, etc.)
- *Table of contents*—details the outline of what is covered in the proposal, very important in large proposals
- *Budget*—organized according to the funding agency's guidelines
- *Budget justification*—explanation of the amount requested in the budget
- *Bio sketch/es*—This is a two-page résumé that includes academic degrees, current and past employment, honors and awards, funding track record as current and past support, and selected earlier publications or published articles during the past three years
- *Resources, equipment, and facilities*—resources available to the project, such as computer equipment and office and laboratory spaces
- *Specific aims*—describes in concrete and practical terms the desired outcome of the study and should be presented in order of importance or chronologically.
- *Significance*—states the background of the study, the intent of the study in terms of accomplishment and importance, and the relevance of the proposed project to biology, science, and health

---

2.6   Data collection, management, and analysis

Data collection refers to the process of preparing and acquiring data. For example, an investigator wants to see if insulin injection and intensive monitoring of blood-glucose levels compared with insulin injection only decreases retinopathy among diabetics. To provide an answer to this clinical research question with retinopathy as the primary end point, data must be collected on the incidence of retinopathy among those in active treatment (insulin administration and frequent blood-glucose level monitoring) versus control (insulin injection only). The data type will be binary, 0 meaning no evidence of retinopathy and 1 meaning evidence of retinopathy. Demographic data will be collected as well, which will allow the investigator to assess the variation in retinopathy with respect to sex, race/ethnicity, and age.

Data collection is an important aspect of any type of research study, including clinical, experimental, and nonexperimental. Inaccurate data collection can impact the results of a study and ultimately lead to invalid results and erroneous generalizations. Data collection requires a data-gathering plan, which will involve a precollection phase, a data collection process—this ensures that data gathered are both defined and accurate, and data management and analysis. Establishing a data collection process should be seen as a fundamental step at the start of any clinical research. It ensures that research can efficiently and accurately collect data enabling the investigator to answer the research question (Figure 2.2).[2]

Understanding the steps in the pre-data collection and data collection processes enables one to ensure accuracy of the data. These steps are as follows:

1   Data collection goals/objectives defined by the investigator during the proposal development phase of the study. The elements in this step include the following:
    a   A brief description of the research
    b   Specific data that is needed, based on the research question, which clearly defines the outcome and independent variables
    c   The rationale for collecting the data—what question will the data answer
    d   What will be done with the data once it has been collected.
        Therefore, clarity with these issues will facilitate the accuracy and efficiency of data collection.
2   Operational definitions and methodology for the data collection plan— the investigator during the proposal development phase of the study should clearly define which data are to be collected and how this will be achieved. For example, in the hypothetical diabetes retinopathy study, the investigator wishes to collect incidence data from all subjects in the study from the third month following the commencement of the study and thereafter every 6 months until the last month of follow-up (24 months) on the development of retinopathy, implying the comparison of the proportion of those with and without retinopathy in the

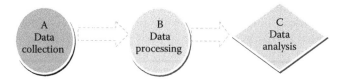

Figure 2.2 **Evidence discovery process.** The illustration of appropriate process in making sense of research data. In making sense of data, investigators must dedicate time to process the data prior to analysis and interpretation. Data processing (B) is crucial since failure to do so may introduce significant bias into the study if indeed outliers and missing data impact the findings from the data.

BOX 2.4   ELEMENTS OF RESEARCH PROPOSAL

- Preliminary results—describes relevant previous works of the investigators as relevant or related to the proposed project
- Methods—overview of design, time frame, and nature of control and study subjects, including selection criteria, design for sampling, and plans for the recruitment of subjects
- Measurements—measurements, such as main predictor variable, outcome variables, potential confounding variables, and so on
- Pretest plans—describes the testing of instruments prior to conducting the study and may include plans for the pilot as well
- Statistical analysis issues—approach to statistical analysis, sample size and power estimations, and specific hypothesis testing
- Quality control and data management
- Time table of study and organizational chart
- Ethical considerations—human subjects and informed consent
- Consultations and arrangement between institutions
- Cited literature
- Appendices

S. B. Hulley et al., *Designing Clinical Research*, 2nd ed. (Philadelphia, Lippincott Williams & Wilkins, 2001).

---

treatment and control groups. Also, investigators should decide what is to be assessed and determine how a numerical value will be assigned, so as to facilitate measurement. For example, in the diabetes retinopathy study, the end point was measured on a binary scale (0, 1), which allows for the assessment of binomial proportion. The scope of the data collection should be formulated by considering these elements while developing the study protocol and proposal: sample size determination, when to begin data collection from baseline data in a prospective design; type of preoperative, intraoperative, and postoperative data if the study was designed to demonstrate the effectiveness of a specific surgical technique in correcting curve deformities for example; and data collection method—medical records, interviews, surveys, and so on. Therefore, failure to address these issues may significantly compromise the analysis and the interpretation of the study results.

Since most clinical research in some subspecialties, such as orthopedics, involves analysis of historical or retrospective data, attention must be paid to the reliability of such data sources.

Data collection must be ensured. This process requires that data collected be performed in a manner that will reflect an appropriate and accurate measurement, which is essential in establishing the internal validity of the study. In addition, repeatability, reproducibility, accuracy, and stability are elements that will inform data accuracy and consistency. *Repeatability* refers to the ability of the investigator or researcher to reach essentially the same outcome multiple times on one particular item with the same equipment.[2,3] For example, if a study is conducted to examine whether or not cervical fusion with instrumentation increases the rate of cervical stability, the outcome measure, being union or fusion, is measured by x-ray. In this case, repeatability refers to the investigator's ability to ascertain fusion on a given subject (subject with fusion) on multiple examinations of the x-ray and nonfusion on a given subject (subject without fusion) on multiple measures. Practically, if the investigator examines the x-ray 5 to 10 times, the measurement is expected to be the same, implying fusion or union on the subject with cervical stability and nonfusion on subjects without cervical stability.

Reproducibility refers to the ability of the investigators to measure the same item with the same equipment (x-ray) and reach essentially the same outcomes (fusion or nonfusion). In addition, the degree to which the measurement system is accurate will generally be the difference between an observed average measurement and the associated known standard value. Finally, the degree to which the measurement system or device is stable is generally expressed by the variation resulting from the same investigator measuring the same item, with the same equipment, over an extended period of time. For appropriate ascertainment of study variables, investigators must reflect and consider the role or impact of these factors (repeatability, reproducibility, accuracy, and stability) in diminishing measurement validity. Because of the need to ensure the validity of measurement, it is often recommended, if feasible, to conduct a pilot, which allows investigators to examine the data collection process and measurement.

Once established or defined, the data collection process must be followed as in the protocol and in line with the information on measurement accuracy from the pilot. The investigator must ensure that the process is executed as planned with consistency and accuracy. For example, if the investigators proposed to study the factors associated with postoperative pancreatitis in CP patients with curve deformities following posterior spine fusion, the measurement scale for the outcome variable could be dichotomous (absence or presence of pancreatitis). In addition, the investigators will establish the criteria for the ascertainment of postoperative pancreatitis, which will be based on serum lipase, amylase, clinical manifestations (symptoms), and imaging (ultrasonography). Consistency and accuracy of data collection require that pancreatitis (outcome variable) be measured as presence = 1 and absence = 0. Further, to be selected as a case, implying subjects with postoperative pancreatitis, the ascertainment criteria must be applied consistently and accurately.

Following data collection, investigators should assess the data collected to determine whether or not the collection criteria were met. In addition, the data collection and measurement system should be logic checked for repeatability, reproducibility, accuracy, and stability. For example, in the previous fictitious postoperative pancreatitis study, investigators should examine the data collection system for these factors prior to the analysis of the data for the effects or role of reactive airway disease and gastroesophageal disease on the development of postoperative pancreatitis. This post–data collection evaluation should lead investigators to determine whether the criteria were met and, if not, to determine the factors that may result in the poor quality data (inaccurate measurement).

2.6.1   Data collection methods

2.6.1.1   Quantitative data collection

Data may be described as set of values for a measured variable. Quantitative data collection refers to a collection method that relies on random sampling and structured data collection instruments that fit diverse experiences into predetermined response categories. This method generates results that are simple to summarize, compare, and generalize. Such data lead to hypotheses testing and subsequent generalization from the sample (study population) to the population (target). For example, a study is designed to examine the effect of maternal exposure to ionizing irradiation and the development of leukemia in offspring (childhood leukemia). The investigators collected data on maternal exposure from mothers (biologic) of children with leukemia and a comparable control, mothers of children without leukemia of the same age with the ages of the cases (children with leukemia). The hypothesis is tested using a test for proportion (chi-square or conditional logistic regression) to determine the odds of exposure in the cases (mothers of children with leukemia) versus the odds of exposure in the control (mothers of children without leukemia). A quantitative data collection may also be illustrated in a clinical trial or randomized controlled trial setting. For example, investigators proposed to examine the effect of a new hormonal agent, semisynthetic MHP (a fictitious agent), in treating polycystic ovarian syndrome. They randomly assigned 50 patients to the new agent (MHP) and 50 patients to current treatment—progesterone—and followed them for five years. The hypothesis is tested to determine the success rate of the new agent in achieving the primary end point (recovery—measured by reduction in cyst numbers by imaging measure). Examples of data gathering strategies for quantitative data include experiments/clinical trials and observing and recording well-defined events (for example, counting the number of patients presenting for fracture treatment at the cast room during the afternoon hours on a specified day), retrieving relevant data from medical records, and survey administration (for example, assessing the need for prostate cancer education for older males by determining their knowledge of prostate cancer risk factors using a face-to-face, closed-ended 10-item structured questionnaire).

Commonly used interview types are face-to-face, telephone, and computer-assisted personal interviewing, which is a form of personal interviewing, but instead of completing a questionnaire, the interviewer brings along a laptop or handheld computer to enter the information directly into the database.

2.6.1.1.1   TYPES OF QUESTIONNAIRES

There are several types of questionnaires in a research project, the choice of which depends on the nature and design of the study. Examples include paper-pencil questionnaires and web-based questionnaires, which is a new and inevitably growing methodology based on the use of the Internet for research.

2.6.1.2   *Qualitative data collection*

Qualitative data collection methods play an essential role in impact evaluation by providing information useful in understanding the processes behind observed results and assessing changes in people's perceptions of their well-being. These methods are characterized by the following attributes:

a   Open ended with less structured protocols
b   More heavily based on iterative interviews
c   Use triangulation to increase the credibility of the findings
d   Nongeneralizable findings

The qualitative methods most commonly used in evaluation can be classified in three broad categories:

1   In-depth interview
2   Observation methods
3   Document review

2.6.2   *Modern data collection techniques*

Other methods of data collection include telephone interviews, focus groups, mail surveys, web/email surveys, fax surveys, disk-by-mail surveys, conference/exhibit surveys, and one-on-one interviews.

All clinical research involves the collection of data, which are recorded in some format for each subject.[3,4] Most data are derived from a source document. Usually, the data need to be transcribed from their original form to another format (e.g., a computer database) where they can be reviewed and analyzed. Whether the data collected are kept in original form, on a personal computer, or transcribed to a paper collection form (a "case report form"), they must be consistent with the source documents or the discrepancies should be explained and documented.

2.6.3   Research data management

Research data management refers to the process of handling a data resource that is valuable to research. Data management is the process of developing data architectures, practices, and procedures dealing with data and then executing these aspects on a regular basis.

Data management involves these processes:

a Data modeling—refers to structure and organization of collected data to ensure efficient storage for analysis.
b Data warehousing—refers to data storage for easy accessibility for analysis and report.
c Data movement.
d Database administration—involves data recovery, integrity, security, availability, performance, development, and testing support.
e Data mining—refers to the process in which large amounts of data are sifted through to show trends, relationships, and patterns.

2.6.4   Data analysis

As it is often observed, not all who use a scalpel are surgeons; in the same manner, not all who handle numbers can adequately make sense of data by applying appropriate analytic models. The skills needed in statistical modeling in clinical and biomedical research involve competent and experienced biostatisticians. We recommend clinicians hire such individuals or seek their consultation prior to the initiation of the research project.

Data (a set of values for a measured variable) analysis is a process of gathering, modeling, and transforming data with the goal of highlighting useful information, suggesting conclusions, and supporting decision making.[5,6] This task involves understanding the study design and the assumptions behind the statistical techniques as well as the limitations of the techniques used. Therefore, knowledge of the basic theory underlying the analysis is essential to the analyst's ability to run the statistical package. The statistical analysis of data is a process with several phases, each with its own goal:

a Data cleaning—process of cleaning erroneous entries to ensure data quality. In cleaning data, it is essential to have duplicate files and not to discard any information at any stage of the cleaning. Also, when altering variables, the original values should be kept in a duplicate dataset or under a different variable name so that information is always cumulatively retrievable.
b Initial data analysis or preanalysis cleaning—involves the use of descriptive statistics to address data quality. Comparison of *distribution* before and after cleaning assesses whether or not cleaning has an effect on the data

system. This process allows for missing data to be assessed—that is, if data are missing at random or if statistical imputation is needed. Finally, data are assessed for extreme observation, and if the distribution is affected, a more robust analytic technique is required or a parameter, such as the median, which is not influenced by extreme values or outliers, is used. *Quality of the measurements* (quality of measurement instrument) may be assessed using homogeneity analysis for internal consistency of measurement or Cronbach's alpha (α) for the reliability of the measurement instrument.[1,2] *Intended purpose to the design* examines whether data gathered for a certain study met the intended design; for example, in a randomized clinical trial, the treatment and control groups could be compared. If the two groups are comparable at baseline, then randomization was achieved; otherwise, propensity analysis could be performed to address the imbalance in the baseline characteristics. For example, Holmes et al.[7] conducted a study on the effectiveness of androgen-deprivation therapy (ADT) in prolonging the survival of older males treated for locoregional prostate cancer. Because of imbalances in study characteristics between those who received ADT and those who did not, they performed a propensity analysis as one of the main analyses to handle the group imbalance prior to the multivariable Cox regression model.[7] Also, the analysis of nonresponse, dropout, or loss to follow-up could be used to assess the implementation of the design. Another area would be *characteristics of the sample*. For example, in the data on the study to assess for the intraoperative factors predisposing to deep wound infection in pediatric patients with neuromuscular scoliosis who underwent posterior spine fusion for curve deformities correction, investigators collected data on age at surgery, height, and weight. If the distributions of these variables are not normal, investigators may transform the data or generate categorical data. In addition, missing data and outliers could be addressed at this stage.

2.6.5   *Hypothesis-specific or main analysis*

The main analysis of the study is that which answers the primary and secondary questions.[1,5,6,8,9] This analysis should be performed to test the hypotheses specifically as proposed in the study. The choice of the test statistic will depend on the scale of measurement of the response or outcome variables, the scale of measurement of the independent variables, the assumptions behind the distribution of the data, the study design, and the clinical relevance of the measure of effect or point estimate.[4-6,8,9] For example, investigators conducted a retrospective cohort study to examine the effectiveness of spine fusion with titanium instrumentation in treating curve deformities in adolescent idiopathic scoliosis. The mean years of follow-up was 2.8, and they obtained baseline and five follow-up measures at immediate, 6 months, 12 months, 18 months, and 24 months. Using the primary end point, thoracic curve angle for correction achievement and maintenance, the statistical technique to determine a statistically significant difference between baseline and postoperative thoracic curve angle was repeated-measure ANOVA. The selection of this test was based on the design, a retrospective cohort study (case-only) that involved repeated measure of outcome or response variables from the same subject, where the same subject is the control (baseline preoperative thoracic curve angle) and case (postoperative thoracic curve angle; *scale of measurement of the outcome variable*, the thoracic curve angle was measured in a continuous case; and *clinical relevance*—the repeated-measure ANOVA generates the mean, SD, ratio of the variances of the mean measures, and the significance level, *p* value). The clinical criteria for loss of correction is an increase in postoperative thoracic curve angle greater than 10°, which is easily determined using a parametric test that produces the mean and SD. In addition, this test allows for adjustment for the confounders, such as age at surgery, sex (variables with clinical or biologic relevance in disease occurrence and treatment outcomes), and other variables that affect curve correction in adolescent idiopathic scoliosis.

The approach to hypothesis-specific analysis in the statistical analysis plan is to present the approach, rationale and assumption, expected or anticipated results, as well as potential pitfalls and alternative strategy (Table 2.1). For example, in testing the hypothesis regarding low birth weight (LBW) and acute lymphocytic leukemia (ALL), the process for the inferential statistics, implying generalizing the findings in the sample data to the population, will involve:

a **Approach:** This step addresses the statistical model or test statistic, mainly logistic regression or z statistics, in examining the proportion as a binomial approximation, given the scale of measurement of the response/dependent or outcome variable (ALL).

b **Rationale and assumption:** (i) The logistic regression model is adequate in examining the association between response/outcome and independent/predictor variable (LBW) if the response is measured on a binary scale (0,1)

Table 2.1 Types of sampling and sampling process

Population and sample	Types of samples	Sampling process
A probability sampling scheme is one in which every unit in the population has a chance of being selected in the sample, implying the same probability of selection—"equal probability of selection" (EPS) design.	**Probability** • Simple random • Systematic • Stratified random • Cluster • Multistage • Multiphase **Nonprobability** • Convenience • Quota • Purposive	• Characterize the population of concern • Specify a sampling frame, a set of items, or events possible to measure • Specify a sampling method for selecting items or events from the frame • Determine the sample size • Implement the sampling plan • Sample and data collection • Review the sampling process

and the independent/predictor/explanatory variables are measured in a qualitative or quantitative scale, (ii) there is no assumption of the shape of the distribution of the variable/s or data, (iii) there is no reference to event or history
data (survival), and (iv) odds ratio (OR) or relative odds (RO) is the measure
of the point estimate and not mean differences or variance-focus analysis.

c **Expected results:** If there is an association between the variables of interest and the predictor is positive, the OR will be expected to be higher than
1.0, where 1.0 implies no association, and if the independent variable
is protective, then the OR will be less than 1.0. Secondly, if the p value
is <0.05, meaning there is a strong evidence against the null hypothesis,
implying the rejection of the null and the acceptance of the alternate
hypothesis, thus the generalization of the findings to the target population as a reflection of the sample as representative. Such inference is
expected when there is: (i) actual difference in the OR, implying difference of a reasonable magnitude (clinically meaningful difference),
(ii) adequate sample size with a sufficient power to detect such a difference should one really existed, and (iii) reasonable difference between
group (exposed versus unexposed) variation (standard error).

d **Potential pitfalls and alternative strategies:** The inability to obtain a statistically significant difference using the p value method of hypothesis testing
remains a function of the sample size, which may occur if the study is under-
powered, and the magnitude of difference or the effect size is marginal. The
alternative approach or strategy is to apply exact logistic regression mode
in compensating for the sparse data or small sample size. Additionally, the
findings may be considered preliminary, while recommending further studies with larger sample size and avoiding to interpret the findings as statistically insignificant but presenting the power analysis in the paper.

2.7   Summary

Clinical research involves a balance between biologic, clinical, and statistical reasoning, which are not incompatible but complementary. As simple as
this may seem, however, it is the willingness of the clinical research team to
embrace these aspects of clinical research that leads to scientific validity of
the study. The result of clinical research is both clinical and statistical, with
the clinical result reflecting the biology of the disease while statistical inference leads to generalization involving the data. The combination of these two
reasoning pathways eventually generates valid scientific inference. However,
it must be noted that biologic and clinical relevance transcend statistical significance, given that a study could be statistically significant but clinically and
biologically irrelevant. In effect, scientific evidence in clinical medicine is not
appraised by p value but by the effect size as reflected by the point estimates.

As earlier described, clinical research commences with study conceptualization, which centers around the biology of the proposed phenomenon and
is often based on the clinical phenomenon observed by clinicians or others in

clinical settings, including epidemiologists. Such conceptualization leads to research question formulation, which is the primary issue to be addressed by the study, as well as hypothesis formulation.

Conducting clinical research involves many areas: clinical, statistical, administrative, funding, and infrastructure. Some of these aspects are not addressed in detail in this book, not because they are not essential, but because of the authors' limited training in the administrative and managerial aspects of clinical research. However, there are good references where readers could enrich their knowledge of this area. A well-designed clinical research study yields data, which are collected using several types of instruments and scales of measurement. Data contain information, and the analysis process generates this information, which is interpreted and presented as findings.

The findings of clinical research are often met with considerable skepticism, even when they have apparently come from studies with sound methodologies that have been subjected to appropriate statistical analysis. While details will be given in chapters to come on the interpretation of clinical research findings, such results should not be reported as "significant" or "nonsignificant" but should be interpreted in the context of the type of study and other available evidence. While the p value is not the measure of evidence, alternative explanations of results, such as bias or confounding, should always be considered for findings with low p values (statistically significant findings). The p value, or significance level, measures the strength of the evidence against the null hypothesis; hence, the smaller the p value, the stronger the evidence against the null hypothesis.[10–13] A significance level of 0.05 need not provide strong evidence against the null hypothesis, but it is reasonable to say that $p < 0.001$ does.[11,13] We recommend the presentation of the precise p value in the results sections of scientific papers and not the arbitrary thresholds.[10,12] The confidence interval (CI) should be included in the interpretation of the results and should not be used as a surrogate means of examining significance at the conventional 5% type I error tolerance of Fisher. The interpretation of the CI should focus on implications (clinical, biologic, and public health importance) of the range of values since this reflects both the point estimate and precision.

Questions for discussion

1 Empirical knowledge can be derived from experience, observation, and data. Discuss the importance of data in making reasonable, accurate, and reliable decisions regarding patient care.
2 Discuss the importance of placing data and theory on an equal scientific platform in clinical research.
3 There is a need for clinicians and other health care professionals to conduct research in order to improve therapeutics. Suppose you are investigating the benefit of a cytotoxic agent in increasing survival of children with neuroblastoma. How will you address the following:
   a Which study design/s will be considered adequate?

b   What is/are the research question/s?
c   What is the primary and secondary outcome or response variable?
d   What is the scale of measurement of the outcome variable?
e   What are the assumptions or rationale for the statistical method/s to be used in the analysis? and
f   How will the result be interpreted?

4   Suppose you are invited to the Center for Disease Control & Prevention (CDC) to discuss the results of your recently published study in a highly reputable pediatric journal on the effect of chemical pollutants on leukemia incidence. How relevant is the significance level in your discussion, which is expected to be informative and constructive in order to identify future research needs?

5   A study is conducted to examine the association between first primary childhood thyroid cancer treated with radiation and second primary thyroid malignancy. Discuss the process of the data analysis to generate the evidence in this context. Will you consider using structural equation model for the anticipated result? Why and why not?

References

1. S. B. Hulley et al., *Designing Clinical Research*, 2nd ed. (Philadelphia: Lippincott, Williams & Wilkins, 2001).
2. L. Holmes, Jr., *Basics of Public Health Core Competencies* (Sudbury, MA: Jones and Bartlett, 2009).
3. J. H. Abrahamson, *Making Sense of Data*, 2nd ed. (New York: Oxford University Press, 1994).
4. J. L. Garb, *Understanding Medical Research: A Practitioner's Guide* (Boston: Little, Brown, and Company, 2000).
5. D. L. Sackett, W. S. Richardson, W. Rosenberg, and R. B. Haynes, *Evidence-Based Medicine: How to Practice and Teach Evidence-Based Medicine*, 2nd ed. (Edinburg: Churchill Livingstone, 2000).
6. D. L. Katz, *Clinical Epidemiology & Evidence-Based Medicine: Fundamental Principles of Clinical Reasoning & Research* (Thousand Oaks, CA: Sage, 2001).
7. L. Holmes, Jr., W. Chan, A. Jiang, and X. Du, "Effectiveness of Androgen Deprivation Therapy in Prolonging Survival of Older Men Treated for Locoregional Prostate Cancer," *Prostate Cancer Prostatic Dis* 10 (2007): 388–395.
8. R. K. Riegelman and R. P. Hirsch, *Studying a Test and Testing a Test*, 2nd ed. (Boston: Little Brown & Company, 1989).
9. B. Dawson-Saunders and R. G. Trap, *Basic and Clinical Biostatistics*, 2nd ed. (Norwalk, CT: Appleton & Lange, 1994).
10. M. J. Gardner and D. G. Altman, *Statistics with Confidence: Confidence Intervals and Statistical Guidelines* (London: BMJ Publishing, 1989).
11. P. N. Hopkins and R. R. Williams, "Identification and Relative Weight of Cardiovascular Risk Factors," *Cardiol Clin* 4 (1986): 3–31.
12. S. N. Goodman, "Toward EvidenceBased Medical Statistics. 2: The Bayes Factor," *Ann Intern Med* 130 (1999): 1005–13.
13. P. R. Burton, L. C. Gurrin, and M. J. Campbell, "Clinical Significance Not Statistical Significance: A Simple Bayesian Alternative to p Values," *J Epidemiol Community Health* 52 (1998): 318–323.

3 Epidemiologic design challenges
Confounding and effect measure modifier

3.1 Introduction

Epidemiologic findings may be factual, biased, and driven by a confounding or effect measure modifier. The disentanglement of these spiders in the web of evidence appraisal renders such studies valid and reliable. We often conceive epidemiology in either simplistic or complex terms, and neither of these is an accurate characterization of epidemiologic studies. To illustrate this, complexities in epidemiology could be observed by considering a study to determine the correlation between exposure to allergens and immunoglobulin G (IgG) concentration in children. Two laboratories measured IgG concentration and one observed a correlation while the other did not. Which is the reliable finding? To address this question, one needs to examine the timing of the blood drawing following exposure to an allergen.

Epidemiologic studies could be easily derailed given the inability to identify and address possible confounding. Therefore, understanding the principles and concepts used in epidemiologic studies design and conduct to answer clinical research questions facilitate accurate and reliable findings in these areas. Another example in a health care setting involves geography and health. The risk of dying in one zip code A was 59.5 per 100,000 and the other zip code B was 35.4 per 100,000. There is a common sense and nonepidemiologic tendency to conclude that there is increased risk of dying in zip code A. To arrive at such inference, one must first find out the age distribution of these two zip codes since advancing age is associated with increased mortality. Indeed, zip code A is comparable to the US population while zip code B is the Mexican population. These two examples are indicative of the need to understand epidemiologic concepts prior to undertaking a clinical research.

Effect measure modifier plays a substantial role in the interpretation and presentation of epidemiologic findings. Consider a study conducted to examine the risk of coronary disease mortality associated with smoking. If the age-specific stratum varies for ages <50 years and >50 years, despite little variation between crude and combined or adjusted risk of dying, then age is an effect measure modifier in the relationship between coronary disease mortality and smoking. The presentation of such result without misleading the scientific audience is to utilize strata-specific inference and where necessary adjust for confounding in the age-specific stratum.

While hypothesis testing is essential in the generalization of findings, epidemiologic findings should benefit more from the presentation of findings using point estimate or effect size. In the context of this random variability of an uncontrolled variation in the data, random error must be quantified. The epidemiologic complexities is experience when researchers do not estimate sample size and power, apply no probability sample nor use disease registry or consecutive sample prior to quantifying the random error in the data.

This chapter attempts to examine the use of confounding, covariate, and mediation by several disciplines involved in population-based research, as well as the simplified notion of confounding, including the rationale for the application of this concept in achieving valid and reliable findings. The effect measure modifier is often interchangeable with interaction, which is not the case. Whereas effect measure modifier reflects biologic interaction as a biologic phenomenon in the process of causation, interaction as used in statistical modeling refers to the application of a product term to examine the multiplicative effect in the data. Confounding per se is not a bias per se, but may lead to a biased estimate in the data. Additionally, bias, which is a systematic error, is introduced, with the notion that while confounding is not bias per se, it may lead to a biased estimate in the data. Finally, examples from published and unpublished data are used to illustrate these concepts.

3.2 Confounding, covariates, and mediation

Confounding refers to the mixing effect of the third variable in the association between exposure (independent/predictor) and disease (outcome/response). To qualify for confounding, a potential confounding variable must meet the some attributes or characteristics namely: First, the confounding variable must be associated with both the risk/predictor variable of interest and the outcome (endpoint). Second, the confounding variable must be distributed unevenly or disproportionately among the study subjects, implying case/control groups or exposed/unexposed groups. Third, the confounding variable must not be on the causal pathway of the exposure (independent/predictor) being considered and the outcome or endpoint of interest.

The concept covariate is not interchangeable with confounding but is used mostly in statistics to refer to another variable that acts similarly like the independent or predictor variable in its relationship with the outcome variable. In epidemiology, the assessment of confounding involves the relation with both the independent and outcome variables. The concept mediation is used often by psychologists to reflect the effect of the third variable in either increasing or decreasing the effect the independent variable on the outcome. While mediation is comparable to epidemiologic confounding, it is not interchangeable as characterized by behavioral scientists.

3.3 Assessment for confounding

Consider the association between heart disease and vegetables/salads. Is extra virgin olive oil (EVOO) a confounder? To determine whether or not EVOO is a confounder, we must assess for the relationship between EVOO and vegetables/salad as well as the relationship between coronary heart disease and EVOO. To be a confounder, EVOO must be associated with the outcome and with the exposure in the source population (Figure 3.1).

While in principle the assessment of confounding may appear to be simple, the application of this concept remains debatable and inconsistent across epidemiologic thinking. Whereas some epidemiologists have applied the measure of random error, p value quantification to assess a variable as a potential confounder, such approach is inadequate and unpractical in assessing the mixing effect of a third variable on the association between the exposure and outcome variable.

```
. tabodds    di_CP R_Ethnic
```

R_Ethnic	cases	controls	odds	[95% Conf. Interval]	
0	187	54823	0.00341	0.00295	0.00394
1	29	11076	0.00262	0.00182	0.00377
2	43	7954	0.00541	0.00401	0.00730
3	38	9104	0.00417	0.00304	0.00574

```
Test of homogeneity (equal odds):  chi2(3) =    11.55
                                    Pr>chi2 =   0.0091

Score test for trend of odds:       chi2(1) =     3.73
                                    Pr>chi2 =   0.0534

. tabodds    di_CP  R_Ethnic,  or
```

R Ethnic	Odds Ratio	chi2	P>chi2	[95% Conf. Interval]	
0	1.000000	.	.	.	.
1	0.767602	1.76	0.1844	0.518827	1.135664
2	1 .584908	7.51	0.0061	1.136770	2.209711
3	1 .223693	1.29	0.2568	0.862778	1.735585

```
Test of homogeneity (equal odds):  chi2(3) =    11.55
                                    Pr>chi2 =   0.0091

Score test for trend of odds:       chi2(1) =     3.73
                                    Pr>chi2 =   0.0534
```

The previous stata output demonstrates the association between cerebral palsy (CP) in children and race/ethnicity (National Health Children's Survey [NHCS], 2012).[5] The data for race/ethnicity were coded as White = 0, Hispanic = 1, non-Hispanic Black = 2, and multiracial = 3. The prevalence odds for all racial/ethnic groups are observed earlier, followed by the odds ratio using White non-Hispanic as the reference group (crude and unadjusted

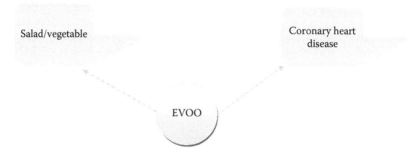

Figure 3.1 **Confounding as the mixing effect of the third variable.** The figure illustrates the confounding effect of EVOO on coronary heart disease.

association). Output also shows the prevalence odds ratio with all the subgroups relative to white non-Hispanics more likely to be diagnosed with CP except Hispanics in this representative sample of noninstitutionalized US children.

The use of stratified analysis of assessing the difference between the crude, raw, and unadjusted estimate and the stratified analysis with the potential confounder by observing the difference in the odds ratio, or hazard ratio, between the crude or unadjusted and the adjusted association is practically appealing since *p* value is not the measure of evidence. By convention, a difference of 10% between the crude and adjusted estimate allows for a variable to be considered as confounding and to be included in the multivariable model. Additionally, if a potential confounder is biologically or clinically relevant such as age and sex, adjustment could be made despite the recommendation of the observed 10% difference between the crude and adjusted point estimate for confounding adjustment. Further, variables established to be confounding, despite this literature claim, require an assessment prior to inclusion in the model for adjustment.

```
. tabodds   di_CP  QPV,   or
```

QPV	Odds Ratio	chi2	P>chi2	[95% Conf. Interval]	
1	1.000000	.	.	.	.
2	0.891786	0.40	0.5280	0.624738	1.272986
3	0.742221	3.18	0.0747	0.534115	1.031412
4	0.589481	9.91	0.0016	0.422599	0.822263

```
Test of homogeneity (equal odds): chi2(3) =    11.70
                                   Pr>chi2 =  0.0085

Score test for trend of odds:     chi2(1) =    11.64
                                   Pr>chi2 =  0.0006
```

We can use stratification analysis to examine the role of potential confounding in the previous relationship between CP and race/ethnicity. The stata output below uses Mantel-Haenzel (M-H) stratified analysis (mhodds var1(outcome) var2 (predictor), by (var 3 – potential confounding)) to fit the model for the analysis.

```
. tabodds    di_CP   QPV,   or
```

QPV	Odds Ratio	chi2	P>chi2	[95% Conf. Interval]	
1	1.000000	.	.	.	.
2	0.891786	0.40	0.5280	0.624738	1.272986
3	0.742221	3.18	0.0747	0.534115	1.031412
4	0.589481	9.91	0.0016	0.422599	0.822263

```
Test of homogeneity (equal odds): chi2(3) =    11.70
                                   Pr>chi2 =   0.0085

Score test for trend of odds:      chi2(1) =    11.64
                                   Pr>chi2 =   0.0006
```

The association between CP and poverty by quartile level is observed on the earlier output. Is there any association between CP and poverty level? How is this assessed from the previous data output?

```
.  mhodds    di_CP R_Ethnic, by (QPV)

Score test for trend of odds with R_Ethnic
by QPV

(The Odds Ratio estimate is an approximation to the odds ratio
for a one unit increase in R_Ethnic)
```

QPV	Odds Ratio	chi2(1)	P>chi2	[95% Conf. Interval]	
1	1.002869	0.00	0.9817	0.78539	1.28057
2	1.111657	0.78	0.3760	0.87940	1.40526
3	1.019044	0.03	0.8588	0.82782	1.25443
4	1.183251	2.44	0.1185	0.95791	1.46160

```
Mantel-Haenszel estimate controlling for QPV
```

Odds Ratio	chi2(1)	P>chi2	[95% Conf. Interval]	
1.079818	1.82	0.1769	0.965931	1.207132

```
Test of homogeneity of ORs (approx): chi2(3)  =    1.43
                                     Pr>chi2  =  0.6987
```

The previous output examines the role of poverty in the association between CP and race/ethnicity in the sample. By observing the crude, combined, and the stratum-specific odds by the level of poverty measured on quartile level with the first quartile as the poorest income group and the fourth quartile as the highest income level group, is income a confounding, effect/association measure modifier, or both?

3.4   Confounding, covariates, and mediation

The terms *confounding*, *covariate*, and *mediation* are not interchangeably used in epidemiology. The terms *consistency* and *standardization* are essential and relevant to the understanding of epidemiologic concepts and application. While confounding differs from mediator or mediation, there remains a statistical mismatch and misclassification as well as interchangeability among psychologists and behavioral scientists. Basically, a confounder is associated with the outcome or endpoint as well as the exposure such as treatment or risk factor (Figure 3.2). Mediator, on the other hand, is associated with the exposure on the causal pathway, leading to the endpoint or outcome (Figure 3.3). From an epidemiologic perspective, a mediator is not a confounder since such an extraneous variable is not expected to be associated with the exposure but on the pathway of the exposure and endpoint/outcome relationship.

Covariates that had been mismatched with confounding by statisticians and often interchangeably used by other disciplines are variables that may influence the outcome per se. In the previous example on the association between coffee consumption and pancreatic neoplasm, subjects' body fat measured by body mass index (BMI) may be a covariate, implying the possible association between BMI and pancreatic neoplasm. Because this concept is easy to be interchangeable with confounding or exposure, it is not widely used in epidemiology (Figure 3.4).

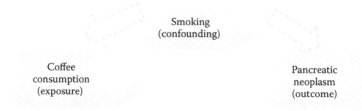

Figure 3.2 **The role of confounding.** The illustration of confounding (smoking) in the association between coffee consumption and pancreatic neoplasm.

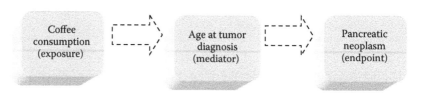

Figure 3.3 **Mediation in clinical research design.** The illustration of mediator (not effect measure modification) age in the association between coffee consumption and pancreatic neoplasm.

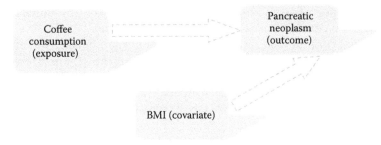

Figure 3.4 **Covariate in clinical research design.** The figure illustrates the application of covariate BMI in the association between coffee consumption and pancreatic neoplasm. In this example, BMI serves as another variable or risk factor or exposure leading to the endpoint, pancreatic neoplasm.

3.5 Types of confounding

If maternal waist circumference is related with maternal age and Down syndrome in their offspring, we can assume waist circumference to be a confounding. However, the direction of waist circumference, a confounding, must be assessed after controlling for its effect in a stratified analysis or regression. The stratification process as will be discussed later is a cross-tabulation of the data on maternal age (exposure) and Down syndrome (outcome/disease) by the potential confounding, namely, waist circumference.

The effect of confounding on the association of interest may be negative or positive and hence the concept, negative and positive confounding. A negative confounding results from the underestimation of the effect of the association, while a positive confounding results in the overestimation of the association. The magnitude of confounding (MC) could be assessed by

$$MC = \frac{RR_{crude} - RR_{adjusted}}{RR_{adjusted}}.$$

The MC could also be assessed by using the starting point, which is the crude point estimate in the denominator:

$$MC = \frac{RR_{crude} - RR_{adjusted}}{RR_{crude}}.$$

This later method of assessing the MC, while almost comparable to the former, is less favored by epidemiologists, since the former is a more accurate (less confounded) measure of effect compared to the crude and hence considered to be the starting value (denominator in the percentage difference estimation).

Other types of confounding include (a) residual, (b) unmeasured, (c) indication/contraindication, and (d) reverse causality.

Residual confounding results from the inability to balance the unequal distribution of the confounding variable between the groups being compared. This phenomenon may occur during the randomization (small/inadequate sample size) process, matching, and most commonly during the stratified or multivariable analysis. Specifically, if a study is conducted on the association between ultraviolet (UV) radiation and melanoma, and age is assessed to be a confounding and adjustment is required to address the distortion by age. The classification of age into two categories such as 0–50 years and >50 years prior to adjustment may result in residual confounding by age, thus biasing the point estimate and the effect size in this relationship. Additionally, confounding variable misclassification may lead to residual confounding, with higher magnitude, given differential misclassification confounding.

In a study on cognitive-related symptoms (CRSs) in sports concussion among children, Holmes et al.[1] observed age at injury as a confounder and utilized three age categories, namely, 2–9, 10–14, and 15–19 years, to adjust for distortion by age in the racial variance in CRS. Despite this apparently stable category, the authors observed that the point estimate in this study may be influence by residual confounding.

Unmeasured confounding refers to a potential mixing effect of the third extraneous variable that was not collected in the process of the study conduct and hence unavailable for adjustment. This situation is very common with secondary or preexisting data. For example, Holmes et al.[2] examined sex variability in pediatric leukemia survival using Survelliance Epidemiology & End Result (SEER) dataset, 1973–2006. The crude result indicated 14% (hazard ratio [HR] = 0.86, 99% confidence interval [CI], 0.80–0.93) survival advantage for females relative to males. After adjustment for age at diagnosis, year of diagnosis, race, number of primaries, tumor cell type, and radiation, there was 12% survival advantage for females (aHR = 0.88, 99% CI, 0.81–0.95). Although the SEER data are considered to be reliable and valid for the conduct of population-based studies involving cancer in the United States, there are significant tumor prognostic factor variables that were not available at the time of the conduct of this study, such as chemotherapy received, income, and education.

Confounding by indication and contraindication is not commonly used in epidemiologic investigation although very commonly encountered. For example, children with asthma are more likely to present with other health conditions and are therefore more likely to be prescribed other medications for other chronic conditions such as antianxiety medication, benzodiazepines. A study investigating the role of anxiety episode in asthma trigger may be confounded by benzodiazepine. Epidemiologic data had indicated the protective effect of diabetes mellitus in prostate cancer (CaP), but such findings were confounded by metformin (diabetes mellitus [DM] controlling/glucose-lowering drug). Bansal et al.[3] performed a meta-analysis of nonexperimental studies on type 2 diabetes (T2DM) and

CaP risk and observed an inverse relationship, implication of protective effect of T2DM on CaP. Holmes et al.[4] using Quantitative Evidence Synthesis illustrated the risk of cancer associated with hyperglycemia, DM, glucose intolerance, and insulin resistance.

```
. tabodds    SEIZURE n_BMICLASS
```

n_BMICL~S	cases	controls	odds	[95% Conf. Interval]	
1	46	2396	0.01920	0.01434	0.02570
2	374	27557	0.01357	0.01226	0.01503
3	98	6236	0.01572	0.01287	0.01919
4	134	5977	0.02242	0.01889	0.02661

```
Test of homogeneity (equal odds): chi2(3) =    26.73
                                   Pr>chi2 =   0.0000

Score test for trend of odds:      chi2(1) =    13.68
                                   Pr>chi2 =   0.0002

. tabodds    SEIZURE n_BMICLASS,or
```

n_BMICLASS	Odds Ratio	chi2	P>chi2	[95% Conf. Interval]	
1	1.000000	.	.	.	.
2	0.706917	4.89	0.0271	0.518954	0.962961
3	0.818557	1.24	0.2662	0.574814	1.165656
4	1.167752	0.81	0.3685	0.832584	1.637845

```
Test of homogeneity (equal odds): chi2(3) =    26.73
                                   Pr>chi2 =   0.0000

Score test for trend of odds:      chi2(1) =    13.68
                                   Pr>chi2 =   0.0002
```

The previous stata output illustrates the association between seizures and body mass index (BMI) in children using BMI percentile, with class 1 as the lowest percentile and class 4 as the highest percentile (>95th). There is a crude association between size and BMI class, relative to class 1, size was more common in 2, 3, and 4 BMI classes.

```
. tabodds    SEIZURE    race,or
```

race	Odds Ratio	chi2	P>chi2	[95% Conf. Interval]	
1	1.000000	.	.	.	.
2	1.276566	6.77	.0093	1.061632	1.535014
3	0.987706	0.02	0.8872	0.832485	1.171869

```
Test of homogeneity (equal odds): chi2(2) =     7.10
                                   Pr>chi2 =   0.0288

Score test for trend of odds:      chi2(1) =     0.32
                                   Pr>chi2 =   0.5711
```

Does race confound the earlier relationship between seizure and BMI? We can examine this using the M-H procedure. The previous stata on tabulation analysis examines the association between race and seizure for possible consideration as a potential confounding. The race variable was coded as White = 1, Black = 2, and other = 3 in the NHCS 2012 dataset.

```
. mhodds   SEIZURE  n_BMICLASS,  by (   race)

Score test for trend of odds with n_BMICLASS
by race

(The Odds Ratio estimate is an approximation to the odds ratio
for a one unit  increase in n_BMICLASS)
```

race	Odds Ratio	chi2(1)	P>chi2	[95% Conf. Interval]	
1	1.250547	14.01	0.0002	1.11236	1.40590
2	1.049465	0.14	0.7088	1.81456	1.35211
3	1.113838	0.73	0.3917	0.87031	1.42551

```
Mantel-Haenszel estimate controlling for race
```

Odds Ratio	chi2(1)	Pr>chi2	[95% Conf. Interval]	
1.196544	12.98	0.0003	1.085259	1.319241

```
Test of homogeneity of ORs (approx): chi2(2)  =   1.90
                                     Pr>chi2  =  0.3869
```

The previous stata output examines the confounding effect of race on the association between seizures and BMI class. Observe the stratum-specific odds ratio for Whites, Blacks, and others to determine effect of race as confounding or association measure modifier. Does the crude OR differ from the adjusted, and by what magnitude? Is race a confounding, association measure modifier, both, or neither?

3.6   Confounding and biased estimate

Confounding may be addressed in both the design and analysis phase of a study. During the design and conduct phase, the commonly used methods are (a) restriction or blocking, (b) matching, and (c) randomization.

In using blocking, the investigator restricts subject selection from a known confounding variable such as sex or age. However, this approach may result in a small study or sample size, limits findings generalization, inability to assess the restricted factor as well as the possibility for residual confounding. To illustrate the application of restriction in addressing confounding, consider a study conducted on the effect of BMI on obstructive sleep apnea among children where investigators excluded girls and children 0–9 years from the sample. While confounding by sex and age is addressed, there is a possibility of residual confounding and limited generalization of such findings to male children of all ages and girls.

At the analysis phase of a study, confounding could be addressed by (a) stratification or stratified analysis and (b) multivariable as well as multivariate analysis. A stratified analysis allows investigators to examine the intended association between the predictor variable and outcome at different levels. For example, imagine a study conducted on the risk of passive or second hand smoking with pediatric asthma with sex as confounding (Table 3.1).

We can estimate the stratum-specific risk ratio (RR) by risk in the exposed (R_e) divided by the risk in the unexposed (R_{ue}):

Mathematically: $RR = a/(a + b)/c/(c + d)$.

Among the male, the $RR = R_e(10/100)/R_{ue} (35/500) = 1.43$, implying a 43% increased risk for asthma among male children whose parents/caregivers are smokers. Among female, the $RR = R_e (36/200)/R_{ue} (25/200) = 1.44$, implying a 44% increased risk of asthma among female children whose parents or caregivers are smokers.

What is the crude estimate of the association? Using the 2 × 2 contingent table, $RR = a/(a + b)/c/(c + d)$; substituting by using the total sample (pool data): Re (46/300)/Rue (60/700) = 1.79, implying a 79% increased risk of asthma in the total sample without sex stratification. With the crude estimate higher than the adjusted estimates for both male and female children, sex remains a confounder in this illustration. With this example, sex is associated with asthma and with smoking, implying the potential for confounding. Additionally, the crude and unadjusted measure of effect is 79% and the adjusted (43% and 44%) for male and female is >10%, which is the minimum difference between the crude and adjusted measure of effect for a variable to qualify as confounding. Further, it is not plausible to consider sex as an effect measure modifier given the "closeness" of the stratum-specific RR (44% versus 43%).

While confounding is not a bias, it may lead to a biased point estimate, implying an effect size or association measure that is pulled toward or away from the null. In effect, clinical and translational research findings must attempt to identify and address confounding at both design and analysis phases or stages. Also, we must note that even after addressing confounding at the design phase of a study, there remains residual confounding of the variable, implying the need for multivariable analysis to further marginalize

Table 3.1 2 × 2 Contingent table on the association between smoking and asthma stratified by sex (hypothetical)

	Male			Female		
	Asthmatic	*Nonasthmatic*	*Total*	*Asthmatic*	*Nonasthmatic*	*Total*
Smoking	10 (a)	90 (b)	100	36 (a)	164 (b)	200
Nonsmoking	35 (c)	465 (d)	500	25 (c)	175 (d)	200
Total	45	555	600	61	339	400

the confounding effect of the matched variable as well as other potential confounding. Further, controlling for confounding should not be based solely on previous studies or literature review but must involve the assessment of the potential confounding variable in determining its confounding or effect measure modification effect or both, prior to adjustment.

3.7   Effect measure modifier

Epidemiologic studies must attempt to provide valid (internal and external) and reliable findings with the intent to inform intervention in controlling disease and population promoting health. Since epidemiologic, clinical, and translational disease findings could be driven by bias, confounding, effect measure modifier, or factual, investigators should attempt minimize bias and confounding as well as identify effect measure modifier and apply a reliable and nonmisleading approach in evidence discovery and interpretation involving an effect measure modifier.

Effect measure modification reflects a situation where the point estimate or the effect of the exposure on the outcome of interest varies by the levels or stratum of the third variable. Consider a hypothetical study on the relationship between hemorrhagic stroke and salicylic acid (aspirin). If the data indicate an 80% risk associated with aspirin (RR = 1.80, 95% CI, 1.45–2.05) in the overall sample of men, and the risk among younger men (<65 years) is 35%, while among older men (>65 years), it is 95%, age remains an effect measure modifier since the age-specific stratum risks substantially differ comparing older with younger men.

One must be very cautious in the presentation of the result with the overall sample since among younger men, the effect on aspirin on the development of hemorrhagic stroke is lower relative to the overall sample (all men), while among older men, the effect of aspirin on the development of hemorrhagic stroke is substantial. Consequently, among older men, aspirin significantly increases the risk of stroke, but not among younger men. In this context, the occurrence of effect measure modification by the third variable, such as age, is indicative of the need to present the data by separate stratum in order to avoid misleading results on the effect of the exposure on the outcome of interest.

Consider another example of hypothetical study on the use of anti-HTN1 (new drug) for the treatment of isolated systolic blood pressure in geriatric patients. Assume that no effect was observed in the total sample (n = 100), and upon sex-specific analysis, isolated systolic was lowered in women (n = 60) and not in men (n = 40). This example illustrates effect modification by sex. While the pool estimate demonstrated no effect or benefit of the hypothetical HTN1 agent in lowering isolated systolic blood pressure, the effect was observed in women (treatment versus placebo). This example clearly indicates the potentials for misleading treatment effect when effect modification is ignored in clinical and translational research data.

Effect modification as a biologic phenomenon could be observed in a situation where some individuals are more predisposed to a disease relative to the general population, given a specific exposure of interest. Consider a hypothetical study on exposure to benzene and acute myeloid leukemia (AML) development. If the risk is 2-fold in the general population of children but 20-fold among children with Down syndrome, the third variable, Down syndrome, modifies the effect of benzene on AML development. Effect measure modifier is a biologic phenomenon that requires description while confounding is a distortion of the factual association as a result of a third variable or imbalance between the group on the magnitude of the third variable that requires balancing or adjustment. As stated earlier, a confounding is expected if the stratum-specific measures of association are comparable or similar to one another but differ from the crude point estimate by 10% or more. Second, effect modification is expected if the stratum-specific point estimate differs substantially from one another. Third, if both confounding and effect measure modifier are expected, the stratum-specific estimate will differ from one another and both will be less than or greater than the crude estimate. Finally, if both effect measure and confounding are observed, data should be presented as effect measure modification by reporting the result separately.

```
. tabodds  DM n_BMICLASS
```

n_BMICL~S	cases	controls	odds	[95% Conf. Interval]	
1	6	2436	0.00246	0.00111	0.00549
2	181	27750	0.00652	0.00564	0.00755
3	62	6272	0.00989	0.00770	0.01269
4	95	6016	0.01579	0.01289	0.01934

```
Test of homogeneity (equal odds):   chi2(3) =    63.70
                                     Pr>chi2 =   0.0000

Score test for trend of odds:        chi2(1) =    62.76
                                     Pr>chi2 =   0.0000

. tabodds  DM n_BMICLASS, or
```

n_BMICLASS	Odds Ratio	chi2	P>chi2	[95% Conf. Interval]	
1	1.000000	.	.	.	.
2	2.648144	5.94	0.0148	1.172814	5.979351
3	4.013393	12.32	0.0004	1.732766	9.295729
4	6.411237	25.61	0.0000	2.802156	14.668692

```
Test of homogeneity (equal odds):   chi2(3) =    63.70
                                     Pr>chi2 =   0.0000

Score test for trend of odds:        chi2(1) =    62.76
                                     Pr>chi2 =   0.0000
```

The previous stata output assesses an association between diabetes and BMI class (described earlier). A dose–response association is observed with diabetes in children: the higher the BMI percentile, the greater the risk of diabetes. Does poverty (described in the earlier quartile) confound this association? Is poverty an effect measure modifier?

```
. mhodds  DM n_BMICLASS, by( QPV)
```

Score test for trend of odds with n_BMICLASS
by QPV

(The Odds Ratio estimate is an approximation to the odds ratio
for a one unit increase in n_BMICLASS)

QPV	Odds Ratio	chi2(1)	P>chi2	[95% Conf. Interval]	
1	1.974922	24.30	0.0000	1.50675	2.58855
2	1.600351	11.12	0.0009	1.21394	2.10976
3	1.327562	5.06	0.0244	1.03725	1.69913
4	1.744348	16.46	0.0000	1.33321	2.28228

Mantel-Haenszel estimate controlling for QPV

Odds Ratio	chi2(1)	P>chi2	[95% Conf. Interval]	
1.628566	52.09	0.0000	1.426558	1.859179

Test of homogeneity of ORs (approx): chi2(3) =   4.85
                                      Pr>chi2 = 0.1830

Observe the crude, adjusted, and stratum-specific odds ratio for poverty level to determine whether or not poverty serves as an effect measure modifier, confounding, both, or neither.

```
. tabodds  DM race,or
```

race	Odds Ratio	chi2	P>chi2	[95% Conf. Interval]	
1	1.000000	.	.	.	.
2	1.288889	3.28	0.0703	0.978432	1.697854
3	0.725072	4.68	0.0306	0.541114	0.971568

Test of homogeneity (equal odds): chi2(2) =   9.30
                                  Pr>chi2 = 0.0096

Score test for trend of odds: chi2(1) =   2.17
                                    Pr>chi2 = 0.1408

```
. mhodds  DM n_BMICLASS, by(  race)
```

Score test for trend of odds with n_BMICLASS
by race

(The Odds Ratio estimate is an approximation to the odds ratio
for a one unit increase in n_BMICLASS)

race	Odds Ratio	chi2(1)	P>chi2	[95% Conf. Interval]	
1	1.632474	37.44	0.0000	1.39530	1.90997
2	1.614440	7.65	0.0057	1.14970	2.26705
3	2.689341	23.56	0.0000	1.80367	4.00991

```
Mantel-Haenszel estimate controlling for race
```

Odds Ratio	chi2(1)	P>chi2	[95% Conf. Interval]	
1.724103	63.28	0.0000	1.507567	1.971741

```
Test of homogeneity of ORs (approx): chi2(2) =    5.37
                                      Pr>chi2 =  0.0683
```

3.8   Interaction: Statistical versus biologic

Statistical interaction which reflects the application of effect measure modification may be complex and challenging to assess. For example, risk difference (RD) may differ across the strata but RR does not in the same situation. This observation signals ambiguity with effect modification since within the same situation, effect modification occurs with RD but not with RR. In effect, it is inaccurate to apply statistical interaction without qualifying the measure of effect, hence effect measure modification and not effect modification.

Consider a hypothetical cohort study on the effect of smoking and lung cancer in those exposed to and not exposed to pesticides. This study indicates no difference in the risk for lung cancer patients exposed to pesticides among nonsmokers (R = 0.83) and smokers (R = 0.83) with an RR of 1.0. With a RD being 0, there is no effect modification by RR or RD, implying that pesticide is not an effect measure modifier in the association between smoking and lung cancer (Table 3.2).

Consider another cohort (hypothetical) on exposure to UV radiation and melanoma and the effect of xeroderma pigmentosum (XP). The risk for melanoma among those with XP is 0.92, while the risk among those without XP is 0.90 (RD, 0.83, 95% CI, 0.79–0.87). There is a substantial difference in RR (RR = 10.15, 95% CI, 6.81–15.1), implying the modifying effect of XP on melanoma development following exposure to UV. With this example the RR effect modification occurs by XP in the association between UV and melanoma (Table 3.3).

Biologic interaction is less complex and is a direct phenomenon that requires the observation of an interaction between two causes if the effect of one is dependent on the presence of the other. For example, while the transformation of prooncogen to oncogens may result in malignancies, this causal

Table 3.2 The effect of pesticides on lung cancer associated with smoking (hypothetical)

	Pesticides exposure	*Nonpesticide exposure*	*Total*
Smokers	500	50	550
Nonsmokers	100	10	110
Total	600	60	660

Table 3.3 The modification effect of xeroderma pigmentosum
on the association between UV radiation and
melanoma (hypothetical)

	Xeroderma pigmentosum	Non-xeroderma pigmentosum	Total
UV exposure	600	22	622
Non-UV exposure	50	220	270
Total	650	242	892

Table 3.4 Triglyceride as effect measure modifier in the
association between LDL and HTN (hypothetical)

	High triglyceride	Low triglyceride	Total
High LDL	290	20	310
Low LDL	20	170	190
Total	310	190	500

pathway is further enhance by immunosuppression as well as the inactivation of the tumor suppressor genes, P53.

Consider a cohort study (hypothetical) to assess the causal role of low-density lipoprotein (LDL) in hypertension (HTN) among young adults. If those with high high-density lipoprotein (HDL) levels are observed to be hypertensive and among those with high triglyceride, the risk for HTN was ninefold. Could this illustrate interaction as a biologic phenomenon, statistical phenomenon or both? This observation clearly describes a biologic interaction in which high LDL predisposes to HTN and triglyceride is in the causal pathway of HTN (Table 3.4).

The risk for HTN among those with high triglyceride is 0.93, while among those with low HDL is 0.10. The RR = 8.9, 95% CI, 5.9–13.5, while the RD = 0.83, 95% CI, 0.78–0.88. The difference in triglyceride-specific stratum varies substantially, indicative of triglyceride as an effect measure (RR) modifier in the relationship or association between LDL and HTN. The pathophysiologic mechanism of HTN involves peripheral resistance, which could result from arterial stenosis. The bioaccumulation of LDL in the blood vessel (arterial lumen) results in plague formation, increasing peripheral resistance and, hence, obstacles to blood flow. This condition is precipitated by high triglycerides, implying interaction as a biologic phenomenon. Can triglyceride be considered a confounding in this association? To examine this possibility, one should examine the crude estimate (HTN and low LDL association) and compare that with the adjusted estimate. A 10% difference in the crude relative to the adjusted is indicative of triglyceride as a confounding variable as well. However, in terms of presentation and interpretation, the finding should be presented separately by the level of triglyceride, given the presence of the biologic and statistical interaction.

```
tabodds  DM  di_SEX,or
```

di_SEX	Odds Ratio	chi2	P>chi2	[95% Conf.	Interval]
1	1.000000	.	.	.	.
2	1.249915	5.54	0.0185	1.037704	1.505523

```
Test of homogeneity (equal odds): chi2(1) =     5.54
                                   Pr>chi2 =   0.0185

Score test for trend of odds:     chi2(1) =     5.54
                                  Pr>chi2 =   0.0185


. mhodds  DM n_BMICLASS, by(  di_SEX)

Score test for trend of odds with n_BMICLASS
by di_SEX

(The Odds Ratio estimate is an approximation to the odds ratio for a one unit
increase in n_BMICLASS)
```

di_SEX	Odds Ratio	chi2(1)	P>chi2	[95% Conf.	Interval]
1	1.415765	13.17	0.0003	1.17339	1.70820
2	2.231546	65.74	0.0000	1.83795	2.70942

```
Mantel-Haenszel estimate controlling for di_SEX
```

Odds Ratio	chi2(1)	P>chi2	[95% Conf.	Interval]
1.764226	68.00	0.0000	1.541530	2.019093

```
Test of homogeneity of ORs (approx): chi2(1) =     10.91
                                     Pr>chi2 =    0.0010
```

The previous stata output considers the potential effect of sex of the child on the association between diabetes and BMI class. There is a relationship between BMI class and sex (male = 1 [54.0%] and female = 2 [48.0%]) in this dataset, with girls being 25% more likely to be diagnosed with diabetes compared to boys (prevalence odds ratio [POR], 1.25; 95% CI, 1.04–1.50). Observe the crude, controlled, and stratum-specific estimates and determine if sex is a confounding effect measure modifier, both, or neither in the association between diabetes and BMI.

```
. tabodds  AS  n_BMICLASS
```

n_BMICL~S	cases	controls	odds	[95% Conf. Interval]	
1	206	2236	0.09213	0.07988	0.10626
2	2545	25386	0.10025	0.09625	0.10442
3	790	5544	0.14250	0.13226	0.15352
4	937	5174	0.18110	0.16892	0.19415

```
Test of homogeneity (equal odds): chi2(3) =    247.25
                                   Pr>chi2 =    0.0000

Score test for trend of odds:     chi2(1) =    234.82
                                   Pr>chi2 =    0.0000


. tabodds  AS  n_BMICLASS,or
```

n_BMICLASS	Odds Ratio	chi2	P>chi2	[95% Conf. Interval]	
1	1.000000	.	.	.	.
2	1.088173	1.25	0.2643	0.938081	1.262280
3	1.546708	28.54	0.0000	1.316341	1.817391
4	1.965702	71.68	0.0000	1.675984	2.305503

```
Test of homogeneity (equal odds): chi2(3) =    247.25
                                   Pr>chi2 =    0.0000

Score test for trend of odds:     chi2(1) =    234.82
                                   Pr>chi2 =    0.0000


. mhodds  AS n_BMICLASS, by (race)

Score test for trend of odds with n_BMICLASS
by race

(The Odds Ratio estimate is an approximation to the odds ratio
for a one unit increase in n_BMICLASS)
```

race	Odds Ratio	chi2(1)	P>chi2	[95% Conf. Interval]	
1	1.323856	128.77	0.0000	1.26124	1.38959
2	1.233155	21.57	0.0000	1.12877	1.34720
3	1.351105	37.42	0.0000	1.22692	1.48786

Mantel-Haenszel estimate controlling for race

Odds Ratio	chi2(1)	P>chi2	[95% Conf. Interval]	
1.310154	185.38	0.0000	1.260183	1.362106

```
Test of homogeneity of ORs (approx): chi2(2)  =    2.37
                                     Pr>chi2  =    0.3058
```

```
. mhodds  AS  n_BMICLASS, by ( QPV)

Score test for trend of odds with n_BMICLASS
by QPV

(The Odds Ratio estimate is an approximation to the odds ratio
for a one unit increase in n_BMICLASS)
```

QPV	Odds Ratio	chi2(1)	P>chi2	[95% Conf.	Interval]
1	1.182909	16.62	0.0000	1.09115	1.28239
2	1.334140	45.66	0.0000	1.22711	1.45050
3	1.414083	84.80	0.0000	1.31355	1.52230
4	1.269969	39.29	0.0000	1.17853	1.36850

```
Mantel-Haenszel estimate controlling for QPV
```

Odds Ratio	chi2(1)	P>chi2	[95% Conf.	Interval]
1.301010	175.38	0.0000	1.251318	1.352677

```
Test of homogeneity of ORs (approx): chi2(3)  =   10.99
                                     Pr>chi2  =  0.0118

. mhodds  AS  n_BMICLASS, by ( di_SEX)

Score test for trend of odds with n_BMICLASS
by di_SEX

(The Odds Ratio estimate is an approximation to the odds ratio
for a one unit increase in n_BMICLASS)
```

di SEX	Odds Ratio	chi2(1)	P>chi2	[95% Conf.	Interval]
1	1.321791	120.87	0.0000	1.25766	1.38920
2	1.385681	105.18	0.0000	1.30194	1.47481

```
Mantel-Haenszel estimate controlling for di_SEX
```

Odds Ratio	chi2(1)	P>chi2	[95% Conf.	Interval]
1.346285	224.70	0.0000	1.294947	1.399658

```
Test of homogeneity of ORs  approx): chi2(1)  =    1.35
                                    Pr>chi2  =  0.2460
```

The previous stata output examines childhood asthma in the NHCS 2012 dataset for a possible association between this condition (asthma as AS) and BMI class. Like in diabetes, a dose–response association is observed here. However, could the crude relationship be confounded by race, poverty (QPL), and sex? Are these variable effect/association measure modifiers, both, or neither in this association?

3.9   Summary

While the primary focus of epidemiology is to assess the relationship between exposure (risk or predisposing factor) and outcome (disease- or health-related event), causal association is essential is assessing intervention and preventive modalities in disease control and health promotions. With appropriate epidemiologic method, we are more capable of providing more accurate and reliable inference on causality and outcomes research. In effect, unless sampling error and confounding are identified and addressed, clinical and translational research findings will remain largely inconsistent, implying inconsequential epidemiology.

This chapter examined the challenges in evidence discovery using epidemiologic methods and designs. Specifically, epidemiologic findings could be factual, confounded, biased, driven by random error, and influenced by inadequate characterization of statistical and biologic interaction, namely, effect modification and effect measure modification. A factual finding does not imply a perfect study given that all studies are driven by some amount of uncertainties but the rigorous ability to minimize bias, control for confounding, quantify random error, and describe effect measure modifier.

As discussed earlier, confounding is a distortion of the association between the exposure and the outcome of interest. Confounding refers to the mixing effect of the third variable in the association between exposure (independent/predictor) and disease (outcome/response). To qualify for confounding, a potential confounding variable must meet the some attributes or characteristics, namely, first, the confounding variable must be associated with both the risk/predictor variable of interest and the outcome (endpoint). Second, the confounding variable must be distributed unevenly or disproportionately among the study subjects, implying case/control groups or exposed/unexposed groups. Third, the confounding variable must not be on the causal pathway of the exposure (independent/predictor) being considered and the outcome or endpoint of interest.

Biological and statistical interactions remain direct concepts and are often unfortunately interchangeably used with effect measure modification. While biologic interaction is a simple phenomenon implying a variable on the causal pathway of predictor and outcome relationship, effect measure modifier as statistical interaction is challenging since RD may remain the same while RR differs by stratum or level of the third variable. Very importantly, while confounding requires an adjustment at design, analysis, or both phases of a study, effect measure modifier remains a variable that needs to be explained and presented based on the levels or strata being considered.

```
. mhodds    AS    n_BMICLASS,   by  ( R_Ethnic)

Score test for trend of odds with n_BMICLASS
by R_Ethnic

(The Odds Ratio estimate is an approximation to the odds ratio for a one unit
increase in n_BMICLASS)
```

R_Ethnic	Odds Ratio	chi2(1)	P>chi2	[95% Conf.	Interval]
1	1.194342	10.06	0.0015	1.07022	1.33286
2	1.333009	120.16	0.0000	1.26623	1.40331
3	1.240188	21.82	0.0000	1.13308	1.35742
4	1.479958	44.67	0.0000	1.31923	1.66027

```
Mantel-Haenszel estimate controlling for R_Ethnic
```

Odds Ratio	chi2(1)	P>chi2	[95% Conf.	Interval]
1.312846	187.81	0.0000	1.262721	1.364962

```
Test of homogeneity of ORs (approx): chi2(3)  =    8.89
                                     Pr>chi2  =  0.0308
```

The previous stata output considers the potential contribution of race/ethnicity on the earlier dose–response nexus between asthma and BMI percentile (discussed earlier). Observe the crude, adjusted, and stratum-specific estimates of the nexus by BMI class and determine if race/ethnicity is a confounding, association measure modifier, both, or neither.

Questions for discussion

1 Since nonexperimental designs are prone to potential confounding, discuss the effect of confounding in epidemiologic investigation. Present at least two examples to illustrate such effect in terms of biased estimate.

2 Suppose a study is conducted to examine the role of environmental pesticides on renal carcinoma, and sex is considered to be a confounding as well as an effect measure modifier. (a) Explain each of these roles in the relationship. (b) How will you present this result?

3 A study is conducted to assess the causal effect of DNA methylation in AML, and race is suggested to be a confounding. (a) How will you assess this in order to confirm the confounding role of race? (b) Can race be an effect measure modifier as well? Please explain.

4 Differentiate between confounding, bias, and covariate. Please provide an example of each in an application, and describe two types of confounding.

References

1. L. Holmes Jr, J. Tworig, K. Dabney et al., "Implication of Socio-Demographics on Cognitive-Related Symptoms in Sports Concussion among Children," *Sport Med Open* 2 (2016): 38. DOI: 10.1186/s40799-016-0058-8.
2. L. Holmes Jr., J. Hossain, M. desVignes-Kendrick, and F. Opara. "Sex Variability in Pediatric Leukemia," *ISRN Oncol* (2012): 1–9. DOI: 10.5402/2012/439070.
3. D. Bansal, A. Bhansali, G. Kapil, K. Undela, and P. Tiwari. "Type 2 Diabetes and Risk of Prostate Cancer," *Prostate Cancer Prostatic Dis* 16 (2013): 151–158.
4. L. Holmes et al. Hyperglycemia, Insulin Resistance and glucose Intolerance Carcinogenesis. Epiresearch.org/poster/search.php
5. 2011/12 National Survey of Children's Health. Maternal and Child Health Bureau in collaboration with the National Center for Health Statistics. 2011/12 NSCH [Stata] Data Set prepared by the Data Resource Center for Child and Adolescent Health, Child and Adolescent Health Measurement Initiative. www.childhealth data.org

4 Epidemiologic case ascertainment
Disease screening and diagnosis

4.1 Introduction

Clinical medicine involves the provider's ability to accurately diagnose a case and provides the treatment needed to be disease-free. The understanding of subclinical and clinical conditions allows for a better characterization and classification of those with the disease relative to those without in the population of interest. The potentials in meeting these demands in clinical medicine and public health transcend the understanding of symptoms and signs of the disease to the application of screening and diagnostic test, with the intent to correctly classify those with the disease (test sensitivity) and accurately rule out those without the disease as disease-free (test specificity).

In benefiting the patient in terms of treatment and the population with respect to primary prevention, clinical medicine and public health require accurate disease ascertainment procedure in terms of screening and diagnostic test. Regardless of the nature of the test, physical examination, neuro-imaging (computed tomography, magnetic resonance imaging, and positron emission tomography), laboratory test (urinalysis, blood test), x-ray, the accuracy of the test is relevant for the assessment of disease etiology, natural history of the disease, and for intervention mapping. This chapter examines the application of screening (detection) and the diagnostic (confirmation) test mainly sensitivity, specificity, predicative values, their reliability and validity, as well as their benefits and limitations in disease ascertainment and prevention. Additionally, the clinical relevance of treatment benefit and harm is described with the number needed to treat (NNT) and the number needed to harm (NNH). Throughout the chapter, test validity is stressed and reflects the ability of the test to accurately classify those with the disease (sensitivity) and rule out those without the disease (specificity).

4.2 Screening (detection) and diagnostic (confirmation) tests

Clinical or medical research involves designs that examine the effect of a test on outcome. Simply, a screening or diagnostic test is beneficial if survival is prolonged among those screened for the disease compared to those who are not screened. Remarkably, the outcome of a diagnostic test is not the mere diagnosis, disease stage, or grade of tumor as in the Gleason Score used in prostate cancer (CaP) clinical assessment but involves the mortality or morbidity that could be prevented among those who tested positive for the disease.

The benefit of a diagnostic test depends on whether or not there are procedures and treatment in place to follow up the true-positives (patients or individuals with the symptoms who test positive for the disease). For example, to determine whether or not screening for prostate-specific antigen (PSA) prolongs survival or reduces the risk related to CaP, investigators may compare the rates of PSA among patients who died of CaP with those of controls who did not (Figure 4.1).

Medicine is a conservative science, and the practice of clinical medicine involves both art and science. The process upon which clinical diagnosis is achieved remains complex, involving history, a review of the system, physical examination, laboratory data, and neuroimaging, as well as probability reasoning. A screening test is performed in individuals who do not have the symptoms or signs of a disease or a specific health condition,[1] for example, the use of PSA in asymptomatic (no signs or symptoms of CaP disease) African-American men, 40 to 45 years of age, to assess for the presence or absence of CaP in this population. A diagnostic test is performed in clinical medicine to acquire data on the presence (+ve) or absence (−ve) of a specific condition.[1,2]

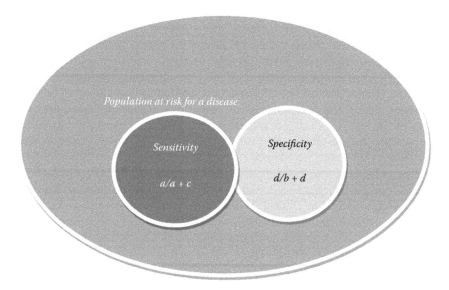

Figure 4.1 **Diagnostic test validity: illustration of the population at risk with those having symptoms correctly classified as diseased (sensitivity) and those without equally correctly classified as disease-free (specificity).** The intersection is indicative of test issues that challenge clinical medicine and public health in terms of treatment and prevention.

The questions are as follows:

- Why conduct a diagnostic test?

A diagnostic test is performed to confirm the presence of a disease following symptoms of an illness (Figure 4.2). For example, a 21-year-old Caucasian female presents with mild fever and frequent and painful urination that is relieved after voiding the bladder. The physician suspects cystitis and recommends urinalysis for bacterial pathogen isolation. The test confirmed *Escherichia coli* (Gram-negative bacterial pathogen). This example is illustrative of a diagnostic test, which simply confirms the diagnosis of bacterial cystitis in this hypothetical illustration.

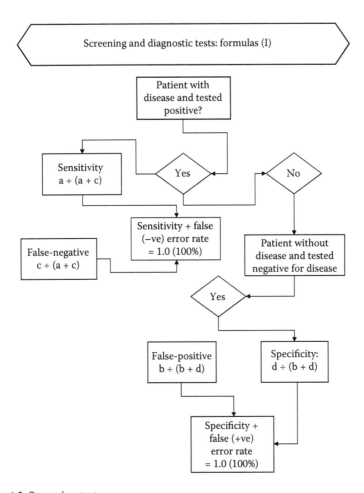

Figure 4.2 Screening test.

- When is a diagnostic test performed? A diagnostic test could also be performed to

  1   Provide prognostic information in patients with a confirmed diagnosis of a disease, such as diabetes mellitus, for example, a blood glucose level,
  2   Monitor therapy to assess benefits or side effects, for example, to assess pseudoarthrosis among patients with adolescent idiopathic scoliosis who underwent spine fusion to correct curve deformities,
  3   Confirm that a person or patient is free from a disease, for example, although not a very reliable marker of CaP prognosis, PSA level to assess CaP remission in men diagnosed with locoregional CaP and treated for the disease with radical prostatectomy and radiation therapy.

- What is a screening test, and what are the possible results?

Screening is an effort to detect disease that is not readily apparent or risk factors for a disease in an at-risk segment of the population. This test can result in four possible outcomes or results:

1   True-positive—positive test with the presence of disease
2   False-positive—positive test in the absence of disease
3   False-negative—negative test in the presence of disease
4   True-negative—negative test in the absence of disease

Diagnostic tests, results, and implications of screening depend on both the prevalence of the disease and test performance. For example, rare diseases are associated with relatively frequent false-positives relative to true-negatives and common diseases are associated with relatively frequent false-negatives relative to true-negatives. A screening test is generally inappropriate when the disease is either exceedingly rare or extremely common.

- What are the measures of the diagnostic value of a screening or test?

Measures of the diagnostic value of a test are its *sensitivity* and *specificity*. These parameters have important implications for screening and clinical guidelines.[3]

Sensitivity refers to the ability of a test to detect a disease when it is present. This measures the proportion of those with the disease who are correctly classified as diseased by the test. Sensitivity = $a/(a + c)$ (Table 4.1).

This implies subjects with true-positive test results (a)/(subjects with true-positive results + subjects with false-negative test results (a + c)). A test that is not sensitive is likely to generate a false-negative result (c). The false-negative error rate is given by the following: False-Negative Error Rate = $Pr(T - | D+) = c \div (a + c)$. This is otherwise termed beta error rate or a type II error. There is a relationship between sensitivity and false-negative error rate: Sensitivity $[a/(a + c)]$ + False-Negative Error Rate = $Pr(T - | D+) = [c \div (a + c)] = 1.0$ (100%).

Table 4.1 A 2 × 2 contingent table illustrating diagnostic test results

Test result	Population (target)	
	Disease	Non-disease or disease-free
Positive	A (true-positive)	B (false-positive)
Negative	C (false-negative)	D (true-negative)

Abbreviations: a = true-positive, b = false-positive, c = false-negative, and d = true-negative. Sensitivity = a/a + c; specificity = d/b + d; positive predictive value (PPV) = a/a + b; negative-predictive value = d/c + d; false-positive rate = c/a + c; and false-negative rate = b/b + d.

Specificity refers to the ability of test to indicate nondisease (disease-free) when no disease is present.

This is the measure of the proportion of those without disease who are correctly classified as disease-free by the test. Specificity is derived by Specificity = d/(b + d).

This implies subjects with true-negative test results (d)/(subjects with true-negative result + subjects with false-positive (b + d). A test that is not specific is likely to generate false-positive results (b). False-positive error rate is calculated as follows: False-Positive Error Rate = Pr (T+ | D−) = b ÷ (b + d).

There is a relationship between specificity and a false-positive error rate: Specificity (d/b + d) + False-Positive Error Rate (b/b + d) = 1.0 (100%).

• What are predictive values?

Predictive values refer to the probability of having the disease being tested for if the test result is positive and the probability of not having the diseases being tested for if the result is negative.[4]

BOX 4.1 THE RELATIONSHIP BETWEEN PREVALENCE, SENSITIVITY, SPECIFICITY, AND PREDICTIVE VALUES

• There is a relationship between disease prevalence, sensitivity, specificity, and predictive values.
• The prevalence simply means the probability of the condition before performing the test (i.e., pretest probability).
• The predictive values refer to the probability of the disease being present or absent after obtaining the results of the test.
• Using the 2 × 2 table, positive predictive value (PPV) is the proportion of those with a positive test who have the disease (a/(a + b)), while the negative predictive value (NPV) is the proportion of those with a negative test who do not have the disease (d/(c + d)).

- The predictive values will vary with the prevalence of the disease or condition being tested for.
- Therefore, the probability of the diseases before (prevalence) and the probability of disease after (predictive value) will be interrelated, with the differences in predictive values driven by the differences in the prevalence of the disease.

- What are the types of predictive values?
  There are two types of predictive values used in diagnostic/screening tests:

1 *Positive predictive value (PPV):* the probability of a test being positive given that the disease is present.
   Mathematically, PPV is given by this equation:

   $$PD+ \text{ or } PPV = a/\{a + [(pT+ | D-)pD-)]\} = a/\{a + b\},$$

   where PD+ = True-positives/{True-positives + False-positives}.
   Using Bayes' theorem, PPV is the probability that an individual with a positive test result truly has the disease, which is the proportion of all positives (true and false) that are classified as true-positives. PPV is thus the probability that a positive test result truly indicates the presence of disease.

2 *Negative predictive value (NPV)*, or PD−, is the probability of disease absence following a negative test result. Mathematically, NPV is given by this equation:

   $$NPV = \text{True-negatives}/\{\text{True-negatives} + \text{False-negatives}\} \rightarrow d/(d + b).$$

   Using the Bayesian theorem: PD− = [Specificity × (1 − Prevalence)]/ {[Specificity × (1 − Prevalence)] + [Prevalence × (1 − Sensitivity)]}.

- What is disease prevalence, and how is it related to PPV?
  Prevalence is the probability of the disease, while sensitivity, in comparison, is the probability of a positive test in those with the disease.

   $$\text{Prevalence} = \{a + c\}/\{a + b + c + d\}.$$

   Using the Bayesian theorem: PD+ = (Sensitivity × Prevalence)/{[Sensitivity × Prevalence] + [(1 − Specificity)(1 − Prevalence)]}. Remember that *sensitivity* remains the probability of a positive test in those with the disease—{a/a = c}.

- What are likelihood ratios (LRs)?

LR is the probability of a particular test result for an individual with the disease of interest divided by the probability of that test result from an individual without the disease of interest. There are two types of LRs: (1) *LR positive* (LR+) refers to the ratio of the sensitivity of a test to the false-positive error rate of the test. Here it is mathematically:

$$LR+ = [a/(a+c)/[b/(b+d)].$$

The *LR+* = Sensitivity/(1 − Specificity).
LR negative (LR−) refers to the ratio of false-negative error rate to the specificity of the test. Here it is mathematically:

$$LR- = \{c/(a+c)\}/\{d/(b+d)\}.$$

The LR− = (1 − Sensitivity)/Specificity.

- What is the measure of the separation between positive and negative tests?
The ratio of LR+ to LR− refers to the measure of separation between the positive and negative test. Here it is mathematically:

$$LR+ \text{ to } LR- \text{ ratio} = LR+/LR-.$$

This is an approximation of the odds ratio, OR = ad/bc using 2 × 2 contingent table. The *odds ratio* is the odds of exposure in the disease/odds of exposure in the nondisease. The odds of disease (lung cancer) = Probability that lung cancer will occur (*P*)/Probability that it will not occur (1 − *P*).

Vignette 4.1 Consider 160 persons appearing in a deep vein thrombosis (DVT) clinic for a lower extremities Doppler ultrasound study. If 24 out of 40 subjects with DVT tested positive for DVT, and 114 out of 120 without DVT tested negative, calculate the following:

1. Sensitivity
2. Specificity
3. False-positive error rate
4. False-negative error rate
5. PPV
6. NPV
7. LR+
8. LR−
9. Ratio of LR+ to LR−
10. The prevalence of DVT

Generate a 2 × 2 contingent table and perform the computation.

Computation: (1) Sensitivity = 24/40 = 0.6 (60%); (2) Specificity = 0.95 (95%); (3) FP error rate = b/(b + d) = 6/120 = 0.05 (5%); (4) FN error rate = c/(a + c) = 16/40 = 0.4 (40%); (5) PPV = 24(a)/30(a + b) = 0.8(80%); (6) NPV = 114(d)/130(c + d) = 0.88 (88%); (7) LR+ = {a/(a + c)} = Sensitivity/{b/(b + b)} (false-positive error rate) → 0.6/0.05 = 12.0; (8) LR− = False-negative error rate {(c/(a + c)/Specificity {d/(d + b)} → 0.4/0.95 = 0.42; (9) LR+ to LR− ratio = LR+/LR− = 12/0.42 = 28.57; and (10) Prevalence of DVT = (a + c)/(a + b + c + d) → 40/160 = 0.25 (25%).

The false-positive error rate (alpha error rate or type I error rate) simply refers to an error committed by asserting that a proposition is *true*, when it is indeed *not true* (false). If a test is not *specific*, this will lead to the test falsely indicating the presence of a disease in nondisease subjects (cell B; see accompanying table). The rate at which this occurs is termed the false-positive error rate and is mathematically given by B/(B + D). A false-positive error rate is related to specificity: FP rate + Specificity = 1.0 (100%).

- What is multiple or sequential testing?
  Multiple or sequential testing refers to the following:

a *Parallel testing* (ordering tests together)—the rationale is to increase sensitivity, but specificity is compromised. There are four possible outcomes in parallel testing:
   1 T1+ T2+ (disease is present)
   2 T1+ T2− (further testing)
   3 T1− T2+ (further testing)
   4 T1− T2− (disease is absent)[2]

   1 Sensitivity (net) = (Sensitivity T1 + Sensitivity T2) − Sensitivity T1 × Sensitivity T2.
   2 Specificity (net) = Specificity T1 × Specificity T2.
   3 Individual tested positive on either test is classified as positive.
   4 Appropriate when false-negative is main concern.
b *Serial testing* refers to using two tests in a series, with test 2 performed only on those individuals who are positive on test 1 (Tables 4.2 and 4.3).[2,5]

4.3   Disease screening: Principles, advantages, and limitations

Population screening refers to early screening and treatment in large groups in order to reduce morbidity or mortality from the specified disease among the screened. Screening for the purpose of disease control or mortality reduction involves the examination of asymptomatic or preclinical cases for the purpose of correctly classifying the diseased as positive and nondiseased as negative.[1,6–8]

Table 4.2 Screening and diagnostic test

Test parameters	Estimation	Interpretation
True-positive (TP)	A (2 × 2 table)	Number of individuals with the disease who have a positive test result
True-negative (TN)	D (2 × 2 table)	Number of individuals without the disease who have a negative test result
False-positive (FP)	C (2 × 2 table)	Number of individuals without the disease who have a positive test result
False-negative (FN)	B (2 × 2 table)	Number of individuals with the disease who have a negative test result
Sensitivity = true-positive rate (TPR)	TP/(TP + FN)	The proportion of individuals with the disease who have a positive test result
1 − Specificity = false-positive rate (FPR)	FN/(TP + FN)	The proportion of individuals with the disease who have a negative test result
Specificity = true-negative rate (TNR)	TN/(TN + FP)	The proportion of individuals without the disease who have a negative test result
1 − Specificity = false-positive rate (FPR)	FP/(TN + FP)	The proportion of individuals without the disease who have a positive test result
Positive predictive value	TP/(TP + FP)	The probability that a patient with a positive test result will have the disease
Negative predictive value	TN/(TN + FN)	The probability that a patient with a negative test result will not have the disease
Likelihood ratio of a positive test result (LR+)	Sensitivity/ (1 − specificity)	The increase in the odds of having the disease after a positive test result
Likelihood ratio of a negative test result (LR−)	(1 − sensitivity)/ specificity	The decrease in the odds of having the disease after a negative test result

Note: This table is based on the following 2 × 2 contingency table, where the disease is represented in the column, while the test results are on the row. *Bayes' theorem* refers to posttest odds, which are estimated by pretest odds × likelihood ratio (the odds of having or not having the disease after testing). *Accuracy of the test* is measured by (TP + TN)/(TP + TN + FP + FN) and is the probability that the results of a test will accurately predict the presence or absence of disease.
Abbreviations: True-positive (TP), false-positive (FP), false-negative (FN), true-negative (TN).

Table 4.3 2 × 2 Contingency table

	Disease (+)	Disease (−)
Test (+)	(A) TP	(B) FP
Test (−)	(C) FP	(D) TN

4.3.1 Diagnostic or screening test accuracy/validity

Diagnostic or screening test accuracy/validity refers to the ability of the test to accurately distinguish those who do and do not have a specific disease.[9] Sensitivity and specificity are traditionally used to determine the validity of a diagnostic test. *Sensitivity* is the ability of the test to classify correctly those who have the disease or specific/targeted disorder. Sensitivity is represented by a/(a + c) in a 2 × 2 contingent table. "SnNout" is used to describe sensitivity, meaning that when "sen"sitivity is high, a "n"egative result rules "out" diagnosis. *Specificity* is the ability of the test to classify correctly those without the disease as nondiseased. Specificity is represented by d/(b + d). "SpPin," which is used to describe specificity, implies that a very high specificity with a positive result effectively rules in the diagnosis.

The predictive value of the test addresses the effectiveness of the test to accurately identify those with the disease and those without. The PPV of the test addresses the question: if the test result is positive in an individual, what is the probability that such individual had the disease? This is estimated as follows: a/(a + b). The NPV addresses the probability of an individual with a negative test being disease-free. This is estimated by d/(c + d). The false-positive error rate is estimated by 1 − Specificity = b/(b + d). The false-negative error rate is estimated by 1 − Sensitivity = c/(a + c). Prevalence = (a + c)/(a + b + c + d). LR+, which is the LR for a positive test, is estimated by sensitivity/(1 − specificity). LR−, which is the LR for a negative test is estimated as follows: (1 − sensitivity)/specificity. The posttest probability is estimated by posttest odds/(posttest odds + 1), where pretest odds are estimated by prevalence/(1 − prevalence) and posttest odds by pretest odds × LR.

Vignette 4.2 Consider a population of 2000 people of whom 200 have unicameral bone cysts and 1800 do not. If 160 with the disease were correctly identified as positive by the test, 40 were not. Of the 1800 who did not have the disease, 1600 were correctly classified as negative. Calculate

1. Sensitivity
2. Specificity
3. PPV
4. NPV

Solution: (1) Sensitivity = a/(a + c); substituting: 160 ÷ 200 = 80%;
(2) Specificity = d(d + b) = 1600 ÷ 1800 = 89%; (3) PPV = a/(a + b) =
160 ÷ 360 = 44.4%; and (4) NPV = d/(c + d) = 1600 ÷ 1640 = 97.6%.

•   What is a receiver operating characteristic (ROC) curve?

The ROC, which is derived from electronics, was used to measure the ability
of the radar operators to differentiate signals from noise. The ROC curve is the
graphic approach to illustrating the relationship between the cutoff point that
differentiates positive and normal results in a screening test and the influence
of this cutoff point and the sensitivity and specificity of a test. This curve is
constructed by selecting several cutoff points and using them to determine the
sensitivity and specificity of the test. The graph is then constructed by plotting
the sensitivity (true-positive) on the Y axis as a function of 1 ROC– specificity
(false-positive rate/proportion) on the X axis [sensitivity versus (1 – specificity)].
The area under the ROC curve provides some measure of the accuracy of the
test and is useful in comparing the accuracy of two or more tests. Simply, the
larger the area, the better or more accurate the test. In interpreting the area
under the ROC curve (0.5 – 1.0), 1.0 is indicative of a perfect test, while 0.5
represents a poor test; this implies that an ideal test is that which reaches the
upper left corner of the graph (all true-positive without false-positive results).

•   What is the relationship between disease prevalence and predictive value?

There is a positive relationship between disease prevalence and predictive
values; thus, the higher the prevalence in the population at risk or screened
population, the higher the PPV.

4.3.2   *Advantages and disadvantages of screening*

Screening is most productive and efficient if it is directed at a high-risk population. It may motivate participants to follow a recommendation after the
screening and seek medical services given positive test results. In terms of
disadvantages of screening, if the entire population is screened and the condition is infrequent (low prevalence), this will imply a waste of resources, yielding few detected cases compared to the effort invested in the screening.

4.3.3   *Issues in early disease detection*

•   What are the benefits of screening?

Early disease detection: The natural history of a disease involves the following stages:

a   A *preclinical phase*, which is the phase that may be termed the *biologic* or
   psychological onset, but the symptoms have not yet occurred.

b   A *clinical phase*, which is the period after which the symptoms occurred.
c   A *detectable preclinical phase*, which is the natural stage of the disease where the disease is detected by screening.
d   *Lead time*, which is the interval by which the time of diagnosis is advanced by screening and early detection of disease relative to the usual time of diagnosis.
e   A *critical point*, which refers to a point in the natural history of the disease in which the condition is potentially curable, implying optimal treatment potential. The inability to identify a critical point in the natural history of a disease, screening, and early detection calls into question the benefit of screening.

The effectiveness of screening includes these elements:

a   Mortality reduction in the high-risk population screened
b   Reduction in case fatality
c   Increase in the percent of asymptomatic cases
d   Minimized complications
e   Reduction in recurrent cases or malignancies
f   Improvement in the quality of life[6,10]

Issues in screening include these elements:

1   Sensitivity and specificity of the screening test as well as the predictive values
2   False-positive test results
3   Cost of early detection
4   Emotional and physical adverse effects of screening
5   Benefit of the screening[6,11]

Biases in disease screening and detection are as follows:

1   Referral bias, also referred to as volunteer bias
2   Length-biased sampling associated with prognostic selection—this bias refers to a selection bias in which screening involves the selection of cases of disease with better prognosis[4,6]
3   Lead-time bias
4   Overdiagnosis bias

•   What is lead-time bias?
   Lead-time bias refers to the apparent increase in survival time after diagnosis resulting from earlier time of diagnosis rather than later time of death.

•   What is length bias?

This is a form of selection bias and refers to the tendency, in a population screening effort, to detect preferentially the longer, more indolent cases of any particular disease.

Vignette 4.3 Consider a new screening program for CaP in County X. The CaP screening program used a test that is effective in screening for early stage CaP. Assume that there is no effective treatment for CaP, and as such, the screening results do not change the natural history or course of CaP. Second, assume that the rates observed are based on all known cases of CaP and that there are no changes in the quality of death certification for CaP. With these assumptions,

a. What will be the influence of this screening test on incidence and prevalence proportion during the first year of this program?
b. What will be the influence of this screening on the case-fatality and mortality rate of CaP during the first year of CaP screening?

Solutions: (a) There will be an increase in both the incidence rate and prevalence proportion. (b) There will be a decrease in the case-fatality rate while the mortality rate will remain constant because of the assumption that changes were not observed with respect to the quality of death certification.

4.3.4   *Disease screening: Diagnostic tests and clinical reasoning*

• What is clinical reasoning?

The process by which clinicians channel their thinking toward a probable diagnosis is classically thought of as a mixture of pattern recognition and "hypothetico-deductive" reasoning.[12,13] The reasoning process depends on medical knowledge in areas such as disease prevalence and pathophysiological mechanisms. Teaching on the process of reasoning, as diagnostic tests provide new information, has included modifications of Bayes' theorem in an attempt to get clinicians to think constructively about pretest and posttest possibilities.[12]

Clinical decision making is guided, by and large, by statistical and epidemiologic principles, as well as biologic and clinical reasoning. The understanding of the former is the purpose of this book, which is not intended to place statistical stability in results interpretation over sound biologic theories and clinical judgment in clinical research conceptualization, design, conduct, and interpretation of results. A sound clinical judgment comes with experience, but such experience, in order not to be biased, ought to be guided by some statistical and epidemiologic principles, including, though not limited to, probability concepts (sensitivity, specificity, and predictive value),

Bayes' theorem, risk, and predisposition to disease. Therefore, since clinical decision making involves some risk acceptance, the understanding of probability serves to guide alternatives to treatment while assessing the risk and benefit of therapeutics.

Vignette 4.4 A 48-year-old Asian-American woman presents with hip fracture. She has a history of metabolic fracture and was previously diagnosed with osteoporosis. The clinical scenario involves the estimation of the probability of hip fracture in this individual, and clinical impression on previous cases indicates the common presentation of this condition in this subpopulation of age with a concurrent diagnosis of osteoporosis. The probability of response to treatment is dependent on the response of similar patients in the past, indicative of statistical reasoning. Although not a very good example to illustrate the application of diagnostic testing, the risk inherent in this case could be seen in the diagnosis of hip fracture resulting in a false-positive or false-negative test result. Also, the natural history of hip fracture may influence the clinical judgment in terms of the planned therapeutics. Clinical reasoning is also brought to question when considering alternative treatment.[14]

As sound clinical reasoning (avoiding biases) continues to shape therapeutics, there remains the necessity of clinicians being able to appraise clinical and scientific literature for evidence, and the volumes of clinical and epidemiologic studies become the basis of clinical decision making. Clinicians must understand how outcome studies are conducted and how the results obtained from these studies can be used in clinical decision making involving care improvement and patient safety. The intent is not to train physicians or clinicians to become statisticians but to refine the already available skills in order to provide evidence-based care that is optimal through the utilization of results from internally (biases, confounding, random error) and externally (generalizability) valid studies.[15,16]

4.4   Balancing benefits and harmful effects in medicine

Clinicians are interested in knowing the impact of treatment or intervention on individual patients. A large impact, relative to a small one, is of interest to both the clinician and his or her patient. The relative risk (RR) and absolute risk (AR) are two concepts that are extrapolated to determine risk in individual patients. The AR reduction (ARR) is used to assess whether the benefit of treatment outweighs the adverse effects.

We present these concepts in detail in the chapter on the measure of disease association and effect, but here, it suffices to provide a basic understanding of RR reduction (RRR), ARR, NNT, and NNH. Simply, the RRR refers to the difference in event rates between two groups, implying a proportion of event rate in the control (ERC) or untreated group.[17] Suppose 40 patients had recurrent cystitis out of 100 patients treated initially with erythromycin (control group), and 30 patients had recurrent cystitis out of 100 patients treated initially with erythromycin plus amoxicillin (treatment group). What is the RRR? The RRR is the AR difference (ARD) (40% to 30%) divided by the ERC group (40%).

RRR = ARD/ERC, where ARD = ERC − Event rate in the treatment group, substituting 40 − 30/40 = 25%. This means that recurrent cystitis was 25% lower in the treatment group compared to the control.

What is the ARR? Also termed *risk difference*, it is the arithmetic difference between two event rates expressed as the ERC minus the event in the treatment (ERT). Substituting, ARR = ERC − ERT = 40% − 30% = 10%.

The NNT simply reflects the consequences of treating or not treating patients, given a specified therapy. NNT may be described as the number of patients who would to be treated for one of them to benefit. Mathematically, NNT is estimated by dividing 100 by the ARR expressed as a percentage (100/ARR).

$$\text{NNT could also be expressed as a proportion} = \frac{1}{\text{ARR}}.$$

As ARR increases, NNT decreases, and inversely, as ARR decreases, NNT increases.

Vignette 4.5 If in hypertensive patients treated for the disease with a diuretic, the risk of stroke is 1.5 and 2.5 among the controls, how many hypertensive patients are needed to be treated (NNT)? What are the estimated ARR and NNT?

Solution: ARR = ERC − ERT. Substituting: 2.5 − 1.5 = 1.0. NNT = 1/ARR, substituting 100/1.0. Therefore, to prevent one incident of stroke, we need to treat 100 cases of hypertension.

The NNH is expressed as the inverse of the AR increase (1/ARI). The NNH represents the number of patients required to be treated for one of them to experience an adverse effect.

$$\text{Mathematically, NNH} = \frac{100}{\text{ARI expressed as a percentage}}$$

NNT could also be expressed as a proportion: 1/ARI.

Vignette 4.6 If the risk of developing postoperative infection in cerebral palsy children with scoliosis is 2.9 among those with rod instrumentation and 1.9 among those who received spinal fusion without instrumentation, examine the risk associated with unit rod instrumentation. What are the estimated ARI and the NNH?

Solution: ARI = Risk in cases (exposed) − Risk in control (unexposed) − Re − Ru. Substituting: 2.9 − 1.9 = 1.0. NNH = 100/ARI = 100/1.0. Consequently, we need to treat 100 patients (spinal fusion) in order for one patient to develop postoperative infection.

4.5   Summary

Clinical research is conducted primarily to improve therapeutics and prevent disease occurrence in clinical settings in contrast to population-based research. This effort involves adequate conceptualization, design process and conduct, analysis, and accurate interpretation of the results, which is achieved through a joint effort of clinician and biostatistician. The selection of patients depends on accurate ascertainment of disease, implying a screening/diagnostic test that is capable of classifying those with the disease as test-positive (sensitivity) and those without as test-negative (specificity). Screening is a particular form of disease detection test and is applied to a population at risk for developing a disease, such as CaP (PSA for older men, 50 years and older), in an attempt to diagnose CaP earlier than the natural history would manifest it. The intent is to diagnose early where CaP is treatable and curable. Diagnostic tests are performed to confirm the presence of a disease following symptoms of an illness.

The prevalence of disease simply means the probability of the condition before performing the test, meaning pretest probability. The predictive values refer to the probability of the disease being present or absent after obtaining the results of the test. Using the 2 × 2 table, PPV is the proportion of those with a positive test who have the disease [a/(a + b)], while the NPV is the proportion of those with a negative test who do not have the disease [d/(c + d)]. The predictive values will vary with the prevalence of the disease or condition being tested for. Therefore, the probability of the disease before (prevalence) and the probability of disease after (predictive value) will be interrelated, with the differences in predictive values driven by the differences in the prevalence of the disease. Sensitivity and specificity are properties of a diagnostic test and should be consistent when the test is used in similar patients and in similar settings. Predictive values, although related to the sensitivity and specificity of the test, will vary with the prevalence of the condition or disease being tested. The difference in the sensitivity and specificity of the test is most likely a result of the test not being administered in similar conditions (patients and settings).[1] The screening test should be highly sensitive (sensitivity) while a diagnostic test should be highly specific (specificity). As a cutoff point between positive and negative result changes, the sensitivity and specificity of the test will be influenced. This relationship is illustrated by the ROC and assesses the extent to which a screening test can be used to discriminate between those with and without disease and to select the cutoff point to characterize normal and abnormal results.

The advantages and limitations of screening remind us of the balanced clinical judgment in recommending large-population screening tests. The common biases in screening include length-bias sampling, lead time, over-diagnosis bias, and volunteer or referral bias (where those screened for the disease are healthier than the general population, thus influencing the conclusion regarding the benefit of screening). These systematic errors are all selection bias and if not considered have the tendency to affect the conclusions regarding the benefits of screening.

Often, clinicians may want to know the benefits or risk of treating a future or potential patient. In assessing the benefit-versus-risk ratio, the NNT, and the NNH are practical alternatives to RR or AR reduction in assessing the treatment effect. NNT remains a concise and clinically more useful way of presenting intervention effect. The NNT simply reflects the consequences of treating or not treating patients, given a specified therapy. The question remains as to which NNT is clinically acceptable to clinicians and patients, which is termed the NNT threshold. To address this question, one must consider the cost of treatment, the severity of preventable outcomes, and the adverse or side effects of the treatment or intervention. NNT may be described as the number of patients who would need to be treated for one of them to benefit. The NNH is expressed as the inverse of the AR increase (1/ARI). The NNH represents the number of patients required to be treated for one of them to experience an adverse effect.

Questions for discussion

1 Suppose there is no good treatment for disease X.
    a   What will be the advantages, if any, in performing a screening trial in this context?
    b   What are the design issues in such a trial if you were to conduct one?
    c   Survival is often seen as a definitive outcome measure in screening trials; would you consider population incidence of advanced disease and stage shifts as possible outcome measures?
    d   Early detection induces a bias in the comparison of survival times that artificially makes screen-detected cases appear to live longer. What is this biased termed, and how would you correct this in order to estimate the true benefit of screening?

2 Suppose that disease A is potentially detectable by screening during a window of time between its onset and the time when it would ordinarily become clinically manifest.

   a   What is lead-time bias?

   b   Would people with a longer window due to person-to-person variability in disease manifestation be more likely to be screened in the window?

   c   Would you expect the "window of screening" to result in length-time bias?

3 Suppose that 82% of those with hypertension and 25% of those without hypertension are classified as hypertensive by an automated blood pressure machine.

   a   Estimate the predictive value positive and predictive value negative of this machine, assuming that 34.5% of the adult US population has high blood pressure. Hints: Sensitivity = 0.82, specificity = 1 − 0.25 = 0.75. Using Bayes' theorem: PV+ = (sen × prevalence)/(sen × prevalence) + (specificity × prevalence). Comment on these results and state which is more predictive, positive or negative?

4 Suppose 8 out of 1000 cerebral palsy children operated on for scoliosis developed deep wound infection and 992 did not, while 10 out of 1000 children who were not treated with surgery developed deep wound infection. What is the RR of deep wound infection associated with surgery? Estimate the RRR. What is the ARR, also termed ARD? What is NNT? Hints: RR = (a/a + b)/(c/c + d); ARR = (c/c + d) − (a/a + b); NNT = 1/(c/c + d) − (a/a + b). What is the 95% CI for ARR and NNT? Hint CI for NNT = 1/UCI − 1/LCI of ARR. Hints: 95% CI for ARR = ±1.96 [CER × (1 − CER)/number of control patients + EER × (1 − EER)/number of experimental or treatment patients].

References

1. D. L. Sackett, W. S. Richardson, W. Rosenberg, and R. B. Haynes, *Evidence-Based Medicine: How to Practice and Teach Evidence-Based Medicine*, 2nd ed. (Edinburg: Churchill Livingstone, 2000).
2. D. L. Katz, *Clinical Epidemiology & Evidence-Based Medicine: Fundamental Principles of Clinical Reasoning & Research* (Thousand Oaks, CA: Sage, 2001).
3. M. S. Kocher, "Ultrasonographic Screening for Developmental Dysplasia of the Hip: An Epidemiologic Analysis (Part II)," *Am J Orthop* 30 (2001): 19–24.
4. J. F. Jekel, L. Katz, and J. G. Elmore, *Epidemiology, Biostatistics, and Preventive Medicine* (Philadelphia: Saunders, 2001).
5. R. K. Riegelman and R. P. Hirsch, *Studying a Test and Testing a Test*, 2nd ed. (Boston: Little Brown & Company, 1989).
6. S. Greenland, "Bias Methods for Sensitivity Analysis of Bases," *Int J Epidemiol* 25 (1996): 1107–1116.
7. G. D. Friedman, *Primer of Epidemiology*, 4th ed. (New York: McGraw-Hill, 1994).
8. D. G. Altman, *Practical Statistics for Medical Research* (London: Chapman & Hall, 1991).
9. P. Armitage and G. Berry, *Statistical Methods in Medical Research*, 3rd ed. (Oxford, UK: Blackwell Scientific Publishing, 1994).
10. B. Rosner, *Fundamentals of Biostatistics*, 5th ed. (Duxbury, CA: 2000).
11. J. A. Freiman et al. "The Importance of Beta, the Type II Error and Sample Size in the Design and Interpretation of the Randomized Clinical Trial," *N Engl J Med* 299 (1978): 690–694.

12. D. L. Sackett, R. B. Haynes, G. H. Guyatt, and P. Tugwell, *Clinical Epidemiology: A Basic Science for Clinical Medicine* (Boston: Little, Brown, 1991).
13. J. Dowie and A. Elstein, *Professional Judgment: A Reader in Clinical Decision Making* (Cambridge: Cambridge University Press, 1988).
14. J. P. Kassirer, "Diagnostic Reasoning," *Ann Intern Med* 110 (1989): 893–900.
15. J. P. Kassirer, B. J. Kuipers, and G. A. Gorry, "Toward a Theory of Clinical Expertise," *Am J Med* 73 (1982): 251–259.
16. A. Tversky and D. Kahnemann, "Judgment under Uncertainty: Heuristics and Biases," *Science* 185 (1974): 1124–31.
17. G. Chatellier, E. Zapletal et al., "The Number Needed to Treat: A Clinically Nomogram in Its Proper Context," *BMJ* 312 (1996): 426–429.

Section II

Epidemiologic concepts and methods

Epidemiology remains a basic science of clinical medicine with the purpose of assessing how diseases, disabilities, injuries, and health-related events are distributed as well as their determinants at population level. With respect to public health, epidemiology occupies comparable position by serving in the assessment arm of the core function of public health. In order to improve the care of the patients we see in clinical medicine, epidemiologic principles and concepts must be understood. Equally, an effective public health effort in controlling disease and promoting health requires factual and rational assessment of the risk and predisposing factors in disease etiology.

Epidemiologic study conduct either nonexperimental (incorrectly termed observational) or experimental or clinical trial (experimental design involving humans) are not simple as often conceived. The complexities of these designs rise from the attributes of subjects or participants given genetic and epigenetic super-variability of humans. And in line with Hippocrates' concept of disease etiology, the knowledge of the underlying cause of disease leads to the treatment and cure of disease, with this etiology including environment. Consequently, it is not epidemiologically sound to ignore these complexities in the design of clinical or translational studies.

As observed earlier, epidemiologic findings are inconclusive but cumulative, with findings or current results/data subject to changes or mutation as new evidence emerge. While studies' replication serves to improve patient and public health, replication of ongoing epidemiologic studies has its challenges, including, though not limited to, the differences among studies on how confounding, effect measure modifier, bias, and random errors were addressed.

This section explains the basic concepts used in assessing disease frequency/occurrence and the measure of effect in human–animal population. Designs are described with examples to allow clinicians to conceptualize studies with background and significance, biologic plausibility, and feasibility.

5 Epidemiology, historical context, and measures of disease occurrence and association

5.1 Introduction

Clinical research yields data and provides benefits for both the individual patients and the specific population of patients. Because clinical research involves a specific patient population, the distinction between epidemiologic and clinical research remains challenging. The design of clinical research is fundamentally observational (nonexperimental) and experimental/clinical trial. Although epidemiologic designs have been termed *observational*, epidemiologic methods are both nonexperimental or observational and experimental, which renders this distinction an imperfect one. These two methods are used in designing clinical research, and the answer to the question about which methods to apply depends on many factors including the research question and hypothesis, the type of data, the level of evidence, the disease or outcome frequency, feasibility, infrastructure, availability of funding, and availability of subjects.

Whatever methods or study design is used, the primary objective of a methodologist or clinical researcher is to obtain valid and reliable evidence from the data. This evidence primarily involves the measurement of disease or outcome/response effect. Common measures of disease effects are relative risk, risk ratio, or rate ratio (relative measures of comparison); rate or risk difference (absolute measures of comparison); population rate difference; attributable proportion among the exposed; attributable proportion among total population exposed; and correlation coefficient and coefficient of determination. While the relative measure of disease effect compares two measures of disease frequency, such as relative risk or odds ratio, and quantifies the strength of relationship or association between exposure (independent, explanatory, or predictor variable) and disease (outcome or response), absolute measure of disease effect describes and quantifies the effect or impact of disease by comparing the difference between two measures of disease frequency, such as incidence rate (IR) or prevalence proportion.

The measure of disease occurrence quantifies both the crude and adjusted rates and the proportion of disease or outcome of interest in a specific patient or community-based population. In clinical research settings, patient groups

Figure 5.1 **Population characterization and prevalence of outcome of interest.** Prevalence of outcome estimation is obtained by (X) ÷ (A), where A is (X) + (Y).

usually consist of those who show improvement after a procedure or medication and those who do not. The proportion of those with improvement measures the occurrence of the outcome of interest and could be characterized as the prevalence or count/frequency of those who showed the preferred outcome (improvement) and is measured by those with improvement divided by the total number of all patients studied (Figure 5.1). In a prospective cohort design, it is possible to measure the incidence of a complication among patients who received surgery (number of new cases of complications/person-time [P-T]). We can also compare the incidence of an outcome/disease in one patient population with that of another patient population, provided the two populations are standardized with respect to confounders, such as age and sex, which allows one to compare the age or sex-adjusted rate, also termed *standardized rate*.

This chapter explains epidemiology as the study of disease/health-related events distribution, determinants, and the application of such knowledge in the improvement of health in a specific population. Since epidemiology is a quantitative science, the measures of disease occurrence and effects are presented briefly. Mention is made of the history of epidemiology as well as the model of disease causation. The sources of epidemiologic data are listed to enable clinicians to explore resources for large data sets in performing community-based studies on issues of clinical importance to therapeutics and preventive medicine/health.

5.1.1   Epidemiology: Basic notion

Epidemiology, which originates from *epidemic*, comes from the Greek word *epi* (upon) and *demos* (people). An epidemic implies the occurrence of disease, disability, and injury beyond the usual or the expected (out of proportion). Although epidemiology has been provided many definitions from its modern and formal inception, it remains a population health science focused primarily on the distribution and determinants of disease, injuries, disabilities, and health-related events at the population level and the application of such knowledge to disease prevention and control. Epidemiology is simply a population-oriented "discipline" that quantifies, locates, and determines causes and mechanisms of health-related states or events and applies this knowledge to prevention and control of health-related events in specified populations. Epidemiology has traditionally been defined as the study of the distribution and determinants of health-related events in the human population[1] and the application of this knowledge to disease, disability, and injury control and prevention. As a basic science of public health, epidemiology is involved in the assessment and monitoring of health status at the population level and the application of these results in disease prevention and control.[1] Specifically, epidemiology deals with measurement of disease occurrence and frequency in the population; identification of when, where, and within which population subgroup health-related events are more or less likely to occur; determination of the causes at the population level; determination of the mechanisms of causation, natural history, and the clinical course of the health-related events; and application of the results to the prevention and control of disease and health-related events.[1,2]

In practical terms, epidemiology is an information science, and like biostatistics, it is not strictly a discipline since it is involved in all aspects of research design, conduct, analysis and interpretation whether or not one is conducting a bench, clinical, or population-based study. Because epidemiologic knowledge is required in intervention mapping and implementation to improve health and population health, epidemiology is a purposive science with the extended role and purpose of controlling disease and promoting health.

5.1.2   Distribution, determinants of health and health-related events, and specified population

The term *distribution* implies the frequency (number, counts, percentage, prevalence) and pattern (time, place, person) of health events in a population. The term *determinants* implies the causes, variables, and factors influencing the health-related events with respect to their occurrences. This aspect of epidemiologic methods involves disease or health-related events quantification (odds ratio, relative risk, risk ratio, hazard ratio, beta coefficient). Specified population implies the collective health of the population/people in a community setting in contrast to clinical medicine, which is concerned with the health of an individual patient. While the primary role of epidemiology is not to control or prevent health-related events, application provides data for public health action in controlling and preventing diseases, disabilities, and injuries.

5.1.2.1   Epidemiology and clinical research

Clinical research often involves investigation into the association between variables, identification of predictors of disease, and prognosis or outcome (response), as well as the effectiveness or efficacy of treatment modalities in a specific set of patients. Epidemiology, as the basic science of public health that deals with the *distribution, determinants*, and *prevention/control* of disease, disabilities, and injuries in human populations, plays a fundamental role in design and inference in clinical research. For example, clinical investigation into the effect of ionizing radiation on thyroid cancer in a pediatric cancer clinic may involve a retrospective cohort or case-control design. Therefore, without a sound knowledge and application of these designs and their measures of association and effect, such studies cannot be properly conducted, implying flawed design, confounding effects, effect measure modifier or interaction, and impaired generalizability. Additionally, epidemiology is involved with the distribution of disease and health/health-related events, implying the frequency (number, counts, percentage, prevalence) and pattern (time, place, person) of health events in a specified population.

Vignette 5.1 The city of Notown, Maryland, with a population of 246,000, normally has an incidence of *salmonella* of 5.0/1000 during the year. In summer 2015, the incidence was 125.0/1000. The occurrence of new cases (incidence) in 2015 clearly illustrates an epidemic of *salmonella* in Notown, Maryland.

5.1.3   Epidemiologic classification: Descriptive versus analytic

While it is inaccurate to classify epidemiology into descriptive and analytic due to the overlapping of these two concepts, such classifications are commonly used for the purpose of classification. Descriptive epidemiology is the basis for analytic epidemiology and remains the basis for hypothesis-generating studies rather than testing. On the other hand, analytic epidemiology aims at hypothesis testing given appropriate sampling technique and sample size (Table 5.1).

Table 5.1 Descriptive and analytic epidemiology

Descriptive epidemiology	Analytic epidemiology
• Disease occurrence data with respect to time, place, and person • Provides information on what, who, when, and where	• Disease causes data with respect to the rate of occurrence, the differences in rates, and why the differences occurred • Provides information on why and how

5.2 Epidemiology, clinical medicine, and public health research

The focus of clinical medicine is to treat disease and maintain health, but clinicians are also required to prevent complications and mitigate the risk factors that result in the development of disease. The understanding of epidemiologic study designs remains an essential part of the practice of medicine. The primary focus of epidemiology is the assessment of disease, disabilities, and injuries at the population level. The knowledge gained from epidemiology is used to design intervention in order to prevent and control diseases, disabilities, and injuries at the population level. Epidemiology is the tool for public health to use in its mission of disease control and health promotion. Epidemiology in public health is therefore an applied science providing analytic input to the understanding of health and health-related issues. The focus of public health is to control and prevent disease, as well as promote health, whereas that of epidemiology is to assess the health condition involving diseases, disabilities, and injuries, as well as health-related states.[3] Epidemiology is essential in clinical research, and its role is significant from conceptualization to statistical inference. Only a well-designed study can yield a reliable clinical data and valid statistical inference. Therefore, no matter how sophisticated a statistical approach to analysis is, such an approach cannot substitute for a well-conceived and designed study that minimizes bias and randomness or variability and confounding at the design phase through blocking, randomization, or matching.

The primary goal of the epidemiologic method in research is to establish an association between disease and exposure, not causal inference. Epidemiologic objectives embrace clinical medicine, as it evaluates both existing and new preventive and therapeutic modalities as well as the manner in which the health care is delivered. Epidemiologic methods enhance disease risk reduction by assessing etiologic factors in disease initiation and progression.

Causal inference is an extension of association and involves several criteria, beyond evidence from a single epidemiologic study. This notion is covered in detail later in the course of this book.

Vignette 5.2 The Maryland State Department of Health is responding to increasing cases of opiate overdose and addiction. The chief epidemiologist proposes to examine the determinants of these overdoses. The epidemiologist's role in this context is that of health-related event assessment, not control and prevention or health promotion per se. However, the knowledge gained from this epidemiologic investigation is intended for intervention to address the epidemic in the state. The director of the department proposes to address the determinants of these heroine or opiate overdose and addiction by starting an intervention to eliminate the risk and predisposing factors including free Naloxone distribution to street heroin addicts; this approach illustrates the disease prevention and health promotion role of public health. With the extended role of epidemiology, this profession is integrative implying the collaboration with other disciplines (transdisciplinary approach to evidence discovery and intervention mapping and evaluation) in advancing the knowledge of population health and the intervention to improve the health of the public. Therefore, given its integrative role in research initiative involving human-animal health, epidemiology is at the core of translational research (Table 5.2).

Table 5.2 The focus of epidemiology, public health, and clinical medicine

Epidemiology (core focus)	Public health (core focus)
• Assessment of diseases, disabilities, and injuries (health phenomena)	• Control and prevention of diseases, disabilities, and injuries, as well as health promotion
• Distribution (frequency) and determinants (risk and protective factors)	• Intervention, design, and implementation to address disease, disabilities, and risk of injuries, and protective factors. • Diagnosis, treatment, and cure of disease at the individual patient level

The primary focus of epidemiology is not to control and prevent diseases and disabilities and promote population health.[3] This is the primary function/role of public health.

BOX 5.1   OBJECTIVES OF EPIDEMIOLOGY

While epidemiology plays a significant role in the core function of public health, its objectives reflects the extent in which knowledge gained from the assessment of health problems at the population level could be used in program planning, implementation and the assurance that essential public health services are provided to the public.

• Identification of the factors that increase individual's risk for disease, disability, injury, or health-related event

---

- Determination of the extent of disease or frequency in the community
- Assessment of the natural history, severity and prognosis of disease
- Examination of the existing and new preventive and treatment measures and modes of health care delivery
- Provision of the scientific basis for decision making on health policies including the regulation of environmental problems in the society

5.3 The history and modern concept of epidemiology

The goal of epidemiology, as indicated earlier, is to identify disease and health-related events in specific populations. This exercise results in the identification of at-risk populations. The steps involved in conducting an epidemiologic investigation are complex and involve education and training. However, the growth of epidemiology has been gradual, with epidemiologic transitions. Simply, epidemiology began with an attempt to identify what causes morbidity and mortality in the human population, and this task continues to be primary. Epidemiologists first determine whether or not there is an association between exposure and disease development or mortality, followed by causal association (Table 5.3).

5.4 Models of disease causation

As indicated earlier, epidemiology is primarily concerned with disease association, implying the relationship between the disease and the potential risk factor or exposure (conceived to result in the disease) (Table 5.4). In considering the purposive role of epidemiology in public health, epidemiologic investigations also are directed at causation and the etiologic role of the exposure in the disease, if the intervention mapping that is intended to be risk-adapted is to lead to the prevention and control of the disease. Causation refers to the process of an event (disease, disability, or injury) occurring as a result of either intrinsic or extrinsic factors acting individually or collectively.[4] The causal action of exposure comes before the subsequent development of disease as a consequence of exposure. This is the basis of a longitudinal study in which exposure data or information refers to an earlier time than that of disease, disability, or injury occurrence.[4] The intrinsic factor in disease causation simply refers to the host factor (organism). Examples of this factor include the immune system as well as the personality, social class membership, and race. The extrinsic factor refers to the environmental factors, which are identified as biologic, social, and physical environments.[4,5]

Table 5.3 History of modern epidemiology

Person	Contribution to disease causation	Time (period)
Hippocrates	• Environmental and host factors in the development of a disease	Circa 400 BC
John Graunt—first epidemiologist, statistician, and demographer	• Quantification of patterns of birth, death, and disease occurrence; bills of fertility, morbidity, and mortality on weekly count of death in London	1662
James Lind—surgeon with interest in epidemiology Edward Jenner— discovered a safer way of preventing small pox	• Conducted one of the earliest experimental investigations on the treatment of scurvy; attributed causes of scurvy to moist air and diet • Smallpox prevention	1747 1749
William Farr— trained physician and self-taught mathematician (Miasmatic theory of disease applied to cholera cause in London)	• Described the state of health of the population, determinants of public health, as well as the application of the knowledge gained to the prevention and control of the disease	Mid-1800s
John Snow— physician	• Established the cause and mode of communication of cholera in London	1854
British Medical Research Council	• Streptomycin tuberculosis trial	1940s
Bradford Hill and Richard Doll	• Smoking as a causative agent in lung cancer	1950
Framingham study	• Foundation stone for cardiovascular risk factors (high blood pressure, elevated serum cholesterol level, physical activities, etc.)	1947–present
Modern epidemiology	• Health determinants at molecular and genetic levels; health determinants at biological and societal levels; penetration of the epidemiologic black box, "Big Data" Administrative Claims Data, Health Services and Health Outcomes, health disparities, epigenetic, socio-epigenomics, socio-genomics, mHealth	Twenty-first century

Table 5.4 Models of disease causation

Model	Description
Ecologic model	• Disease occurs as a result of the interrelationship between biological, social, and physical factors.
Epidemiologic triangle model	• Disease is caused by an imbalance between the host (intrinsic factor), agent, and environment.
Web of causation model	• Diseases do not occur as a result of a single isolated factor but as a result of multiple factors interacting to predispose to disease (e.g., coronary artery disease, which is associated with diet, smoking, physical inactivity, estrogen replacement therapy, stress).
Wheel model (man/ environment interaction)	• This model stresses the genetic makeup as the most prominent determinant of a disease. • Ignores the agent in the causation of the disease, places the gene at the core of disease causation, and incorporates social, biologic, and physical environments in the interpretation of disease process.
Causal pie (multicausality)[a]	• Disease occurrence requires the joint action of component causes as "sufficient cause"; multitude of component causes.

[a] One of the most frequently used models, which claims that to understand the disease process, the environmental, the host, and the agent factors must be understood.

5.5 Measures of disease frequency, occurrence, and association

In epidemiological investigations, the occurrence of cases of disease is related to the "population at risk," which is the population that gave rise to the cases. Several measures of disease frequency are in common use. The measures of disease frequency or occurrence, and association in epidemiology include prevalence, incidence, *ratios, proportion*, and *rates*. Specifically the measures of disease occurrence refer to the distribution of disease, health-related events or outcomes of interest, implying the "distribution" aspect of epidemiology characterization or definition. For example, the number of patients with sepsis, reflects the frequency, incidence, and prevalence of sepsis count, new cases and all cases diagnosed during a specific period, respectively. The measure of effect or association on the other hand attempts to quantify the "determinants" of events by observing the effect or impact of the predictor or risk factor on the outcome of interest. For example, the association between opioid use and sepsis in hospitalized patients with nosocomial infection reflects the impact of the risk factor (opioid use) and outcome (sepsis). Such determinants measure include odds ratio or relative odds, risk ratio, and hazard ratio. Rates as used in epidemiology involve incident rates, mortality rates, attack rates (ARs), and fatality rates. However, attack and fatality

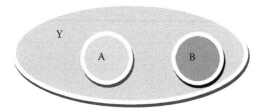

Figure 5.2 **Estimation of ratio.** Y is the total sample, A and B are subsamples used in ratio estimation.

rates are not accurately characterized in traditional epidemiology texts since these measures do not reflect time such as P-T exposure/contribution. The basic measures of disease frequency in epidemiology are incidence and prevalence.

5.5.1   *Ratio*

Ratio is one number (X) divided by another (Y). For example, the sex of adults attending a blood pressure screening clinic could be compared in this way (e.g., male/female; male/male + female). For example, if among 1000 patients screened for hypertension (HTN) and 300 were female (A) while 600 were male (B), what is the sex ratio of diagnosed HTN in this patient sample? The male-female ratio for HTN is 2:1, implying for every one female diagnosed with HTN, two male patients were diagnosed. This estimate is obtained by: (B) ÷ (A), substituting: 600 ÷ 300 = 2. Epidemiologically, males are twice as likely to be diagnosed with HTN relative to females. These data are relevant for HTN prevention in the first place by targeting the population at greater risk, mainly men (Figure 5.2).

5.5.2   *Proportion*

Proportion is a type of ratio, but the numerator is included in the denominator. The distinction between a ratio and proportion, therefore, implies that the proportion represents the relationship between X and Y. Proportion reflects the prevalence of the condition or issue of interest and could be characterized as chance or simple/unconditional probability in a broad sense (Figure 5.3).

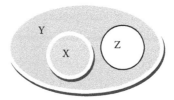

Figure 5.3 **Proportion estimation.** Y is the denominator and includes X and Z, while X is the subpopulation with the outcome of interest and Z without the outcome of interest.

$$\text{Proportion} = \frac{\text{Presence of outcome of interest}\,(X)}{\text{Total sample}\,Y\,(X+Z)}$$

Consider a cross-sectional study on children food insecurity where investigators surveyed 1000 (Y) families and observed 500 (X) families with food insecurity. What is the proportion of families with food insecurity in this sample? Fifty percent of the families have food insecurity, which is estimated by:

$$\frac{\text{Presence or true positive for food insecurity}\,(X)}{\text{Presence and absence of food insecurity (total sample or population at risk)}\,(Y)}$$

$$\text{Substituting:}\quad \frac{500\,(X)}{1000\,(Y)}.$$

5.5.3 Rate

Rate is a type of proportion and is a measure of the occurrence of events in a population over time. Time is therefore an integral part of the denominator in rate. Mathematically, this appears as follows:

Rate = Number of cases or events occurring during a given time period/

Population at risk during the same time period $\times 10^n$.

Vignette 5.3 During the first 12 months of Nostate's surveillance for AIDS malignancy (AM), the health department received 2166 case reports that specified sex: 1000 cases were in females, 1166 in males. How will you calculate the female-to-male ratio for AM? In addition, how will you calculate the proportion of males with AM?

Ratio computation: Identify the number of AM cases of female (X) and the number of AM cases of males (Y). Compute the ratio by using the basic formula: X (cases in female)/Y (cases in males). Substituting for X and Y → 1000/1166 = 0.86:1. Therefore, there was less than one female patient for each male patient who reported for AM to the health department.

Proportion computation: Identify the number of AM cases of females (X) and the number of AM cases of females and males (Y). Compute the proportion by using the basic formula: (cases in females)/Y (cases in females and males). Substituting for X and Y → 1000/2166 = 0.46. Therefore, less than 5 out of every 10 AM cases were in females. Ratios and proportions are used to characterize populations by age, sex, race, exposure, etc. Rates, ratios, and proportions are used to describe morbidity, mortality, and natality health and human conditions.[4]

5.5.4   *Measures of disease occurrence*

The measure of disease occurrence in epidemiology compares disease frequency. These measures include *risk*, *IRs*, period prevalence, cumulative incidence (CI), and prevalence proportion. *Risk* refers to the probability that an individual or group of persons will develop a given disease. For example, if the total number of persons in a population (Notown) equals T, and D represents the number of people out of the T population who develop the disease (AM) during the period of time, the proportion D/T represents the average risk of developing AM in the population during that period.

5.5.4.1   *Formula for risk*

The *basic formula for risk* computation is D/T = number of subjects developing the disease or the event of interest during a time period/number of subjects followed for that time period (Figure 5.4). Mathematically:

$$\text{Risk} = \frac{\text{Number of cases or individuals with the disease or health-related events during a time period}}{\text{Number of subjects/people followed during the time period}}.$$

5.5.4.2   *Average risk or CI*

The *average risk* of a disease in a population is interchangeable with the *incidence proportion* as well as the *CI* of the disease. CI is the proportion of the population that becomes diseased or presents with the event of interest over a specified period of time.

5.5.4.3   *Average risk or CI computation*

The average risk of getting a disease over a period of time, which is the probability of getting a disease, is the adequate measure when there are few or no losses to follow-up. The basic formula for CI or average risk is as follows: number of new cases of disease or event of interest or related health factor/ number in the population of interest, over a specific time period (Figure 5.5).

$$\text{AVERAGE RISK (AR) or CI} = \frac{\text{Number of new cases(NC)}}{\text{Total Population at risk(TP)}}.$$

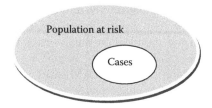

Figure 5.4 Illustration of risk as a proportion with cases as numerator (white circle) and the total population as a denominator (gray + white circle).

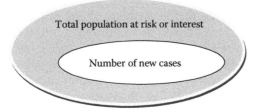

Figure 5.5 Demonstration of average risk (AR) or cumulative incidence (CI) as a proportion with new cases as numerator and the population of interest or at risk as denominator.

5.5.4.4 IR or incidence density computation

The IR is the measure of disease frequency that utilizes CI or average risk and ignores the concept of competing risk, thus underestimating the point estimate. Rates can be used to estimate risk only when the period of follow-up is short and the rate of the disease over that interval is relatively constant. IR takes into account the competing risk by modeling the disease occurrence with the P-T of observation. The IR or *incidence density* (ID) is the occurrence of new cases of disease or events of interest that arise during P-T of observation (Figure 5.6).

Incidence rate density = Number of new cases

÷ (Population at risk × time during which cases were ascertained).

How is ID or incidence rate computed?
IR measures the incidence when the population at risk is roughly constant. The basic formula for IR is:

$$\frac{\text{Number of subjects developing the disease or events of interest (new cases)}}{\text{Total time experienced by the subjects followed (P-T) of observation}}.$$

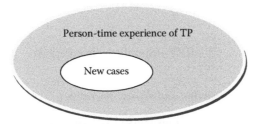

Figure 5.6 Demonstration of incidence density with incident or new cases as numerator (white circle) and the person time experience of cases and noncases/cases in remission within a specified time period (gray + white circle).

Vignette 5.4 Consider that in Newcity, 35,000 women were at risk for postmenopausal breast cancer and contributed 250,000 person-years of follow-up. If there were 1500 incident cases during the 10-year follow-up, what would be the ID for breast cancer in this population?

Computation: Identify the number of cases during the time period (A) and identify the total P-T of observation (follow-up) (B). Apply the basic formula, A/B. Substituting → 1,500/250,000 = 600.0 per 100,000 per year.

Incidence rate density = Number of new cases ÷ Total person years at risk

This formula measures incidence when the population is not constant, since incidence measure is complicated by changes in the population at risk during the period when cases are ascertained, for example, through births, deaths, or migrations. This difficulty is overcome by relating the numbers of new cases to the *person years at risk*. The denominator (person years at risk) is calculated by adding together the periods during which each individual member of the population is at risk during the measurement period.

5.5.4.5   *CI estimation from ID/IR*

Whereas CI represents a frequency estimate, ID is a force or impact of the risk factor on disease development in the population of interest. The CI is the ratio or proportion of incident cases to the population at risk at the initiation of the period of observation assuming there is no loss to follow-up. Please note that time is not a component of the denominator in CI. While CI mirrors ID, there is no time in the denominator of CI, but the time period of observation is necessary in the estimation and understanding of ID. In effect, IR estimates, force, momentum, speed, intensity of the risk factor in question that leads to the case. The CI is related to IR by the formula $CI = IR \times T$, where T is the specified period of time. Risk is related to IR and is mathematically given by $Risk = IR \times T$.

$$CI = (IR) \times (\text{Specified Time Period})$$

5.5.5   *Prevalence proportion and disease prevalence*

The *prevalence proportion* (*P*) measures the frequency of the existing disease (disease status). Two types of prevalence measures are common in epidemiology: *point prevalence* (proportion of the population that is diseased; new cases, current cases, old cases) at a single point in time and *period prevalence* (proportion of the population that is diseased during a specified duration of time), for example, during the year 2006. The denominator for the point prevalence is the estimated population at the point in time, whereas the denominator of the period prevalence is the estimated population at mid-interval.

5.5.5.1   *Factors influencing disease prevalence*

Prevalence is influenced by time, implying that the longer the duration of the disease, the greater or higher the prevalence (Figure 5.7). Prevalence is also influenced by both IR and disease duration. The relationship between prevalence and IR is given by $P = IR \times D$, where D is the duration of the disease or the event of interest (applicable to low disease prevalence, i.e., less than 10%).

When the prevalence of the disease is not low, the relationship between the prevalence and IR is given by ID/1 + ID, where I = incidence and D = the duration of the disease.

$$\text{Prevalence } (P) = \text{Incidence rate } (IR) \times \text{Duration } (D)$$

5.5.5.2   *Formula for point prevalence and period prevalence*

The basic formula for *point prevalence* is as follows:

$$\frac{\text{Number of existing cases of disease or event of interest}}{\text{Number in total population, at the point in time}}.$$

Period prevalence is given by the following formula:

$$\frac{\text{Number of existing cases of disease or event of interest}}{\text{Number in total population (estimated population at midinterval)}}.$$

5.5.5.3   *Uses of incidence and prevalence data*

Epidemiology generates information for public health and clinical medicine decision making. Information generated from prevalence studies such

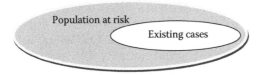

Figure 5.7 Point prevalence illustration with population at risk and existing cases (old, new, current) as the denominator (gray) and existing cases as numerator (white).

Table 5.5 Uses of incidence and prevalence data in public health

---

Prevalence
- Important and useful in the planning and monitoring of public health services (facilities, personnel, manpower)
- Expresses the burden of health-related events in a specified population
- Useful in determining the extent of the health-related events
- Substitution for the calculation of the impact of the health-related events in the absence of incidence data
  - Not a good estimator of incidence
- Point prevalence is useful in tracking changes of health-related events in a population over time.

Incidence
- Important in estimating disease etiology
- Provides direct measure of disease/disability/injury rate or risk
- Allows for hypothesis testing on the magnitude of the effect of the risk factor(s) on the outcome of the health-related event (disease/disability/injury)

---

as cross-sectional are useful in program planning in public health services or quality assurance and training in clinical medicine setting for healthcare improvement. Similarly, incidence data that are generated from prospective cohort or clinical trials point to the direction of factors that determine the observed effect and are primarily useful in assessing etiology (Table 5.5).

5.5.5.4   Limitations of prevalence data

Prevalence data tend to produce a biased picture of health-related events, such as disease, favoring the inclusion of chronic over acute diseases. Second, cause and effect are measured simultaneously. Third, they cannot be used for causal inference, and finally, the prevalence is determined from one survey, whereas incidence requires at least two sets of observations (records/data) of the same subject.

5.5.6   Proportionate mortality and morbidity

Proportionate mortality (PM) refers to the fraction or proportion of deaths observed in a specified population over a specified period of time due to different causes. Mathematically, each cause is expressed as a percentage of all deaths, with the sum of causes approximated at 100%. This measure is useful in describing the burden of death in a population given specific cause. Holmes et al.[6] conducted a study to examine racial and ethnic disparities in in-hospital pediatric mortality in a specific population. The PM was used to assess specific causes of death among in-hospital mortality. This analysis used the total number of deaths as the denominator and death from specific cause as a numerator. The PM for respiratory diseases was estimated by using the number of children who died from any respiratory condition, such as respiratory failure, divided by the total number of in-hospital deaths and multiplied by 1000.

Mathematically, PM is calculated as follows:

$$\frac{\text{Specific cause of death}}{\text{In-hospital total number of deaths} \times 1000}.$$

As part of the results, 80 deaths (in-hospital) were observed over a two-year period, and using these data, PM was computed, which indicated the highest in-hospital proportionate mortalities in respiratory diseases (20/80; 25%, 250 per 1000 deaths) and cardiovascular disorders (19/80; 23.8%, 238 per 1000 deaths). The respiratory-disease-related mortalities were acute respiratory failure (8.8%, 88 per 1000) and acute and chronic respiratory failure (5%, 50 per 1000), and the cardiovascular-disease-related mortalities were cardiac arrest (3.8%, 38 per 1000) and ventricular septal defect (2.5%, 25 per 1000). Gastrointestinal disorders, mainly necrotizing enterocolitis in newborn, were associated with 11.3% (113 per 1,000), and malignancy accounted for 8.8% (88 per 1,000). Other conditions included pneumonitis due to food inhalation (5%, 50 per 1000), subdural hematoma (2.5%, 25 per 1000), septicemia due to gram-negative pathogenic microbes (2.5%, 25 per 1000), complications of bone marrow transplant (2.5%, 25 per 1000), epileptic grand mal seizures (3.8%, 38 per 1000), and congenital anomalies (2.5%, 25 per 1000).

Holmes et al. illustrated the use of PM in their study of pediatric cerebral palsy patients discovered dead during sleep (DDDS) between 1993 and 2011. Of the 177 patients who expired during this period, 19 were DDDS resulting in a PM of 114.5 per 1000. The study also indicated proportionate morbidity in the comorbidity associated with DDDS.[7]

Proportionate morbidity reflects the number of cases of a specific disease in a specified population, divided by the total number of observed disease over a specified period. PM had been used to characterize the number of cases in a subpopulation of cases of a specific disease divided by the total number of cases during a specified period of time. For example suppose 5250 adults were hospitalized during 2014 for several diseases in a comprehensive tertiary hospital. The hospitalization included asthma (650), chronic obstructive pulmonary disease (COPD) (450), congestive heart failure (CHF) (300), pneumonia (550), metabolic disorders including diabetes mellitus (DM) (400), uncontrolled hypertension (elevated blood pressure) (414), cancer (800), stroke (900), infection (500), fractures (300), psychiatric conditions (195), substance and chemical dependency (105), and angina pectoris (86). The proportionate morbidity for uncontrolled HTN during 2014 is 414/5250 = 7.89%, implying that 8 out of every 100 patients were hospitalized for uncontrolled HTN. The PM for stroke is 900/5250 = 0.17 = 17.14%; stroke hospitalization in this hypothetical situation in 17 per 100 patients. Holmes et al.[8] conducted a study on racial and ethnic disparities in pediatric asthma admission and readmission. Using proportionate morbidity with subpopulation count divided by the total number of children admitted with asthma ($n = 1070$) during 2010 and 2011 and indicated the proportionate morbidity to be highest among whites (40.9%) and blacks (40.5%), intermediate among others (16.7%), and lowest among Asians (0.6%), American Indians/Alaska Natives (0.3%) and Hawaiian Natives/Pacific Islanders (0.3%).[8]

5.6 Measures of disease association or effect

There are many steps in epidemiologic investigation, one of which is the association between the exposure and disease development. Measures of disease association include but are not limited to commonly used point estimates in epidemiologic research. These measures can be absolute or relative, such as risk difference and relative risk, respectively. The application of such measures depends on multiple steps, which involve an association in the first place and the establishment of factual association by eliminating random error, confounding, and effect measure modifier as the possible explanation of such association. Commonly used measures of disease association include but are not limited to odds ratio, relative risk, risk ratio, coefficient, and hazard ratio.

5.6.1 Types of rates (crude, specific, adjusted)

5.6.1.1 Crude rates

Crude rates are based on the actual number of events in a population over a given time period.

Crude rates computation:

Examples of crude rates are birth rate, infant mortality rate, fetal death rate, maternal mortality rate, etc (Table 5.6). Crude birth rate is computed by the basic formula:

$$\frac{\text{Number of live births within a given period}}{\text{Population size at the middle of that period} \times 1000 \text{ population}}.$$

Table 5.6 Crude rates—example and basic formula for rate estimation

Crude rate	Formula	Interpretation
Birth rate	Number of live births within a given period/population size at the middle of that period × 1000 population	• Projects population changes • Affected by number of women of childbearing age
Infant mortality	Number of infant deaths among infants aged 0 to 365 days during the year/number of live births during the year × 1000 live births	• Used for international comparison • Low rates reflect balanced health needs
Postneonatal mortality rate	Number of infant deaths from 28 to 365 days after birth/number of live births minus neonatal deaths × 1000 live births	• Low rates reflect environmental events, infectious disease control, and adequate nutrition

From the strict epidemiologic characterization of rate, these health events describe the proportion and not rates since time is not involved in the denominator. Caution should be exercised in the interpretation of these health parameters as rates.

Crude rate (proportion) = Number of live births ÷ (Population size × 100)

Vignette 5.5 Consider a population of Newcountry to be 280,000,000 during 1996, and the number of babies born was 4,500,000 during the same period. The crude birth rate will be as follows: Number of live births (A)/Population size (B) × 1000. Substituting for A and B → 4,500,000/280,000,000 × 1000 = 16.07 per 1000.

In epidemiology, the rate is often incorrectly used to refer to proportions or ratios, as in these illustrations.

Vignette 5.6 Consider a population of 200,000 people of whom 40 are diagnosed with pancreatic neoplasm (PN) in 2005, and during the same time period (2005), 36 died from PN. How will you calculate the mortality rate in 2005 in this population and the case fatality rate in this population?

Computation: Mortality rate as a result of PN: 36/200,000 = 0.00018 (0.018%) or 18.0 per 100,000. Case fatality as a result of PN: 36/40 = 0.9 (90%).

5.6.1.2 Specific rates

Specific rates refer to a particular subgroup of the population defined, such as age, sex, social class, and race. An example of specific rate is age-specific rate. Age-specific rate refers to the number of cases per age group of population during a specified time period.

Vignette 5.7 Consider that in No-county during 2006, there were 1100 deaths due to bronchial carcinoma (BC) among the 55 to 74 age group, and there were 35,000,000 persons in same age group. What will be the age-specific BC death rate in this age group?
Specific rate computation:

Computation: Using the formula Number of deaths (BC) among those aged 55 to 74 years (A)/Number of persons aged 55–74 years during 2006 (B) × 100,000, substituting → A/B × 100,000; 1,100/35,000,000 × 100,000 = 3.14 per 100,000.

5.6.1.3   Adjusted rate

Adjusted rate refers to summary measures of the rate of morbidity and mortality in a population in which statistical procedures have been applied to remove the effect of differences in the composition of the various populations, such as age, for the purpose of comparison. Two methods of rates adjustment are most commonly used in public health: *Direct method* is used if age-specific death rates in a population to be standardized are known and a suitable standard population is available. *Indirect method*, or standardized mortality ratio (SMR), is used when the age-specific death rates are unknown or unstable.

Direct method: Multiply the age-specific rate by the number of persons. Sum the expected number of deaths in each age group to determine the total number of expected deaths. The age-adjusted rate is

$$\frac{\text{Total expected number of deaths}}{\text{Number of deaths in the standardized or combined population} \times 100,000}.$$

The result, the adjusted death rate, ensures that the observed differences in the death rates between the two populations compared are not due to age, gender, or sex.

Vignette 5.8 Using Table 5.7, consider the age group in years, the age-specific death rates per 100,000 in populations X and Y, and the number in the United States in 1998 (census population estimates). Determine which population has excess mortality.

Computation: Multiply A by C to obtain D, expected deaths for population X. Multiply B and C to obtain E, expected death for population Y. Obtain the age-adjusted rate for population X by summing the total in column D and dividing by the total in column C, then multiplying by 100,000. Repeat the steps in 3 for population Y. Subtract the rate in X (702.56 per 100,000) from Y (815.15 per 100.000). The excess age-adjusted mortality rate is 112.6 per 100,000.

Indirect age-adjusted rate computation:

Indirect age-adjusted rate (SMR) is calculated by

$$\frac{\text{Observed number of deaths } (A) \times 100}{\text{Expected number of deaths } (B)}.$$

Table 5.7 Age-specific mortality rates for populations X and Y

Age group	Population X (age-specific rates per 100,000) (A)	Population Y (age-specific rates per 100,000) (B)	US population (1998 census estimate) (C)	D (expected death for population (X))	E (expected death for population (Y))
<5 years	149.19	181.40	18,989,257		
5–19	43.44	36.78	58,712,947		
20–24	165.97	178.23	100,919,429		
45–64	521.18	725.04	57,241,131		
>65 years	4,011.94	4,517.68	34,385,239		
Total	417.91	1,060.94	270,248,003		

Source: Data from National Center for Health Statistics, Division of Data Services.

Vignette 5.9 Consider the number of observed deaths in Notown from angina pectoris to be 1200 during 2005. If the expected number of deaths is 2000, what is the SMR?

Computation: SMR = A/B × 100. Substituting → 1200/2000 = 0.6 (60%).

5.7   Measures of disease comparison

Measures of disease comparison are interchangeably used with measures of association or effect. These measures are listed below in this chapter (Table 5.8). Next, we present the formula to enable clinicians to apply these crude measures of effect in understanding these basic epidemiologic approaches to disease association.

A   Absolute measure reflects difference that is computed through subtraction. We can determine this by subtracting one number from the other. For example, if infant mortality in blacks is 11 per 1000 live births and for whites is 4 per 1000. The absolute risk difference in infant mortality comparing black to white children is 7 per 1000 live births. This measure provides information about public health impact of an exposure.

B   Relative measure reflects difference that is computed through division. This measure is obtained by dividing one number from another. Using the previous example, the relative risk for infant mortality comparing black to white children is 2.75, implying that black children are almost 3 times as likely to die before their first birth day compared to whites. This measure provides information about the strength of the relationship between exposure (independent variable) and outcome (disease, disabilities, or injuries).

C   Absolute measures of comparison are risk difference, rate difference, IR difference, CI difference, and prevalence difference.

D   Relative measures of comparison are risk ratio, rate ratio, relative rate or relative risk, IR ratio, CI ratio, and prevalence ratio.

E   Rate versus Risk. Risk is the accumulated effect of rate occurring during some specified time period. Risk has no time dimension, and the reference population in risk is the population unaffected at the beginning of the period of observation. Risk as explained earlier is a proportion with the numerator characterized as cases, and the denominator as the population at risk. If we observe a group of 60 children (N) in a weight management clinic with overweight/obese (body mass index > 25 kg/m^2) from 2010 and 10 of them developed type 2 DM in 2015, the 5-year risk of type 2 DM is estimated by

Table 5.8 Measures of comparison/association

Measure	Formula	Explanation
Rate or risk ratio	RE/RU, where RE = risk or rate in the exposed and RU = risk or rate in the unexposed	Measures the strength of association between exposure and the disease (outcome)
Attributable proportion among total population	(RT − RU)/RT × 100, where RT = incidence rate (IR), cumulative incidence (CI), or prevalence proportion (PP) in the total population and RU is the IR, CI, or PP in the unexposed population	Measures the excess proportion of disease in the total population, assuming the exposure is causal and implying that the proportion of a disease in a total population that would be eliminated if the exposure were eliminated
Attributable proportion among the exposed	(RE − RU)/RE × 100	Measures the proportion of disease among the exposed, assuming the exposure is causal and implying the proportion of disease among the exposed that will be eliminated if the exposure is eliminated
Population rate difference	RT − RU or RD × PE, where RD = IR difference, CI difference, or PP difference; and PE = proportion of population that is exposed, and RD = RE − RU	Measures excess rate or risk of a disease or outcome in the total population
Rate or risk difference	RE − RU	Measures rate or risk of disease or outcome among the exposed population
Attack rate	ND/TP, where ND = number of people at risk in whom a certain outcome develops, and TP = total number of people at risk	Compares the risk of outcome in groups with different exposure

$$R = \frac{\text{New cases (n)}}{\text{Total number of overweight/obese children (N)}}.$$

F *AR*, although not specifically a rate but a proportion, is the CI of a disease during an outbreak or transient epidemic (Figure 5.8).[4] AR is estimated by the following:

$$\frac{\text{Diseased (exposed and developed an illness)}}{\text{Diseased and Non-diseased (all exposed to the suspected agent of contamination)} \times (\text{multiplier [100]}) \text{ during a time period}}.$$

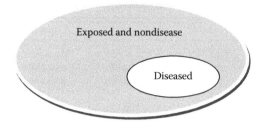

Figure 5.8 Attack rate illustrating exposed and diseased versus exposed nondiseased, with diseased as the numerator (white) and nondiseased plus diseased as denominator (gray + white).

G   *Secondary AR* (SAR) is the proportion of individuals exposed to the primary case (primary cases), who themselves develop the disease (secondary case).[4]

$$SAR = \frac{\text{Number of new cases in group minus initial case(s)}}{\text{Number of susceptible persons in a group-Initial case(s)}}$$

Vignette 5.10 Consider data on primary and secondary attack from salmonella pathogen. Is this a rate or ratio?

Solution: Because time is not involved in the denominator, this measure of disease is strictly not a rate but a risk (proportion).

5.7.1   *Survival/history/event measure*

Survival measures estimate the probability of not expiring or remaining alive for specified period of time, termed survival time which is time to event. Survival for cancer often utilizes a five-year survival as a measure of remission. Consider a study (hypothetical) on the effectiveness of an agent A (antineoplastic) in childhood neuroblastoma, where patients were followed for five years. If 600 entered the study in 2010 and 100 expired at the end of the study in 2015, the five year survival is as follows:

$$\frac{\text{Newly diagnosed patients with neuroblastoma on antineoplastic agent A-Number of death by 2015}}{\text{Newly diagnosed patients with neuroblastoma on agent A}}.$$

Using this formula, the five-year survival for childhood neuroblastoma is this sample is 600 − 100 ÷ 600 = 0.83. In this sample of patients a five year survival was 83%, implying 17% risk of dying from neuroblastaoma (Figure 5.9).

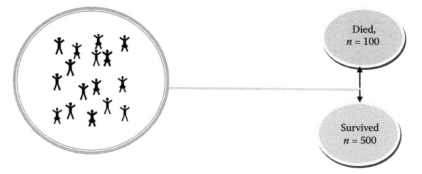

Figure 5.9 Survival or time to event experience illustrating the number of patients who expired and those survived in a specified time from follow-up.

5.8   Sources of epidemiologic data

Data are available for epidemiologic studies, with sources ranging from vital statistics to National Institutes of Health and other US Health and Human Services agencies. These preexisting data enable retrospective analysis of cross-sectional or prospectively collected data. The use of these data sources, while recommended, requires caution in the interpretation of their results. Therefore, like with most preexisting data, data validity and reliability remain an issue in terms of internal and external validity of the findings derived from these data sources (Table 5.9).

5.9   Summary

Epidemiologic objectives remain the identification of populations at risk and the application of such knowledge to disease prevention and control. Clinical medicine is comparable given that the clinicians have an obligation to prevent death in the process of treating disease and preventing complications following treatment, thus maintaining health. Within this context, epidemiologic principles and methods are applied by clinicians in the process of minimizing therapeutic complications, prolonging survival, and maintaining health.

The measures of disease occurrence reflect the distribution aspect of epidemiology implying counts, frequency, incidence, and prevalence of the event or outcome of interest. This aspect involves descriptive epidemiology, namely disease distribution by place, person, and time. Another aspect of distribution involves the epidemiologic triad or triangle, which claims the interaction between host, agent, and environment for disease occurrence (Figure 5.10). Epidemiologic investigation requires a careful consideration of the host factors such as the immune system, agent (infectious pathogen, contaminated water), and the environment (temperature, physical ambience, air pollution, gas stations, farm, and pesticide).

The objective of clinical research is to provide valid and reliable evidence regarding therapeutics, screening, diagnostics, and prevention and depends on the design as well as the statistical methods used to generate these results.

Table 5.9 Sources of epidemiologic data

Sources	Description
Vital statistics	• Provides information for births, deaths, marriages, and divorces
US Census	• Provides information on complete counts of US population every ten years • Types of information include race, sex, age, and marital status (all samples) and income, education level, housing, and occupation (representative samples)
National Health Interview Survey	• Provides data on major health problems, such as acute and chronic disease conditions, impairment and injuries, and utilization of the health services, such as dental care • Useful in examining annual changes in disease and disability conditions
National Health and Nutrition Examination Survey (NHANES)	• Provides information on the health and diet of the US population based on home interview and nutritional examination
Behavioral Risk Factor Surveillance System	• Survey of random sample of US population by phone interviews on behaviors affecting health and well-being (exercise, smoking, obesity, alcohol, automobile seat belt use, and drinking and driving)
National Notifiable Diseases Surveillance System	• Provides information on most communicable diseases, including HIV/AIDS, botulism, gonorrhea, human and animal rabies, etc.
Vital Statistics	• Provides information for births, deaths, marriages, and divorces
Surveillance, Epidemiology, and End Results Program (SEER)	• National Cancer Institute database that provides information on trends in cancer incidence, mortality, and survival • Information includes patient demographics, primary cancer sites, pathology, first mode of therapy, and severity of the disease
World Health Statistics Annual	• Provides information on international morbidity and mortality
Cancer Incidence of Five Continents	• WHO's international agency for research and cancer that provides information on cancer incidence and mortality globally (estimated 170 cancer registries in 50 countries)
National Occupational Hazards Survey and National Occupational Exposure Survey	• Provides data on workers exposed to chemical, physical, and biologic agents
Surveillance of AIDS and HIV Infection	• Provides information on HIV/AIDS incidence and prevalence, as well as cumulative incidence

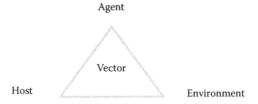

Agent

Vector

Host   Environment

Figure 5.10 **Epidemiologic Triad.** The measure of disease effect or association reflects the determinant, namely the implication of a predictor variable in the event or disease occurence. The risk ratio, hazard ratio, and relative odds or odds ratio remain reliable measures of disease effects or association.

Clinical research designs are broadly classified as observational or epidemiologic and experimental or clinical trials if conducted in human populations, but this distinction remains inaccurate since experimental designs are also observational with respect to outcome or endpoint. This (clinical) evidence is presented as measures of effects of disease, treatment, procedure, or screening, etc. These effects are described as absolute or relative measures of comparison. Absolute measures of comparison describe and quantify the differences between two measures of disease frequency, while relative measures of comparison describe and quantify ratios of two measures of frequency, as well as the strength of association or relationship between exposure and the outcome of interest. For example, the rate difference measures the excess rate of outcome or disease among the exposed patient population, while relative rate compares the rate in the exposed with the unexposed and indicates the strength of the relationship between the exposed and the disease or outcome. The rates of disease or outcome obtained from clinical studies may be compared across different study populations, but the reliability of such comparisons requires adjusted rates (for example, age-adjusted rate), also termed *standardized rate*.

Understanding the interpretation of these measures is essential to the application of the findings in clinical research to the improvement of patient care. Therefore, although sound statistical methods and inference are highly relevant in clinical results, it is important to give due consideration to the epidemiologic methods or the principles of the design of an investigation, since valid evidence cannot be obtained unless the design is sound and accurate. Finally, because clinical research or epidemiologic studies are often entangled with confounding, caution is required in the interpretation of measures of disease occurrence or effects where these factors are not adjusted and illustrated in the crude or raw measures of association.

Questions for discussion

1   Read the study report by Holmes et al.[7] on androgen-deprivation therapy and the prolongation of survival of older men diagnosed and treated for locoregional prostate cancer. Comment on the research design,

hypothesis, statistical methods, and inference. Does this study represent the role of epidemiology in clinical medicine, public health, or both?

2   Suppose you are conducting a study on the incidence of cerebral palsies in children (aged 0 to 4 years) exposed to maternal can beverage consumption during gestation, and a similar study is conducted in a different center with children (aged 12 to 21 years).

   a   What is the measure of effect of can beverage consumption?

   b   What is the problem in comparing these two IRs?

   c   How will you perform a valid comparison in this case?

   d   Is the association in this case causal?

3   One way to measure the effect of disease is by relative risk or odds ratio. What is the distinction between these two measures? Comment on the advantage of one over the other in determining the direct association between exposure and disease.

4   In a hypothetical study of the relationship between polycystic ovarian syndrome (POS) and endometrial carcinoma, 80 out of 280 with POS had developed endometrial carcinoma, compared with 600 out of 4000 control women, who had endometrial carcinoma at some time in their lives.

   a   Compute the odds ratio in favor of never having been diagnosed with POS for women with endometrial carcinoma versus control.

   b   What is the 95% CI for this association?

   c   What can be concluded for these data?

   d   Is there an association between POS and endometrial cancer based on these data?

5   Briefly discuss the role of epidemiology in the practice of clinical medicine. What is the role of epidemiologic findings in the formulation of health policies and guidelines on disease prevention?

References

1. J. M. Last, *A Dictionary of Epidemiology*, 3rd ed. (New York: Oxford University Press, 1995).
2. R. S. Greenberg et al. *Medical Epidemiology*, 4th ed. (New York: Lange Medical Book, 2005).
3. D. A. Savitz, *Interpreting Epidemiologic Evidence* (New York: Oxford University Press, 2003).
4. J. Mausner and S. Kramer, *Epidemiology—An Introductory Text*, 2nd ed. (Philadelphia: Saunders).
5. B. MacMahan and D. Trichopoulos, *Epidemiology, Principles & Methods*, 2nd ed. (Boston: Little, Brown, 1996).
6. L. Holmes Jr., P. Oceanic, K. Dabney. Lower in-Hospital Mortality Albiet Racial/Ethnic Disparities. JANMA (in press).
7. A. F. Karatas, E. G. Miller, and L. Holmes Jr. "Cerebral Palsy Patients Discovered Dead during Sleep: Experience from a Comprehensive Tertiary Center," *J Pediatr Rehabil Med* 6 (2013): 225–231.
8. L. Holmes Jr, F. Kalle, L. Grinstead, F. Dabney et al. "Health Disparities in Pediatric Asthma: Comprehensive Tertiary Care Center Experience," *JNMA* 107 (2015): 1–7.

6   Epidemiologic study designs
Overview

6.1   Introduction

In the previous chapter, epidemiology was presented as a nonexperimental or observational science concerned with the distribution, determinants, or etiology of disease and health-related events in the human population and the application of such knowledge to the prevention and control of disease, injury, and disabilities in specific populations. But epidemiologic investigations go beyond the nonexperimental approach. The process of how diseases, disabilities, injuries, and health-related events are quantified remains essential to epidemiology, implying sound conduct of clinical trials (experimental design involving humans). Depending on the nature of the disease occurrence, several epidemiologic designs are available for the quantification of occurrence/frequency and the association or measure of effect. These measures of occurrence and effect were presented in a previous chapter.

Epidemiologic designs are used in clinical research. The selection of an appropriate design is essential to the results, since no matter how sophisticated the statistics used in the analysis of the data are, a study based on unsound or flawed design principles will generate an invalid result. There are two broad classifications of study designs: nonexperimental, also loosely termed observational, and experimental or clinical trial if the experiment is conducted on humans. What distinguishes these methods is the process of assignment or allocation of subjects to the study arms. Whereas clinical trial or experimental design allocates subjects or eligible participants to the treatment or control arm of the study, based on the equipoise (collective uncertainty about the advantage or superior benefit of one treatment arm versus its alternative or control arm) principle, nonexperimental designs do not involve subject allocation to the exposure or nonexposure arm but merely observe the exposed as well as the unexposed for the occurrence of the outcomes of interest (prospective cohort design if there is follow-up or cross-sectional in the absence of follow-up), such as symptoms, disease, or death.

The clinical trial remains the gold standard in terms of research design, if appropriate sample size is used because of its distinctive features of randomization and placebo-control. These features minimize baseline variability between the treatment and control groups, yielding a more accurate result on the effect of the treatment. But there is a price to these advantages, mainly enrollment issues, the high cost of conducting the trial, and ethical considerations. Therefore, in spite of the advantages of a randomized, placebo-controlled clinical trial, this design may not be feasible in certain contexts, requiring the use of the nonexperimental design.

Traditionally, there are two primary types of nonexperimental design cohort studies, in which study subjects are characterized by their exposure status and followed for a period of time to ascertain the outcome of interest, and case-control studies, in which study subjects are characterized by their disease status and the presence of exposure is ascertained in the cases as well as the controls or comparison group, who are comparable to the cases but do not have the disease of interest (Figure 6.1).

Whereas cohort design provides information on the outcome of interest, case-control generates data on the exposure distribution among the cases and control groups. Cross-sectional and ecologic designs are other traditional designs often employed in epidemiologic methods. The former assesses the relationship between disease or outcome of interest and exposure among a well-defined group or population at a point in time. This design measures the prevalence of the exposure or exposures of interest in relation to the disease prevalence of interest—for example, if a study were to be conducted using the US National Health Interview Survey to assess the factors associated with ethnic/racial disparities in hypertension. Since information on the exposure and outcome was collected prior to the design of the study and there was no follow-up of participants, cross-sectional design remains a feasible approach to providing information on the disease prevalence (hypertension) in relation to exposure prevalence (exercise, diet, education, marital status, etc) (Figure 6.2). The ecologic design examines the association between exposure and disease at a group level and does not use individual (case) data as the unit analysis.

The most appropriate design depends on many factors:

a The nature of the research question and hypothesis to be tested
b The current state of knowledge regarding the hypothesis to be tested or the research question to be answered
c The frequency of the exposure and disease in the specific population (rare disease for case-control and rare exposure for cohort design)
d The expected magnitude of association between the exposure and outcome of interest
e Subject availability and enrollment
f Financial and human resources
g Ethical consideration if a clinical trial is planned

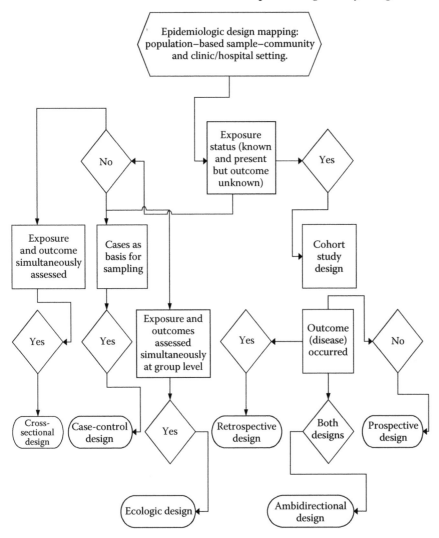

Figure 6.1 Choice of epidemiologic design.

h   Whether or not all, some, or no data were collected prior to the planning and design of the study

However, regardless of the design used, there are advantages and limitations in these designs in terms of the level of evidence (internal and external validity). Therefore, the intent is to increase the validity of the study by minimizing bias (selection, information and measurement), assessing effect measure modifier, controlling confounding, and increasing precision by minimizing random error (Figure 6.3).

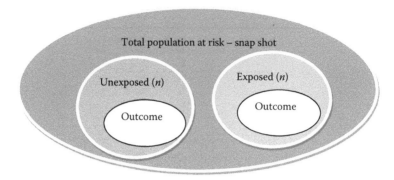

Figure 6.2 **Cross-sectional design illustrating simultaneous examination of exposure and outcome.** The effect of the exposure is assessed by identifying the number of outcomes in the exposed relative to those in the unexposed.

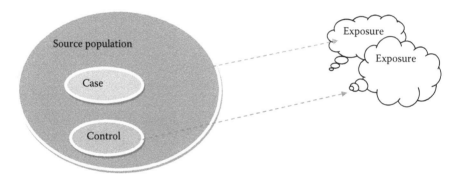

Figure 6.3 **Case-control design.** Illustrates the control and case groups from the source population and the assessment of the exposure status among the case and the controls to determine if the exposure produced the cases or not.

BOX 6.1   EPIDEMIOLOGIC UNDERSTANDING OF DISEASE DISTRIBUTION

- *Epidemic*—refers to occurrence of disease or health-related event in a community (city, county, state, nation) in excess of what is usually or normally expected—for example, the H1N1 virus (swine, bird, human, flu) in Mexico and the United States during the months of April and May 2009.
- *Pandemic*—refers to an epidemic that occurs all over the world. The H1N1 could be loosely termed pandemic (Mexico, United States, Canada, Europe).

> • *Endemic*—refers to the habitual presence of a disease or health-related event within a given geographic area. A classic example of this is Burkett's lymphoma, a tumor that was predominant in certain part of Africa.

This chapter presents the overview of epidemiologic study designs. The appropriate design depends on the research question and the level of evidence. The ecologic nonexperimental design and the measures of effect are presented in detail. Ecologic fallacy, which is the application of ecologic findings on the individual level, is explained.

6.2   Nonexperimental versus experimental design

Observational or nonexperimental studies are research designs in which investigators do not assign study subjects to the study groups/arms but passively observe events and determine the measures of association/ magnitude of effect (Figure 6.4). The purpose is to draw inferences about possible causal relationship between exposure and some health outcome, condition, or disease.[1] These studies are broadly characterized as descriptive and analytic—the observational analytic designs are so traditionally identified but remain inappropriate characterizations (analytic designs have descriptive components as well as the description of incidence of disease over time). They are cross-sectional, case-control, and cohort and the several hybrids of these designs (nested case-control, case-cohort, etc). *Cohort studies* are observational or nonexperimental designs, which commence with the identification of the exposure status of each subject and involve following the groups over time to determine the outcome in both the exposed and unexposed. And like most epidemiologic studies, cohort designs are intended to allow inferences about exposure influence on the occurrence of the disease or outcome of interest.[2] Whereas sampling (selection of study subjects) in *case-control* is based on the disease or health outcome, in cohort designs, sampling is performed without regard to the disease or health outcome but exposure status.[1] In comparison to *cross-sectional*, which is an "instant cohort" design, sampling (study population selection) is done without regard to exposure or disease status.[1,3] *Ecologic* studies are sometimes characterized as analytic because of their abilities to assess the effect of the exposure at the group level on the outcome, using the correlation coefficient. However, it is not uncommon to go through an introductory epidemiology text and not see mention of an ecologic design, and when it is discussed, it is classified as descriptive design. Therefore, the classification of epidemiologic designs into analytic and descriptive remains a meaningless classification and should not be stressed (Table 6.1).

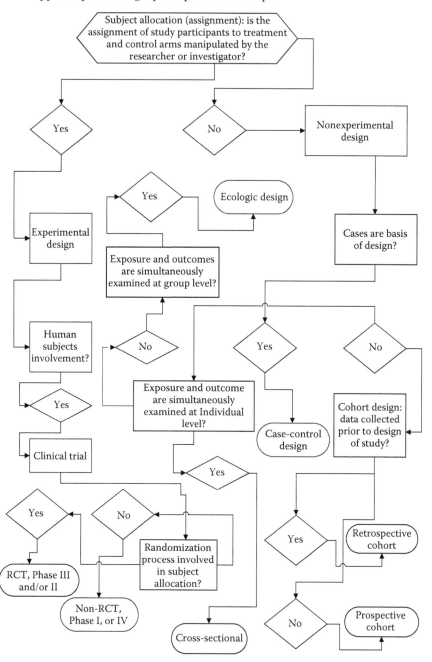

Figure 6.4 Study designs—experimental versus nonexperimental (observational).

Table 6.1 Classical types of epidemiologic design

Design types and examples	Description
Experimental/clinical trial	Subjects are assigned to study arms by the investigator—active manipulation of participants but not outcome. Used when feasible because of ethical considerations to examine the effect screening, diagnosis, therapeutics, and preventive practices on health.
Nonexperimental Design	Does not involve subjects' allocation or assignment to the arms of the study.
a Cohort design—commences with exposure status, has follow-up, and determines the outcome b Case-control—commences with disease and examines exposure distribution in cases and controls c Cross-sectional—snapshot examination of exposure and outcome without follow-up d Ecologic-group-level analysis	Used to assess the etiology, effects of treatment on disease, screening, diagnosis and prevention. Classical examples are cohort, case-control, cross-sectional, and ecologic designs.

BOX 6.2   TRADITIONAL EPIDEMIOLOGIC DESIGN

- Cohort studies are traditionally classified as (a) prospective and (b) retrospective depending on the temporal relationship between the initiation of the study and the outcome (occurrence of disease or event of interest).
- A design is considered the retrospective cohort, which is also termed historical cohort or nonconcurrent prospective study, if the exposures and the outcomes of interest (disease, for example) have already occurred prior to the initiation of the study.
- In the prospective design, the exposure, which defines the cohort, has occurred in the exposed group prior to the initiation of the study but the outcome (disease) has not occurred. In this context, both groups are followed to assess the incidence rate of the disease, comparing the exposed to the unexposed.
- Both designs compare the exposed to the unexposed groups to assess the measure of effect. However, the main distinction between these two designs is the calendar time. In the retrospective design, as illustrated in this vignette, exposure to radiation is ascertained from birth data (medical record) and the outcome (thyroid cancer) at the beginning of the study (no follow-up).

- Cross-sectional studies, also called surveys and prevalence studies, are designed to assess both the exposure and outcome simultaneously. However, since exposure and disease status are measured at the same point in time (snapshot), it is difficult, if not impossible, to distinguish whether the exposure preceded or followed the disease, and thus cause-and-effect relationships are not certain, lacking temporal sequence.
- Ecologic designs examine group-level data in order to establish the relationship between exposure and outcomes.
- A case-control design classifies subjects on the basis of outcome (disease and non-disease or comparison group) and then looks backward to identify the exposure. This design could be prospective as well.
  - In this design, the history or previous events for both case and comparison groups are assessed in an attempt to identify the exposure or risk factors for the disease.

Epidemiologic research is not simple to conduct given the genetic heterogeneity of humans and the potential for confounding. Nonexperimental or observational studies are entangled with confounding, which is described throughout this book. To disentangle these confounding effects, a stratified or stratification analysis is conducted. This is the analysis of disease-exposure relationships in separate subgroups of the data, where the subgroups are defined as potential confounders. Consider a study to examine the relationship between selenium intake and the development of prostate cancer. If the family history is a known confounder, the effect or point estimate may be obtained with stratified analysis using the Mantel–Haenszel method. A confounder could be positive if it is negatively related to both exposure and disease or negative if it is positively related to the disease and negatively related to the exposure. Specifically, a confounder is positive if, after adjustment, the adjusted risk or odds ratio is lower than the raw or crude risk or odds ratio, and vice versa, for a negative confounder.

6.2.1 *Disease outbreaks determinants*

The prevalence of a disease or health-related event is dependent on several factors, including susceptible individuals and at risk as well as those who are not susceptible and, consequently, not at risk (Figure 6.5). Nonsusceptibility in such populations may be associated with immunity provided by individual vaccination or herd immunity as well as hereditary or genetic basis. Herd immunity reflects disease resistance given a large population immunization. In addition, the incubation period influences disease transmission. The incubation period is the window (disease-free period following exposure to an infectious pathogen) between infection (contact/exposure to pathogen) and infectivity (symptoms manifestation).

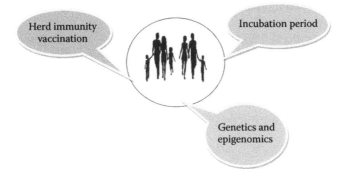

Figure 6.5 Factors influencing disease outbreak.

6.3　Descriptive and analytic epidemiology

Epidemiologic investigation can broadly be classified into descriptive and analytic. While this classification is not very accurate since all analytic epidemiologic work requires descriptive epidemiology. Basically, the notion of descriptive reflects who develops the disease or the health-related event, where does the disease occur (geographic locale) and when does the disease occur (time and seasonality). This notion of descriptive epidemiology affirms the concept of diseases not occurring randomly but have a pattern of distribution, namely, person, place, and time (Figure 6.6). Descriptive epidemiology is essential for clinical medicine, thus allowing the patterns of disease occurrence to be used in hypothesis generation for analytic epidemiologic studies

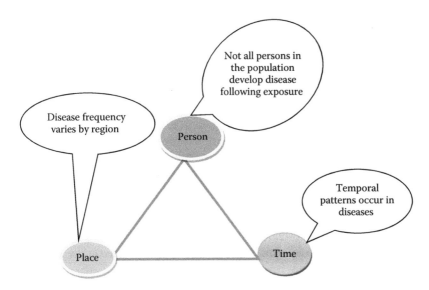

Figure 6.6 Descriptive epidemiology illustrating the PPT: person, place, and time.

towards the understanding of diseases determinants as risk and predisposing factors.

Analytic epidemiologic studies are conducted to assess disease determinants, implying the use of such designs to identify possible association and causal associations where feasible. These studies involve hypothesis testing and are characterized as inferential studies. The explanations of the descriptive patterns of diseases are provided by analytic studies, which are efficient in facilitating and improving disease surveillance initiatives.

6.4   Summary

Clinical research is conducted to yield valid and reliable evidence concerning screening, diagnosis, therapeutics, and preventive practices. This research requires efficient designs as well as statistical methods or techniques to generate results and draw inference from the data. The classical or traditional designs are experimental or clinical trial, in which the investigator allocates subjects or participants to the study arms, and observational or nonexperimental, in which the investigator merely observes subjects who are exposed or unexposed until the occurrence of the outcome of interest (cohort study).

The nonexperimental designs are further classified into cohort design, which commences with the exposure status and follows participants in order to determine the occurrence or incidence of the outcome of interest; case-control design, which commences with the disease status, selects a comparable control from the same population that produced the cases, and determines the distribution of the exposure of interest; cross-sectional design, which is a snapshot of the specific population that examines the prevalence of the disease of interest in relation to the prevalence of exposure/s; and ecologic design, which assesses the relationship between the exposure and outcome of interest at a group level and does not involve individual-level analysis as applicable to cohort, case-control, and cross-sectional classic designs.

Questions for discussion

1 Appropriate designs in conducting clinical research are necessary for the well-being of future patients but are not always in the best interest of the current patient. Suppose a study is planned to assess twice dosing versus one-time dosing of an agent to improve pulmonary function, and both clinical trials and observational designs are feasible for such conduct. Please address the following:
   a Which design would you prefer to use? Comment on your response.
   b Suppose your preference is a clinical trial; under what principle will you sign up your patients for this study? Comment on the application of equipoise and uncertainty in the clinical trial.
2 Suppose a study is proposed on the association between pregnancy and multiple sclerosis (MS) in women. What design should be chosen

to demonstrate the risk of developing MS that is associated with pregnancy? What will you consider as an appropriate measure of effect in this design? Comment on how you will determine your referent group if subjects with more than one pregnancy will be recruited in the study.

3 A study is conducted to examine the association between selenium and the development of prostate cancer. Using the following data, investigate the relationship between prostate cancer and selenium while controlling for the history of prostate cancer in the family. Among those with a family history of prostate cancer ($n = 1000$), 24 of those who did not use selenium had prostate cancer while 776 did not, and among those who used selenium, 6 had prostate cancer while 194 did not. Among those without a family history of prostate cancer ($n = 3000$), 9 of those who did not use selenium had prostate cancer while 891 did not, and among those who used selenium, 20 had prostate cancer while 2080 did not. Construct a 2×2 table for the confounding variable.

    a What is the odds ratio associated with selenium and prostate cancer?
    b Is there a relationship between selenium and prostate cancer?
    c Is family history a positive or negative confounder? Explain.

4 Epidemiologic designs are traditionally termed *observational*. Do you agree with this classification? Can you identify flaw or flaws in the continued us of this notion.

5 Epidemiologic textbooks and some epidemiologists continue to classify epidemiology into analytic and descriptive. Comment on the complexities and overlap in this classification.

6 Differentiate between latent disease and incubation period. Discuss the importance of incubation period in disease outbreak such as the Ebola virus in South Saharan Africa. Also comment of the role of herd immunity with respect to the proportion of the population immunized and the population disease resistance.

References

1. D. A. Savitz, *Interpreting Epidemiologic Evidence* (New York: Oxford University Press, 2003).
2. H. Morgenstern and D. Thomas, "Principles of Study Design in Environmental Epidemiology," *Environ Health Perspect* 101 (Suppl 4) (1993): 23–28.
3. L. Holmes, Jr., *Basics of Public Health Core Competencies* (Sudbury, MA: Jones and Bartlett, 2009).

7 Ecologic studies
Design, conduct, and interpretation

7.1 Introduction

Ecologic studies are sometimes not understood in epidemiologic or medical settings due to the limited or low frequency of its utilization in evidence discovery. Ecologic designs reflect investigations in which the unit of observation is the group and the analysis is performed on the group and not individual level. This design is feasible in assessing an association when the exposure and outcomes are available on the group level. In this context, ecologic studies may serve the purpose for generating hypothesis for individual-level studies. Often, data are available on aggregate measure of the exposure and outcome of interest. Additionally, causal association with ecologic design is difficult to establish. Assuming that prostate cancer (CaP) mortality is higher in zip code 19810 with lower level of pesticide exposure relative to 19960 with higher pesticide exposure, does this design imply the protective effect of CaP mortality by pesticide exposure? Such an inference cannot be drawn given the reality of population dynamics in terms of migration since CaP mortality in 19810 may be due to CaP patients or individuals moving to 19810 from 19960 and other zip codes with higher levels of pesticides. Also, such a design restricts the individual-level data on confounding in addressing the confounding effect of comorbidity, income, education, etc., factors observed to influence CaP mortality.

This chapter describes ecologic design as group level or aggregate data study design, presenting hypothetical and real-world examples (Figure 7.1). The different types of ecologic designs are presented as well as ecologic fallacy. The advantages and limitations of ecologic design are addressed, notably confounding as a mixing effect of the third variable in the association between the exposure and the outcome of interest. The advantages include public access data, low-cost data acquisition, and the feasibility of evaluating community-level intervention.

7.2 Ecologic studies: Description

Ecologic designs, also called group-level ecologic studies, correlational studies, or aggregate studies, obtain data at the level of a group or community often by making use of routinely collected data.[1,2] Second, if the population,

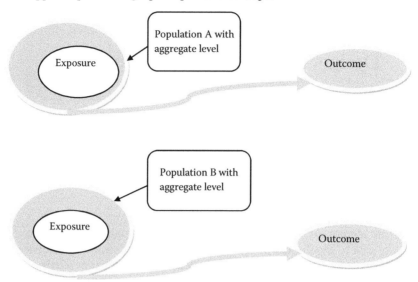

Figure 7.1 Ecologic study design illustrating aggregate level exposure by two groups or populations and the assessment of outcome.

rather than the individual, is the unit of study and its analysis, such a study is correctly characterized as ecologic. This design involves the comparison of aggregate data on risk factors and disease prevalence from different population groups in order to identify associations. Because all data are aggregate at the group level, relationships at the individual level cannot be empirically determined but are rather inferred. Thus, because of the likelihood of an ecologic fallacy, this type of study provides weak empirical evidence.[1]

Basically, the focus of ecologic studies is the comparison of groups, and not individuals, implying the missing of individual data on the joint distribution of variables within the group. This focus places the need for ecologic inference about effects on group levels.[1] The questions is: Why conduct an ecologic study given critique of this method among some epidemiologists? The rationale involves feasibility and data reliability and accuracy in generating testable hypothesis. Ecologic studies are conducted given no initial data on a health problem, no individual-level data, data are available at group-level, and limited research resources and time (rapid conduct).

The advantages of ecologic design include its ability for hypothesis generation for individual-level data design and analysis and it is inexpensive and requires a short period for its conduct. The required data for ecologic studies may be obtained from published literature or public access database, rendering the conduct less time-consuming and inexpensive. While ecologic fallacies had been observed to be the main disadvantage of ecologic design, individual-level studies are not completely immune from ecologic fallacies, implying careful ascertainment of the exposure and disease variables in the conduct of ecologic studies.

Ecologic designs are used to for geographical comparisons of diseases such as the correlation between childhood brain cancer in certain regions in the United States, implicating clusters in some regions relative to the state. If in the same region, there is a low consumption of extra virgin olive oil, a hypothesis can be generated on the association between brain cancer and extra virgin olive oil. However, care must be exercised in the interpretation of such ecologic studies given the potentials for confounding such as age, sex, socioeconomic status, education, access to primary care, etc. Ecologic studies are also useful in assessing time and secular trends in disease. While rates of acute conditions such as bronchiolitis fluctuates over time, chronic disease rates tend to remain stable over time. Ecologic studies may be used to generate hypothesis if disease rates illustrate a correlation with environmental changes. For example, increasing rates of upper respiratory disorders in children during summer may be due to carbon monoxide car emission during the summer months. Migrant studies remain a typical example of ecologic designs for hypothesis generation. These studies provide the opportunity to examine genetic, environmental, and gene–environment association or determinant of disease. For example if a migrant population in the United States (i.e., Asians) are observed to have a higher incidence of CaP in the United States compared to Asians in Asia, the higher rate of CaP among Asians in the United States may be due to environmental condition in the United States. Also, the observed higher incidence of CaP among Asians in the United States may be due to selective emigration from Asia, implying those who were more susceptible to prostatic adenocarcinoma or hormonally related malignancies in general. Race/ethnicity, mortality, chronic obstructive pulmonary disease, and occupation illustrate correlation. African Americans have higher age-adjusted mortality compared to whites and are more likely to be employed in a low-paying job which correlates with higher mortality. On the basis of these correlations, hypothesis on the association between COPD incidence and low paying jobs could be generated.

BOX 7.1   ECOLOGIC DESIGN

Ecologic design or aggregate study refers to an observational study in which all variables are group measures, implying the group as the unit of analysis, in contrast with either a case-control or prospective cohort design, where the unit of analysis is the individual level measures.

May be classified on two dimensions, namely, exploratory versus analytic, and whether subjects are grouped by place (multiple-group model), time (time-trend model) or place and time (mixed model).

H. Morgenstern, "Ecologic Studies in Epidemiology: Concepts, Principles, and Methods," Annu Rev Public Health *16 (1995): 61–81.*

7.2.1   Conducting an ecologic study

To conduct an ecologic study, we need to have aggregate information on groups or subpopulations on the dependent or outcome variable of interest and the independent, explanatory, or predictor variable. For example, to determine the effect of alcohol consumption on stroke, we can obtain information on the prevalence of stroke in populations A, B, and C and then determine alcohol consumption in these three populations. Finally, we correlate alcohol consumption and stroke prevalence in these three populations. If alcohol is a risk for the development of stroke, the population with the highest alcohol consumption will be associated with the highest prevalence of stroke. Alternately, if alcohol consumption per capita is protective, then the population with the highest alcohol consumption will be associated with the lowest prevalence of stroke.

BOX 7.2   TYPES OF ECOLOGIC DESIGNS

- Exploratory—refers to the design where there is no specific exposure of interest or the exposure of potential interest is not measured during the investigation phase of the study
- Etiologic—refers to the design where there is a measurement of the primary variable or exposure of interest, which becomes part of the analysis
- Multiple-group design—involves the comparison of rate of disease among regions during the same period, with the purpose of identifying spatial patterns that may be suggestive of environmental etiology
  - This may be etiologic or exploratory in nature.
- Time trends—also called time series, refers to the ecologic design that compares disease or specific events occurrence over time in a geographically defined population
  - Like multiple-group design, this may be etiologic or exploratory in nature.
- Mixed designs—refers to the combination of the basic features of multiple-group designs and time series. This design could be exploratory or etiologic.

K. J. Rothman, Modern Epidemiology, *3rd ed.*
(Philadelphia: Lippincott, Williams & Wilkins, 2008).

7.2.2   Importance of ecologic data

One situation where ecologic data are particularly useful is where a powerful relationship that has been established at the individual level is assessed at the ecologic level in order to confirm its public health impact. If a risk factor is a major cause of a condition (in terms of population attributable fraction as well as the strength of association), then a lower presence of that factor in a population should presumably be linked to a lower rate of the associated outcome.

7.2.3   Examples of ecologic studies in epidemiologic evidence discovery

A study on CaP mortality and dietary practices and sunlight levels as environmental risk factors for geographic variability in CaP rate was conducted using ecologic design. CaP mortality rate was compared in 71 countries. The per capita food consumption rate and sunlight levels were correlated with age-adjusted mortality rate in CaP. The study indicated an increase CaP mortality rate with total animal fat calories, meat, animal fat, milk, sugar, alcoholic beverages, and stimulants consumption, but inverse correlation with increased sunlight level, soybeans, oilseeds, onions, cereal grains, and rice.[2] Caution must be exercised in the application of these aggregate data in clinical decision making regarding the recommendation of these food products and sunlight exposure. Like all aggregate or group-level data, the geographic variation in lifestyle and potential CaP confounders remain to be assessed. Additionally, countries may differ in the presence of effect measure modifiers, which may explain part of the observed correlation in these data.

7.3   Statistical analysis in ecologic design

The estimate of effect of exposure/s on disease or health-related events involves not just a correlation coefficient but a predictive parameter.[3-5] To estimate the effect or association, we have to regress the group-specific disease or outcome rates (Y) on the group-specific exposure prevalence (X). Therefore, the linear regression model remains useful in estimating the effect or association in ecologic studies. The prediction equation in this context is represented by $Y = \beta_0 + \beta_1 X_1$, where β_0 is the intercept on the Y axis (coefficient without the effect of the exposure) and β_1 is the slope. The predicted outcome rate ($Y_x = 1$) in a group with the exposure or entirely or mostly exposed is $\beta_0 + \beta_1(1) = \beta_0 + \beta_1$, and for the group that is less exposed or unexposed, the predicted rate for ($Y_x = 0$) is $\beta_0 + \beta_1(0) = \beta_0$. Consequently, the estimated rate difference is $\beta_0 + \beta_1 - \beta_0 = \beta_1$, while the rate ratio is $(\beta_0 + \beta_1)/\beta_0 = 1 + \beta_1/\beta_0$.

BOX 7.3   ECOLOGIC FALLACY AND INFERENCE

- Ecologic studies are based on the average or aggregate effect of exposure on a group, and not individual risk.
- The inability to determine if the individuals who are part of the group are at risk due to the group variable exposure of interest renders such designs noncausal or rather very limited in causality.

- The average effect of fat consumption in geographic locale, while it may show an association with average or cumulative incidence of breast cancer in regions with high fat consumption, may not necessarily link individuals with high fat with breast cancer.
- Because of the possibility of other risk factors at individual level influencing the outcome, ecologic studies are limited in causal inference as well as in temporal sequence.
- Ecologic fallacy implies invalid, unreliable, and unreasonable inference on individual risk factor in a disease causation given the group level assessment of the outcome as a function of exposure.
  - Despite this fallacy, this design provides the initial step in examining the relationship between the exposure of interest at group level and the prevalence of the outcome, disease of interest, or health-related event of interest.
- Hypothesis generating on the basis of ecologic design requires appropriate interpretation and inference.

7.4   Ecologic evidence: Association or causation?

Data from ecologic designs indicate association and not causation. However, etiologic studies are often based on initial ecologic investigations.

Biological pathway: The association involves a possible biological mechanism. For example, extra virgin olive oil consumption (group-level) and female breast cancer mortality rate among women in the five selected countries (hypothetical). The biologic pathway reflects the inhibition of abnormal cellular proliferation given extra virgin olive oil consumption. These data showed an inverse correlation between extra virgin olive oil consumption and breast cancer mortality, implying that countries with high extra virgin olive oil consumption have lower breast cancer mortality rates (Figure 7.2).

Group level: The association is based on group-level exposure in the countries examined. For example, women who consume extra virgin olive oil may be exposed to vegetable and fruit consumption, as well as a physically active lifestyle, than women who do not; and breast cancer had been associated with vegetable and fruit consumption as well as physical activities.

Contextual: The association involves biological mechanism as well as ecologic or group level exposures (Figure 7.3).

7.5   Limitations of ecologic study design

Despite several practical advantages of ecologic studies, there are methodological issues that limit causal inference, including ecologic fallacies and cross-level bias, unmeasured confounding, within-group misclassification, lack of

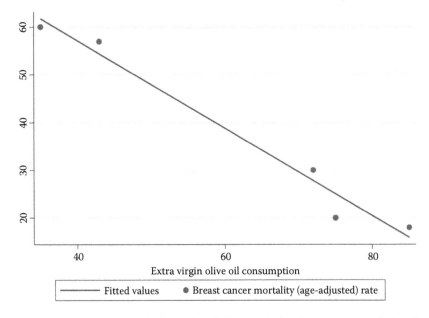

Figure 7.2 Hypothetical ecologic study of the association between extra virgin olive oil and breast cancer mortality (age-adjusted) rate in five countries.

BOX 7.4   ADVANTAGES AND DISADVANTAGES OF ECOLOGIC STUDY DESIGN

- Low cost and convenience
- Measurement limitations of individual-level studies
- Design limitations of individual-level studies
- Interest in ecologic or aggregate effect
- Simplicity of analysis and presentation of results

K. J. Rothman, Modern Epidemiology, *3rd ed.*
(Philadelphia: Lippincott, Williams & Wilkins, 2008).

---

adequate data, temporal ambiguity, colinearity, and migration across groups.[6] Ecologic fallacies typically represent the absence of association observed at one level of grouping to correlate to effect measure at the group level of interest. Specifically, ecologic bias or fallacies refer to the absence of an association at the individual-level data despite the observed association at the group level. Additionally, study limitation using this design reflects geographic variability in the ascertainment of exposure and disease, implying the need for the uniformity of the exposure and disease exposure across geography.

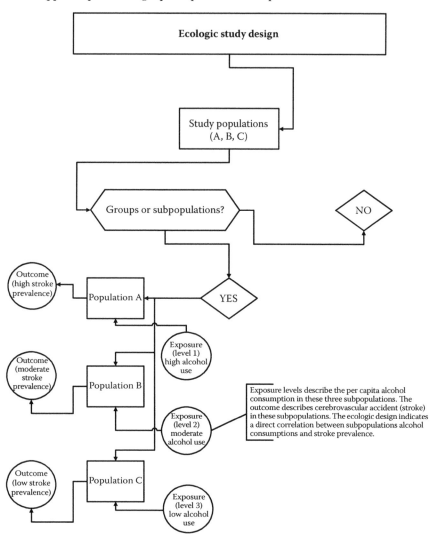

Figure 7.3 Design of ecologic study.

7.6   Summary

Ecologic design assesses the relationship between the exposure and outcome of interest at a group level and does not involve individual-level analysis as applicable to cohort, case-control, and cross-sectional classic designs. These *designs* are feasible when group-level data are available and inference is required on such a level and not at individual-level risk. It is analytic since the measure of effect, being the correlation coefficient, is an essential inference when provided with the coefficient of determination. Since individual data are not assessed in ecologic design, an inference about individual risk from such a design remains invalid, leading to an *ecologic fallacy*.

The analysis of ecologic design involves different measures of effect and association and includes the correlation coefficient but mainly predictive parameters, namely, the linear regression model. While the linear regression model is appropriate in the analysis of ecologic research data, temporality (cause-and-effect association) and confounding remain major issues in the interpretation and application of ecologic findings in public health policy formulation as well as in intervention mapping.

Unlike other nonexperimental designs, it is extremely difficult, if not impossible, to assess and control for confounding. Additionally, unmeasured confounding and the inability to assess effect measure modifier or biologic interaction may render ecologic data misleading to the scientific audience. Therefore, while there is a need to conduct ecologic studies, caution is required in the interpretation and application of such findings in clinical and public health decision-making.

Questions for discussion

1 A study is planned to investigate the benefits of agent X in drinking water (agent X is measured at group level) and the risk of developing dental caries in children.
  a Which design should be used if individual-level data are not available?
  b What are the advantages and disadvantages of ecologic design? Comment on ecologic fallacy.
  c What is the measure of effect or association in ecologic design, and how is it interpreted?
2 Suppose you are required to examine the effect of maternal education on learning abilities in Sweden, Norway, Finland, Austria, Australia, the United Kingdom, and the United States, and there are no data on individual cases. How will you begin to conceptualize the study? What design will be most feasible to draw an inference on the association between maternal education and learning disabilities in children?
3 Consider a study to determine whether or not there is an association between extra virgin olive oil consumption and breast cancer. If data are obtained from several countries on extra virgin olive oil consumption and the incidence of breast cancer, what design could be feasible is assessing this relationship? Second, on the basis of these aggregate data, what sort of causal inference could be drawn if any? Comment on the distinction between biologic and ecologic causality.
4 Suppose you are required to assess poverty among children and education attainment in adulthood and data are only available in different countries on poverty level and mathematical skills in children. What design should be feasible in this case? What will be the measure of effect? Comment on the association between education and poverty, and discuss the implication of this with subsequent health status of children.

References

1. K. J. Rothman, *Modern Epidemiology*, 3rd ed. (Philadelphia: Lippincott, Williams & Wilkins, 2008).
2. C. H. Hennekens and J. E. Buring, *Epidemiology in Medicine* (Boston: Little Brown & Company, 1987).
3. D. A. Savitz, *Interpreting Epidemiologic Evidence* (New York: Oxford University Press, 2003).
4. S. Greenland, "Epidemiologic Measures and Policy Formulation: Lessons from Potential Outcomes," *Emerg Themes Epidemiol.* 2 (2005):1–4.
5. J. L. Colli, A. Colli, "International Comparison of Prostate Cancer Mortality Rates with Dietary Practices And Sunlight Levels," *Urol Oncol Semin Orig Investig* 24 (2006): 184–194.
6. H. Morgenstern, "Ecologic Studies in Epidemiology: Concepts, Principles, and Methods," *Annu Rev Public Health* 16 (1995): 61–81.

8   Case-control studies
Design, conduct, and interpretation

8.1   Introduction

Case-control studies are traditional to epidemiology and refer to a design that compares subjects or patients ascertained as diseased or with the specific outcome of interest, with comparable subjects or patients who do not have the disease or outcome, and examines retrospectively (most cases) to determine the frequency of the exposure or risk factor in each group, with an attempt to assess the relationship between the exposure/risk factor and the disease/outcome. As simple as it may appear in conceptual terms, implying the cases as the basis of design upon which controls are sampled, this design is very challenging in terms of the selection of comparable controls from the source population. These sampling difficulties, which may create noncomparable controls, render evidence from this design unreliable as controls may not reflect similar experiences or other exposure experiences of the cases (differences in related risk factors that may not be known—unknown confounding). In the previous chapter, ecologic epidemiologic design with a focus on multiple groups and group-level analysis was presented. In this chapter, an attempt is made to present individual-level design with individual-level analysis. While randomized placebo-controlled clinical trials (RCTs) are the gold standard of clinical research in determining therapeutic benefits, thus providing evidence to guide clinical or surgical practice, they are not always feasible or ethical. Randomization of study participants into treatment and control ensures the balance of baseline prognostic factors and implies that the differences between the groups compared result from the trial or intervention and are not confounded by baseline differences between them. Despite the advantages of RCT, ethical issues remain potential obstacles to the application of this design in clinical research, requiring epidemiologists or investigators to use nonexperimental designs that are feasible in addressing the research questions. In addition, nonexperimental studies are efficient in clinical epidemiology, population science, or medicine since they could be used in assessing a wider range of exposures relative to RCTs.

  Case-control studies are classically retrospective designs in which investigators identify and enroll cases of the disease or outcome of interest and sample the source population (control or comparison group) that generated the cases. Since case-comparison studies are relatively inexpensive and faster to conduct, the availability of cases, as in rare diseases, should suggest the application of this design. There are limitations to this design, but this should not discourage the use of a well-designed case-control study in examining the exposure status of those with and without the outcome or disease of interest especially while exploring rare outcomes or when the induction or latent periods are long, as in malignancies. Therefore, investigators should prefer case-control design when limited information is available on disease etiology or exposure. This approach allows investigators to generate information on the exposure distribution, thus indirectly comparing the rate of the disease or outcome in exposed and unexposed groups.

This chapter describes the notion, design process, measures of association or effect, and strengths and limitations of case-control design (Figure 8.1). First, case-control is presented along with the variants of this design. Second, the notion of case-control as a prospective design is mentioned, but not discussed in detail due to the scope of this book. For example, if all the cases did not occur at the time of the study initiation and new cases are included as

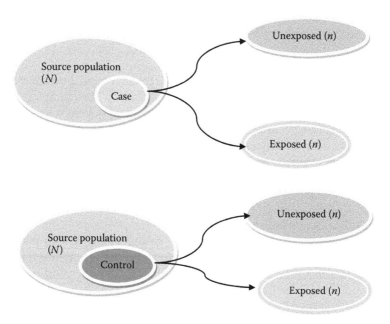

Figure 8.1 **Case-control design.** Illustration of exposure status determination based on the cases and the controls from the source population. The challenge in this design remains that of comparable selection of the control since the comparison group must come from the same population that produced the cases (source population). Despite controlling for potential confounding from the design phase (matching) or utilizing stratified or multivariable analysis to control for confounding at the analysis phase, residual confounding and misclassification bias, especially differential, may substantially affect the validity of case-control data in improving patient care and enhancing public health effort to control disease and promote health.

the study progress, such design represents prospective case-control. However, while this notion of prospective case-control is not widely used among epidemiologists, the inclusion of incident cases in an ongoing case-control studies represent an "ambidirectional case-control" design. Next, the limitations of case-control are discussed with the intent to describe the inherent inadequacies of this design despite its widespread use in epidemiologic studies, especially in the context of rare disease. Finally, the recommendations are made to reflect how to report the method and results in case-control designs (Figure 8.2).

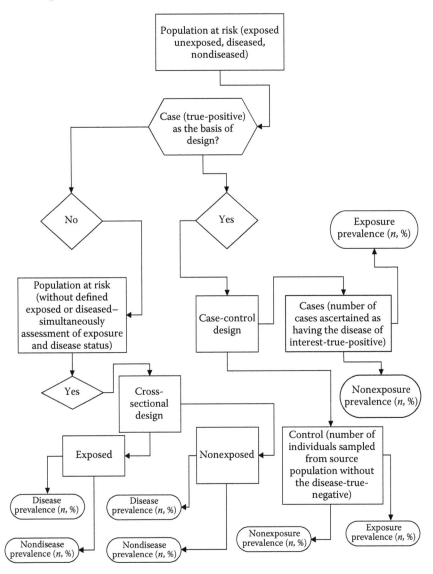

Figure 8.2 Case-control and cross-sectional designs.

8.2 Basis of case-control design

A traditional case-control study represents nonexperimental designs that begin with cases who have the disease or experience events of interest and the selection of the control subjects without the disease or events of interest from the source population. These controls are comparable with the cases except for the outcome of interest.[1–3] In terms of directionality, this design uses outcome to determine the exposure and is mainly retrospective with respect to timing, rendering temporal sequence difficult to properly ascertain; sampling is based on the outcome.[4] In a case-control study, patients who have developed a disease are identified, and their past exposure to suspected etiological factors is compared with that of controls or referents who do not have the disease.[5,6] This design allows the estimation of odds ratios (ORs) (but not attributable risks).[7,8] For example, a case-control study was conducted to examine the association between intraoperative factors and the development of deep wound infection. The investigators retrospectively ascertained 22 cases for over a period of 10 years and sampled controls from the source population (patients with neuromuscular scoliosis who underwent spine fusion for curve deformities correction).

Case-control studies had been shown to be efficient in assessing many exposures, indicating its unique strength; however, caution must be exercised in determining the association of the exposures with the disease. A study with 12,461 cases and 14,637 controls on obesity (body mass index [BMI], hip, waist, and waist-to-hip ratio) and the risk of myocardial infarction indicated a graded and highly significant relationship with waist-to-hip ratio, but not with BMI. This association persisted after adjustment for age, sex, region, and smoking, indicative of the relevance of waist-to-hip ratio in the obesity and diseases relationship.

Another example involved the association between neck circumference and childhood asthma severity in which children with asthma severity (cases) were compared with those with low and moderate asthma (control) with respect to neck circumference as exposure. Data were also collected on hip, waist, and calculated waist-to-hip ratio. Investigators utilized the electronic medical records to identify children diagnosed with asthma severity as cases ($n = 11$) and obtained controls using stratified systematic sampling technique to obtain age matched controls (children with mild and moderate asthma, $n = 44$, 1:3 ratio). With the age-adjusted neck circumference, cases were compared with controls for differences in exposure experience (unpublished paper). This example reflects the use of hospital-based control by selecting controls from the hospital who may not represent the source population where the cases were obtained. However, an alternative to hospital-based design, such as sampling the controls from the population where the hospital is located, may not provide a comparable control if the hospital has a proven quality outcomes and low cost (value care), implying the referral of cases nationally and globally.

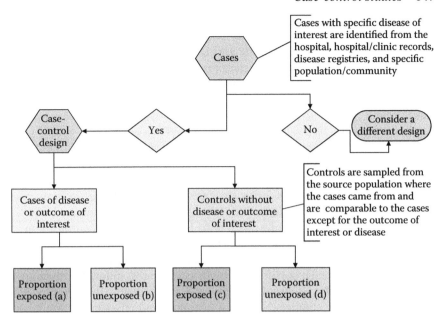

Figure 8.3 Case-control design.

Case-control presents a unique issue in the ascertainment of exposure since the controls may not have similar or comparable exposure with the cases if the source population where the cases originated differs from the control as in the example of hospital-based or clinic-based case-control study on asthma severity and neck circumference (Figure 8.3). Epidemiologists are challenged with uniformity in the ascertainment of exposure and the balance between the exposure experiences of the controls if the controls differ from the cases.

8.2.1   Cases ascertained in case-control studies

8.2.1.1   Selection of cases

The starting point of most case-control studies is the identification of cases.[9] This requires a suitable case definition as in the previous example of deep wound infection. In addition, care is needed so that bias does not arise from the way in which cases are selected. A study of deep wound infection after posterior spine fusion in children with neuromuscular scoliosis might be misleading if cases were identified from hospital admissions and admission to hospital was influenced not only by the presence and severity of neuro-muscular scoliosis but also by other variables, such as medical or a specific health insurance. In general, it is advantageous to use incident (deep wound infection) rather than prevalent cases, since prevalence is influenced not only by the risk of developing the disease of interest but also by factors that determine the duration of illness. Please recall that the prevalence proportion = I × D, where I is the incidence rate and D is the mean duration of illness.[9,10] This formula is applicable when the prevalence of the disease is small, less than 10%.[10] It is adequate because with small prevalence, prevalence proportion will approximate the prevalence odds.[9,10] Furthermore, if a disease has been present for a long time, then premorbid exposure to risk factors may be harder to ascertain, especially if assessment depends on subjects' recall.

In the previous example, deep wound infection case ascertainment was based on the combination of signs and symptoms, physical and microbiologic examination, and results of these diagnostic tests. Investigators should apply existing standard criteria to define the cases with as much accuracy as possible in avoiding selection and misclassification bias. With standard criteria for case ascertainment, the next step is to identify cases and enroll them in the study by gathering data on them. The sources of data in this case were the medical records. In typical case-control studies, other sources of data include patients' rosters, death certificates, birth certificates, magnetic resonance imaging, computed tomography, x-ray, positron emission tomography, etc. It is important to recognize the role of accuracy and efficiency in the ascertainment of the cases. Depending on the research question, incident cases may be preferred to prevalent cases. Therefore, if the intent is to study risk factors, it is preferable to study incident cases, since prevention cases reflect factors that affect the disease duration and not the factors that cause the disease itself. However, regardless of the cases used in case-control studies, investigators should apply caution in the interpretation of the results. Therefore, it is important to point out if the factors studied affect the disease etiology, its duration, or a combination of the two. A 2 × 2 contingent table could be used to illustrate point estimate or association and effect in a case-control design (unmatched design). The odds of the exposure in the case relative to the control is provided by cross product exposed/case (a) and control/noncase (d) divided by the cross product exposed/noncase (false-positive) and nonexpose/case (false-negative). Mathematically, the measure of effect or association in case-control design is given by ad × bc.

8.2.1.2 Selection of controls in case-control studies

Usually, it is not too difficult to obtain a suitable source of cases, but selecting controls tends to be more difficult, since the control must be comparable to the cases, except for the disease status or outcomes of interest. Controls are expected to come from the same source population as the cases and are expected to meet these two requirements:

1 Within the constraints of any matching criteria, their exposure to risk factors and confounders should be representative of that in the population "at risk" of becoming cases—that is, people who do not have the

disease under investigation but who would be included in the study as cases if they had.

2 The exposure/s status of controls should be measurable with similar accuracy to those of the cases.[11] Geographic variation and temporal factors must be considered in the ascertainment of cases and control if different geographic locales are involved in cases and controls sampling. Specifically, the diagnostic criteria, implying disease ascertainment may differ from one location to another.

BOX 8.1 HYBRIDS OF CASE-CONTROL STUDIES

I. Nested case-control
- A case-control study conducted within a cohort study
  - Involves an ongoing study with a defined cohort
- Random sampling of cases and controls are very feasible

II. Case-cohort
- Applicable where source population is a cohort and every individual in the cohort has an equal opportunity of being selected as a control
  - Person–time contribution of the cohort is not relevant
- Efficient when the measure of effect of interest is incidence proportion ratio or average risk
- Mathematically: Re (incidence proportion among exposed subcohort) = De/Ne, where De is the number of the diseased among the exposed and Ne is the total population of the exposed. Likewise, Ru (incidence proportion in the unexposed subcohort) = Du/Nu, where u = unexposed.
- Incidence proportion ratio = Re/Ru
  - To be reliable as design to measure the incidence proportion ratio, the ratio of the number of exposed controls (Re) to the number of the exposed subcohort (Ne) should be similar to the ratio of the of the number in the unexposed control (Ru) to the number of unexposed subcohort (Nu).

III. Density case-control
- Can be used to estimate risk ratio—if the ratio of person-time denominators Te/Tu is accurately estimated by the ratio of exposed to unexposed controls (De/Du)
- Involve the selection of controls such that the exposure distribution among them is the same as it is among the person-time in the source population—density sampling
- This sampling provides for estimation of incidence rate or incidence densities (Table 8.1).

Table 8.1 Case–control design: strengths and limitations

Strengths (advantages)	Limitations (disadvantages)
• Efficient for rare diseases (desirable design) • Efficient for diseases with long induction and latent periods • Adequate for evaluating multiple exposures in relation to a disease (desirable when little is known about exposure variables in a given disease) • Rapid and inexpensive relative to prospective cohort design	• Recall and selection bias due to the retrospective nature of design • Difficult to assess temporal sequence between exposure and disease or health-related events if exposure changes over time • Information bias and poor information on exposure (retrospective nature of design) • Inefficient for rare exposure

8.2.1.3   Sources of controls

There are two commonly used sources of controls:

1   General or source population: Controls selected from the general or source population have the advantage that their exposures are likely to be representative of those at risk of becoming cases. However, assessment of their exposure may not be comparable with that of cases, especially if the assessment is achieved by the subject's recall, as cases are more likely to recall factors that may be related to their illness relative to healthy controls.

2   Hospital-based control: If controls are selected from a group of patients with a disease that is different from the disease of interest in the case-control study, then controls are more likely to recall the exposure. Therefore, measurement of exposure can be made more comparable by using patients with other diseases as controls, especially if subjects are not told of exact focus of the investigation. However, their exposures may be unrepresentative. For example, a case-control study of prostate cancer (CaP) and an agent used to enhance erectile function could give quite erroneous findings if controls were taken from the impotence clinic. If other patients are to be used as referents, it is safer to adopt a range of control diagnoses rather than a single disease group. In that way, if one of the control diseases happens to be related to a risk factor under study, the resultant bias is not too large.

When cases and controls are both freely available, then selecting equal numbers will make a study most efficient. However, the number of cases that can be studied is often limited by the rarity of the disease under investigation. In this circumstance, statistical confidence can be increased by taking more than one control per case. There is, however, a law of diminishing returns, and it is usually not worth going beyond a ratio of four or five controls to one case.[11]

8.2.1.4 Ascertainment of exposure

A wide variety of exposures are involved in disease causation or association and include but are not limited to lifestyle, environment, job, occupation, heredity or genes, diet, alcohol, and drugs. In any of these exposure circumstances, information is required on the source, nature, exposure frequency, and duration of exposure. Many case-control studies ascertain exposure from personal recall, using either a self-administered questionnaire or an interview. The validity of such information will depend in part on the subject matter. People may be able to remember quite well where they lived in the past or what jobs they did. On the other hand, long-term recall of dietary habits is probably less reliable. For example, in a study of the relation between intraoperative factors and deep wound infection, the information for the cases and control were ascertained by searching their medical records. Provided that records are reasonably complete, this method will usually be more accurate than one that depends on memory. Occasionally, long-term biological markers of exposure can be exploited. Biological markers are only useful, however, when they are not altered by the subsequent disease process. For example, serum cholesterol concentrations measured after a myocardial infarction may not accurately reflect levels before the onset of infarction.

8.2.1.5 Case-control analysis—measure of effect or association

The statistical techniques for analyzing case-control studies are discussed in previous chapters. The odds of exposure, given the disease (cases), and the odds of exposure, given nondisease (control), are computed as follows:

The odds of case exposure = exposed cases/all cases
÷ unexposed cases/all cases.

Mathematically this appears as follows:

Odds (of exposure) ratio (or) = AD/BC

where AD and BC represent the cross products from the 2 × 2 contingency table.

(A/A + B) ÷ (B/A + B) = A/B

The odds of control exposure, implying odds of exposure in the control group = C/D, are

$$\text{Odds ratio (OR)} = \text{Odds of case exposure/Odds of control exposure}$$
$$= (A/B) \div (C/D) = A*D/B*C.$$

Because the two groups are sampled separately, rates of disease, disability, or injury in the exposed or unexposed groups cannot be calculated, nor can relative risk be measured directly. However, the OR or relative odds (RO) can be computed; it is the primary measure of association in case-control design. Because of the sampling used, the total number exposed is not $a + b$, and the risk in exposed subjects is not $a/(a + b)$.

It is important to note that the attempt at event (exposure or outcome) estimate is not to directly derive disease incidence in the exposed and unexposed groups but to estimate the odds of exposure in the cases and in the controls. Additionally, if the controls are sampled from all subjects initially at risk, then this design can directly estimate the risk ratio, but if controls are sampled from those who are still disease-free at the time where all cases are obtained (end of follow-up, no more new cases), then it is possible to estimate the OR for the disease (odds of disease ratio). Finally, if the controls are sampled (time matching of controls with the case ascertained) from those still at risk at the time that each case is ascertained, then it is possible to estimate the rate ratio.

8.3 Variance of case-control design

Nested case-control is advantageous to the classic case-control in that it minimizes and eliminates recall bias; it ensures or reduces the uncertainty with the temporal sequence, thus making it easy to determine whether the exposure preceded the disease; and it is relatively inexpensive and rapid, compared to prospective cohort design.[9,12–14] Nested case-control is limited in that the non-diseased may not be fully representative of the original cohort because of loss to follow-up or death. The OR is a good estimate of relative risk, except when the outcome is very frequent (high prevalence).

BOX 8.2   CASE-COHORT DESIGN

Density case-control studies require that the control series represent the person–time distribution of exposure in the source population. Epidemiologists establish this representativeness by sampling controls in such a way that the probability that any person in the source population is selected as a control is proportional to his or her person–time contribution to the incidence rates in the source population. Regarding case-cohort study:

- It is a case-control study in which an individual selected as a control may also be a case.
- Every person in the source population has the same chance of being included as a control regardless of how much time that individual has contributed to the person–time experience of the cohort.
- Each control participant represents a fraction of the total number of individuals in the source population, rather than a fraction of the total person–time.
- The point estimate is similar to that of the density case-control study, but the estimated odds represent the risk ratio, while the odds estimated in the density case-control study is a measure of the rate ratio.

8.3.1 OR in case-control and cohort designs

The odds and probability (case-control versus cohort design): Odds differs from probability (*P*) but is related by the following equation:

$$\text{Odds} = P \div (1 - P).$$

For example, if the probability of the diseased being exposed is 80% (0.8), the odds of the diseased being exposed is 4.0, which is 80/20 ($P/1 - P$).

In a cohort design, the probability that the exposed will develop a disease is a/a + b and the odds that a disease will develop in the exposed is a/b ($P/1 - P$). The probability that the disease will develop in the unexposed is c/c + d; similarly, the odds of the disease developing in the unexposed is c/d ($P/1 - P$). The OR (*incidence rate ratio*) in cohort design is presented mathematically in the following:

$$\text{Incidence Rate Ratio (IRR)} = A/B \div C/D = A*D/B*C.$$

These are the odds that an exposed person develops a disease divided by the odds that a nonexposed person develops the disease.

Consider a hypothetical case-control study to examine the association between renal carcinoma and cigarette smoking (Figure 8.4). The sample consisted of 1200 subjects, of whom 400 were cases (renal carcinoma) and 800 were controls. Of the 400 cases, 224 were exposed to cigarette, while 176 were not; and among the controls, 352 were cigarette smokers and 448 were not. Based on these data, can we estimate the prevalence of renal carcinoma in the population of interest or the targeted population? Is there an association between cigarette smoking and renal carcinoma?

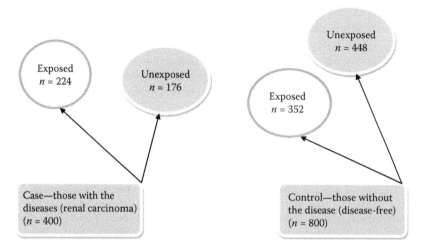

Figure 8.4 Hypothetical case-control design on the association between cigarette smoking and renal carcinoma.

The prevalence of renal carcinoma is 400/1200 = 33%. Recall the prevalence of disease or health-related event is given by the simple or unconditional probability (# of success/total number of events).

Mathematically,

$$\text{Prevalence of renal carcinoma} = \frac{\text{All cases of renal carcinoma (a+c)}}{\text{The total population (a+b+c+d)}}.$$

However, this is not a true prevalence proportion since the denominators in this context is dependent on the investigator's choice of the number of controls from the source or referenced population (Table 8.2).

The proportion of the exposed among the cases is given by

$$\frac{\text{Cases who smoked cigarette (a)}}{\text{Cases who smoked plus those who did not (a+c)}}.$$

Table 8.2 Estimation of the proportion exposed in case and control design as well as the odds of exposure in the case versus the odds of exposure in the control group

	Renal carcinoma (case)	*Non-renal carcinoma (control)*	*Total*
Cigarette smoking (exposed)	a (224)	b (352)	a + b
Nonsmoking (unexposed)	c (176)	d (448)	c + d
Total	a + c	b + d	–
Proportion exposed	a/a + c	b/b + d	–

Table 8.3 Odds ratio from a matched case-control study using 2 × 2 contingency table

	Control exposed	*Control unexposed*	*Total*
Case exposed	a	b	a + b
Case unexposed	c	d	c + d
Total	a + c	b + d	a + b + c + d

The proportion of exposed among the control is given by

$$\frac{\text{Controlled who smoked cigarette (b)}}{\text{Cases who smoked plus those who did not (b+d)}}.$$

8.3.2 Measure of disease effect or association obtained in matched case-control

In Table 8.3, a = both cases and control are exposed; b = case exposed but control unexposed; c = case unexposed but control exposed; and d = case unexposed and control unexposed. a and d are concordant pairs.

Assuming 1:1 matching, the OR is given by this equation:

Odds ratio (1:1) Matched pair = b/c (Discordant pairs),

where B (case exposed and control unexposed) and C (case unexposed and control exposed) are the discordant pairs, implying exposed case divided by unexposed case.

8.3.3 Interpretation of OR in case-control study

Suppose a case-control study was conducted to examine the association between postnatal steroid use and cerebral palsy, and investigators obtained an OR of 3.6. What does this mean? Simply, the odds of the use of postnatal steroid for children with cerebral palsy is over three times greater than the odds for the use of postnatal steroid among the control (children without cerebral palsy) in the study.

Consider another example of a case-control study on the association between measles–mumps–rubella (MMR) vaccination and autism. With 96 cases, investigators sampled 192 matched controls (year of birth, sex, and general practitioners). Investigators used conditional logistic regression model to assess the association between MMR vaccination and autism. The adjusted OR for MMR (vaccinated versus nonvaccinated) after adjusting for mother's age, medication during pregnancy, gestation time, perinatal injury, and Apgar score was 0.17 (95% confidence interval [CI], 0.06–0.52).[13] What is the basic interpretation of this result? First, the odds of developing autism was

83% lower among children vaccinated with MMR compared to unvaccinated children. In addition, the 95% CI (unadjusted type I error level tolerance for multiple comparison/multivariable logistic regression) does not include 1, implying a statistically precise point estimate.

While interpretation of association in nonexperimental epidemiologic studies may be straightforward, that is not the case in case-control designs. Specifically, the observed point estimate or association or no association may be due to (a) selection bias, (b) information bias (exposure), and (c) confounding (assessment and adjustment).

8.4   Scientific reporting in case-control studies: Methods and results

The scientific statement on the reporting of observational (nonexperimental) studies, termed Strengthening the Reporting of Observational Studies in Epidemiology (STROBE), recommends the result section to include participants (numbers potentially eligible, study sample, actually analyzed participants, flow diagram to reflect eligibility, and actual sample); descriptive statistics, mainly participants characteristics (demographic, clinical, social); as well as missing data on all variables examined. Additionally, the numbers in each exposure category or summary measures of effect (OR) should be reported as outcome data. Further, the main result should include unadjusted or crude (raw) and, where applicable, the adjusted estimate and their precisions (95% CI), including the confounders included in the adjusted model, including the rationale for their inclusion. Other reports such as subgroups, interaction, propensity and, sensitivity analysis should be presented in the result section.

STROBE recommended the method section to report on the design used in conducting the study, study setting (location or site), participants (eligibility criteria, data source, sampling method), variables, data sources and measurement, sample size and power estimation, and statistical analysis. The statistical analysis should include the description of all methods used (summary statistics, crude and adjusted), methods for subgroup and interaction analysis, as well as explanation for missing data if applicable.[15]

Vignette 8.1 Case-control (hypothetical) A study was conducted to examine the role of selenium in the development of CaP. There were 15 cases of older men with localized incident CaP and 15 controls (older men without prostate or any other malignancy) (Table 8.4). The proportion of cases and controls who ingested selenium as a daily supplement was estimated from the data. Among cases of CaP, 3 reported having had selenium supplement daily during the past five years,

Table 8.4 Hypothetical data on selenium use and prostate cancer
development

Study ID	Age	Race/ethnicity	Exposure (selenium use)	Disease (CaP)
001	50	1	1	1
002	45	2	0	1
003	60	3	0	1
004	70	4	0	1
005	66	1	0	1
006	65	2	1	0
007	48	1	1	0
008	50	2	1	0
009	55	1	0	0
010	63	2	0	1
011	43	1	0	1
012	67	2	0	1
013	75	3	0	1
014	64	3	0	1
015	65	1	1	0
016	48	2	1	0
017	50	4	0	1
018	55	1	1	1
019	63	1	1	1
020	43	1	0	1
021	67	1	0	1
022	65	1	1	0
023	48	2	1	0
024	50	1	1	0
025	55	2	1	0
026	63	2	1	0
027	43	2	0	0
028	67	2	1	0
029	59	1	1	0
030	61	2	0	1

Data code: Age is in years, race/ethnicity; Caucasian = 1; African American = 2;
Hispanic = 3; Asian = 4, 0 = absence of exposure or outcome, and 1 = presence of exposure or outcome.

while 13 did so among the controls. On the basis of these data, is there an association between routine selenium intake and the development of CaP?

Using STATA statistical software, we are able to obtain the frequency of the cases of CaP and controls who took selenium. The syntax tab exposure (0,1) disease(0,1) generates the frequency distribution of the exposure within the disease status (case/control).

To examine the association between selenium intake and CaP, we can use the software again by entering the appropriate syntax: cc outcome (var) exposure (var).

BOX 8.3   CASE-CONTROL DESIGN ANALYSIS

. cc diseasecap exposureseleniumuse

	Exposed	Unexposed	Total	Proportion Exposed
Cases	3	13	16	0.1875
Controls	12	2	14	0.8571
Total	15	15	30	0.5000

	Point estimate	[95% Conf. Interval]	
Odds ratio	.0384615	.0032135	.3452271 (exact)
Prev. frac. ex.	.9615385	.6547729	.9967865 (exact)
Prev. frac. pop	.8241758		

chi2(1) =   13.39 Pr>chi2 = 0.0003

The data indicate a significant reduction in prostate cancer risk, given the effect of selenium, an antioxidant. The odds ratio (OR) or relative odds (RO), which is the sample estimate, and CI, the precision estimate, are both indicative of a clinically meaningful effect of selenium. Can the observed effect be generalizable, given the p value as the evidence against the null hypothesis of no effect of selenium? With $p = 0.0003$, there is a significant evidence against the null hypothesis of no effect at 0.05 significance level (type I error tolerance level).

The syntax in Box 8.3 generates the OR, 95% CI, and the p value. The odds of developing CaP are significantly lowered by selenium intake according to these data. Selenium is associated with a 99.6% decrease in CaP development, OR = 0.04, 95% CI, 0.003–0.35, p = .0003.

BOX 8.4A CASE-CONTROL ANALYSIS
USING AGGREGATE DATA

. cci 3 13 12 2

	Exposed	Unexposed	Total	Proportion Exposed
Cases	3	13	16	0.1875
Controls	12	2	14	0.8571
Total	15	15	30	0.5000
	Point estimate		[95% Conf. Interval]	
Odds ratio	.0384615		.0032135	.3452271 (exact)
Prev. frac. ex.	.9615385		.6547729	.9967865 (exact)
Prev. frac. pop	.8241758			

chi2(1) =   13.39 Pr>chi2 = 0.0003

We can also determine the odds of exposure among the cases and controls by using the frequency (aggregate data) without the entire data. The STATA syntax cci three (selenium intake and developed CaP), twelve (do not take selenium and develop CaP), two (do not take selenium and do not develop CaP), and thirteen (do take selenium and do not develop CaP) allows us to perform this computation (Box 8.4).

BOX 8.4B ASSOCIATION BETWEEN DIABETES
AND SMOKING ASSESSING FOR CONFOUNDING
OR EFFECT MEASURE MODIFIER

. cc DM SMK

	Exposed	Unexposed	Total	Proportion Exposed
Cases	40	5	45	0.8889
Controls	33	33	66	0.5000
Total	73	38	111	0.6577
	Point estimate		[95% Conf. Interval]	
Odds ratio	8		2.641341	28.70063 (exact)
Attr. frac. ex.	.875		.6214044	.9651576 (exact)
Attr. frac. pop	.7777778			

chi2(1) =   17.97 Pr>chi2 = 0.0000

This stata output indicates a case-control design on the association between diabetes and smoking (hypothetical study). There is a statistically significantly eightfold predisposition to diabetes as a result of exposure to smoking in this sample data (OR or RO = 8.0; 95% CI, 2.64–28.70; $p < 0.001$). As a crude association, there is a potential for confounding by sex or sex could be an effect measure modifier in this association. The following stata output indicates the assessment for confounding and effect measure modifier. By observing the crude and adjusted point estimates, there is reasonable evidence of confounding by sex (OR = 8.0 [crude] versus OR = 8.14 [adjusted]), implying a >10% difference. Likewise, sex is an effect measure modifier given the significant different in the stratum specific (male, OR = 6.6 versus female, OR = 11.5) in the association between smoking and diabetes (below).

```
. mhodds DM SMK, by (Sex)

Maximum likelihood estimate of the odds ratio
Comparing SMK==1 vs. SMK==0
by Sex
          Sex|Odds Ratio   chi2(1) |P>chi2       [95% Conf. Interval]

            1|  6.645833    8.65   |0.0033       1.54467    28.59327
            2| 11.523810    6.94   |0.0048       1.14883   115.59444


        Mantel-Haenszel estimate controlling for Sex

        Odds Ratio     chi2(1)      P>chi2       [95% Conf. Interval]
        8.149109       15.59        0.0001       2.351149   28.244906

Test of homogeneity of ORs (approx): chi2(1) = 0.16
                             Pr>chi2 = 0.6865
```

8.5 Summary

Epidemiologic studies are essentially nonexperimental (observational), experimental, and ecologic. Nonexperimental studies are conducted when RCTs, "the gold standard" of clinical research, are not feasible or are unethical. The choice of nonexperimental designs depends on several factors, some of which are research design and hypothesis to be tested, financial constraint, time, disease frequency, and exposure frequency.

Case-control studies are warranted when the disease is rare, as in when the induction and the latent periods of the disease are long, as observed in malignancies. Although these designs do not estimate the risk directly, if well designed, they could approximate the risk of the disease by comparing the exposure risk or odds in the diseased (case) and the nondiseased (control).

Hybrids or variance of case-control studies in include case-cohort, nested case-control, density case-control, cumulative case-control, case only, case cross-over, and case specular, also termed *hypothetical case-control*. The choice of a particular hybrid design depends on the research question and the manner in which the cases occurred, as well as other conditions that characterize the case. For example, the attempt to examine risk factors implying incident cases reflects the need to consider nested case-control.

The major limitation in case-control design is selection bias since the controls are sampled from the source population and should be comparable to the cases except for the outcome of interest or the disease. The efficiency of this design depends on careful selection of controls, as well as the accuracy in the measurement of the exposure. In addition, because the controls are healthy subjects in most circumstances, these subjects are less likely to recall their exposure experience and recall bias minimization is required for a valid epidemiologic inference from case-control designs.

Questions for discussion

1 Read the study by Yusuf et al.[12]
   a Comment on the eligibility criteria and the analysis used in the implication of waist-to-hip ratio in myocardial infarction risk.
   b Is the analysis used by authors to determine the graded association between waits-to-hip ratio and MI appropriate?
   c Do you consider the appropriate design for this study to be ecologic? Why and why not?
2 Consider a hypothetical study performed to assess the association or relation between education and cervical cancer. A total of 780 sample (case and control) were studied. Among cases (400), 119 had cervical cancer and were never educated (never attended school), while among controls (380), 64 had cervical cancer and were never educated (never attended school). Using the 2 × 2 table, calculate the OR and the 95% CI. Also use chi-square to determine whether or not the relationship is statistically significant at 5% type I error tolerance.
3 Suppose you conducted a case-control study on the association between artificial sweeteners, namely, saccharin and bladder cancer. The data showed of 600 total sample, 500 were diagnosed with bladder cancer and 450 were exposed to saccharin, while among controls, 60 were exposed to saccharin.
   a On the basis of these data, is it possible to create a 2 × 2 table?
   b Is there any association between the exposure and the diseases?
   c What may possibly explain the lack association if data point to that direction?
   d Do you consider sampling insufficiencies to account for this crude result?
4 Suppose among 200 children with cerebral palsy, 125 had feeding difficulties, and among 180 controls, 75 had feeding difficulties. Test the hypothesis that feeding difficulties are associated with cerebral palsy.
   a Compute the OR relating cerebral palsy to feeding difficulties in children.
   b Provide a 95% CI for the estimate.
   c What can you conclude from these data?

References

1. L. Gordis, *Epidemiology*, 3rd ed. (Philadelphia: Elsevier Saunders, 2004).
2. K. J. Rothman, *Epidemiology, An Introduction* (New York: Oxford University Press, 2002).
3. C. H. Hennekens and J. E. Buring, *Epidemiology in Medicine* (Boston: Little Brown & Company, 1987).
4. M. Elwood, *Critical Appraisal of Epidemiological Studies in Clinical Trials*, 2nd ed. (New York: Oxford University Press, 2003).
5. A. Aschengrau and G. R. Seage III, *Essentials of Epidemiology* (Sudbury, MA: Jones & Bartlett, 2003).
6. R. H. Friis and T. A. Sellers, *Epidemiology for Public Health Practice* (Frederick, MD: Aspen Publications, 1996).
7. M. Szklo and J. Nieto, *Epidemiology: Beyond the Basics* (Sudbury, MA: Jones & Bartlett, 2003).
8. J. J. Schlesselman, *Case-Control Studies: Design, Conduct, Analysis* (New York: Oxford University Press, 1982).
9. L. Holmes, Jr., *Basics of Public Health Core Competencies* (Sudbury, MA: Jones and Bartlett, 2009).
10. K. J. Rothman, *Epidemiology: An Introduction* (New York: Oxford University Press, 2002).
11. R. S. Greenberg, *Medical Epidemiology*, 4th ed. (New York: Lange, 2005).
12. S. Ounpuu, S. Hawken, S. Yusuf et al., "Obesity and the Risk of Myocardial Infarction in 27,000 Participants from 52 Countries: A Case-Control Study," *Lancet* 366 (2005): 1640–1649.
13. D. Mrozek-Budzyn and R. Majewska, "Lack of Association Between Measles–Mumps–Rubella Vaccination and Autism in Children: A Case-Control Study," *Pediatr Infec Dis J* 29 (2010): 397–400.
14. J. L. Colli and A. Colli, "International Comparison of Prostate Cancer Mortality Rates with Dietary Practices and Sunlight Levels," *Urol Oncol Semin Orig Investig* 24 (2006): 184–194.
15. J. P. Vandenbroucke, E. von Elm, D. G. Altman, et al., Strengthening the reporting of observational studies in epidemiology (STROBE): Explanation and elaboration. *PLoS Med* 4 (2007): e297. [PMC free article] [PubMed].

9   Cross-sectional studies

Design, conduct, and interpretation

9.1   Introduction

A cross-sectional design (CSD) is a nonexperimental epidemiologic design that is feasible and ethical when randomized clinical trial cannot be conducted and other nonexperimental designs are less feasible or inefficient. This design basically assesses the association between diseases or health-related events and other variables or factors of interest as potential risk factors in a defined population at a particular time. Contrary to the sampling method involved in case-control design, cross-sectional studies obtain data on exposure and disease status at the same time, implying the prevalence measure and not disease incidence data.

While the outcomes of CSDs are determined at the same time as the exposure or intervention, this design remains effective in quantifying the prevalence of disease or risk factors, especially in the circumstance where resources is limited to apply other designs. Appropriate sampling is optimal to inference, and this applies to CSD as well. In effect, the *sampling frame* used for the sample selection and the response rate in CSD determines the extent of its generalizability. Consequently, if epidemiologists select random sample in the conduct of cross-sectional study (CSS), then the sample will be representative, yielding a reliable inference. Additionally, the response rate should be reasonable to reflect sample representation as well, implying an unbiased sample (equal and known probability of being selected). What should clinicians or those conducting CSS aim to accomplish in an attempt to address sampling representation? Clinicians could minimize low response rate by (a) using telephone and mail prompting, (b) second and third mailing of surveys, (c) offering reasonable incentive, and (d) communicating clearly the importance of the study to potential participants. Clinicians should be cautious of biased response, which may be associated with recall bias on participants without the outcome of interest. For example consider a CSS on passive smoking and asthma where door-to-door survey is conducted during the working hours. The groups more likely to be interviewed are women, girls, mothers, children, and elderly and asthma is more likely to be higher in this group, biasing the outcome assessment in a given population.[1] CSS designs are conducted in a situation where multiple exposures could be explored, implying that the investigators need to gather lots of data without a threat to loss of follow-up as experienced in longitudinal or cohort studies. Additionally, CSS is recommended in clinical or public health setting for public health and healthcare planning, examining predisposing factors to disease, and generating hypothesis for multiple and complex disease etiology.

CSDs are limited by the following:

- Lack of temporal sequence—disease and exposure sequence
- Biased identification of cases—a high proportion of prevalent cases of long duration and a low proportion of prevalent cases with short duration
- Healthy worker survivor effect bias—those employed are healthier relative to those who remain unemployed

Because nonexperimental studies can yield valid epidemiologic evidence on the relationship between exposure and disease, a well-designed cross-sectional study can address important clinical research questions regarding disease prevention, treatments, and possible etiology.

9.1.1 Basis of a cross-sectional study

Whereas cohort studies (prospective) are designed to measure the incidence (new events or changes) of a disease or an event of interest, cross-sectional studies assess the prevalence and hence focus on existing states.[2] Thus, no matter the frequency of data collection from a specified population, unless data are collected more than once from the same population, such a design cannot be termed longitudinal or concurrent. CSD remains a snapshot of exposure and outcome (response).

CSDs can also be used for causal association, because prevalence, as pointed out earlier, reflects both the incidence rate and the duration of the disease. As a result, these studies yield associations that reflect both the determinants of survival with the disease as well as the disease etiology.[2–4]

9.1.2 Feasibility of cross-sectional design

A cross-sectional design, as shown in Figure 9.1, is used to measure the prevalence of health outcomes, health determinants, or both in a population at a point in time or over a short period. Such information can be used to explore disease risk factors.[3] For example, Essien et al. (2007) conducted a study to examine the demographic and lifestyle predictors of the intention to use a condom in a defined population.[5] The prevalence of the intent to use a condom was the response or outcome, while demographic and lifestyle variables were the predictors, independent or explanatory variables, and were both measured at the same time from a survey instrument. Since exposure (demographics and lifestyle) and outcome (intent to use a condom) were measured simultaneously for each subject, the cross-sectional qualified the design used by these authors. In this study, the authors first identified the population of persons for the study and determined the presence or absence of the intent to use a condom and the lifestyle and

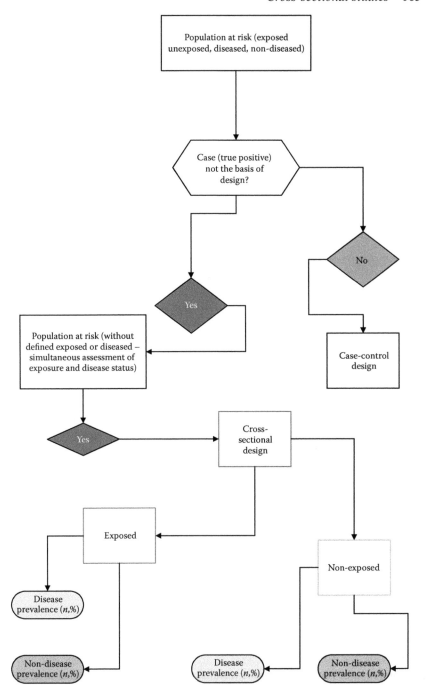

Figure 9.1 **Cross-sectional design.** The figure illustrates a cross-sectional design as a snapshot, implying an instant cohort study.

demographics for each subject. Using a 2 × 2 table, they compared the prevalence of lifestyle and demographic features in those with the intent to use a condom and compared it with those without the intent to use a condom: (A/A + C) ÷ (B/B + D). A CSD represents a snapshot of the population at a certain point in time.

Because of the inability to establish a cause-and-effect relationship, any association in this design must be interpreted with caution.[6,7] Second, bias may arise because of selection into or out of the study population. Due to the issues arising from lack of temporality (cause-and-effect relationship), cross-sectional studies of causal association are best conducted to examine accurate disorders, clinical conditions with little disability, or presymptomatic phases of serious and chronic disorders.

BOX 9.1   CROSS-SECTIONAL VERSUS CASE-CONTROL

- Cross-sectional studies, also called surveys and prevalence studies, are designed to assess both the exposure and outcome simultaneously.
- However, since exposure and disease status are measured at the same point in time (snapshot), it is difficult, if not impossible, to distinguish whether the exposure preceded or followed the disease, and thus cause-and-effect relationships are not certain, lacking temporal sequence.
- No matter how frequent a cross-sectional study is conducted, it does not represent a longitudinal study since one is unable to ensure a repeated measure from the same sample from baseline.
- A case-control design classifies subjects on the basis of outcome (disease and nondisease or comparison group) and then looks backward to identify the exposure.
  - This design could be prospective as well.
- In this design, the history or previous events for both cases and comparison groups are assessed in an attempt to identify the exposure or risk factors for the disease.
- If properly designed with a representative sample, both cross-sectional and case-control designs can generate valid and reliable results (Table 9.1).

Unlikely inaccurately thought any sample provided is representative could be used to provide a generalizable result from both designs. For example, the fact that only older women with chronic kidney disease (CKD) are studied with respect to hypertension as a predisposing factor does not render the results unreliable provided inference is drawn on older women. The problem is assuming that hypertension predisposes to CKD in young women and men who were not in the sample studied.

Table 9.1 Strengths and limitations of cross-sectional design

Strengths (advantages)	Limitations (disadvantages)
• Generalizability, given that the sample is usually obtained from large population • Relatively inexpensive • Relatively easy to conduct • Rapid • Assessment of multiple outcomes and exposures or risk factors • No loss to follow-up	• Inability to assess temporal sequence between exposure and disease or health-related events if exposure changes over time • Preponderance of prevalent cases, indicative of survivorship • Healthy worker survival effects, implying association or prevalence odds/risk ratio reflecting survival after the health-related event rather than the risk of developing the event or disease

CSDs could also be used in planning health care.[1,2,8,9] For example, a prostate cancer epidemiologist planning a chemoprevention intervention with micronutrient supplements in reducing the incidence rate of prostate cancer among African-American men in Texas might wish to know the prevalence of prostate cancer in this subpopulation by age and other factors, so that he or she could address the chemoprevention intervention accordingly.

Relative prevalence – PE/PU—Using 2×2 table a/(a + b)/c(c + d).
Prevalence odds ratio – ad/bc

Vignette 9.1 Cross-sectional design Consider a study that is interested in the possible association between low serum lycopene level (exposure) and prostate cancer (disease). The population is surveyed and the serum lycopene is determined for all subjects and prostate-specific antigen for prostate cancer is performed; both exposure and outcome are determined at the same time.

Could this constitute a cross-sectional design? Calculate the prevalence risk ratio if 20 of the 60 men with low serum lycopene levels had prostate cancer while 10 of the 80 men with high serum lycopene levels had prostate cancer.

Computation: Prevalence risk ratio: a/a+b / c/c+d. Substituting →
20/80/10/90 = 0.25/0.11 = 2.27.

A CSS was conducted using health fair survey to examine the prevalence of chronic disease among participants who take part in at least 45 minutes of daily exercise versus those who do not during the past 12 months. The data obtained are summarized in the 2×2 table in Table 9.2.

Table 9.2 The association between physical activities and chronic disease (hypothetical)

	Physical activity (≥45 minutes)	Physical activity (<45 minutes)	Total
Chronic disease (+)	45	100	145
Chronic disease (−)	155	35	190
Total	200	135	335

The prevalence odds ratio = odds in the exposed/odds in the unexposed = AD/BC = 45*35/100*155 = 1575/15,500 = 0.10. The crude estimate indicates a protective effect of physical activity >45 minutes per day for chronic disease. Thus those who exercise according to this hypothetical data were 90% less likely to be told that they had any form of chronic disease. We can determine the statistical stability of these data by quantifying the random error (p value) and precision (95% confidence interval [CI]).

Prevalence odds ratio from a cross-sectional design

```
. cci 45 100 155 35

                                                                  Proportion
                      Exposed     Unexposed  |    Total         Exposed
         ------------+------------------------+--------------------------------
             Cases  |      45          100    |      145          0.3103
          Controls  |     155           35    |      190          0.8158
         ------------+------------------------+--------------------------------
             Total  |     200          135    |      335          0.5970

                      Point estimate          |    [95% Conf. Interval]
         ------------+------------------------+--------------------------------
        Odds ratio  |      .1016129           |    .0591176      .1739905 (exact)
     Prev. frac. ex.|      .8983871           |    .8260095      .9408824 (exact)
     Prev. frac. pop|      .7328947           |
                                  chi2(1)  =     87.33 Pr>chi2 = 0.0000
```

The STATA output indicates a statistically stable inference, $p < 0.0001$, 95% CI, 0.060–0.17 (precision). Since older individuals are more likely to have chronic disease and are less likely to exercise, age may be a confounding or effect measure modifier in the relationship between physical activity and chronic disease. Therefore, the observed inference may be misleading without assessing for confounding or the modifying effect of age.

Prevalence odds ratio (POR), Cross-sectional design – Association between diabetes (DM) and family history of hypertension (FMH)

```
. cc    DM FMH
                                                           Proportion
                   | Exposed      Unexposed  |   Total      Exposed

         Cases     |   33            12      |    45        0.7333
         Control   |   22            44      |    66        0.3333

         Total     |   55            56      |   111        0.4955

                     Point estimate          [95% Conf. Interval]

      Odds ratio   |          5.5     |     2.218368      13.92918 (exact)
  Attr. frac. ex.  |     .8181818     |     .5492181      .9282083 (exact)
  Attr. frac. pop  |           .6     |

                    chi2(1) =    17.13  Pr>chi2 = 0.0000
```

The stata output indicates an almost six-fold predisposition to diabetes, given family history of hypertension. Simply, among those with the disease (diabetes), the odds of exposure is 5.5 compared to 1.0 for those without the disease (diabetes) (OR = 5.5, 95% CI, 2.22–13.93). This point estimate represents a clinically meaningful exposure effect of FMH as a function of DM development and is statistically significant, ($p < 0.0001$). Specifically, in this sample of patients with and without the disease of interest, there is a statistically significant association between FMH as exposure and diabetes as an outcome based on the point estimate (OR, 5.5). However does this imply that the observed estimate from the sample (OR, 5.5) is extreme or more extreme than would be expected if, indeed, there is no association between DM and FMH? To address this question of the evidence against the null hypothesis in order to generalize this estimate or draw inference from the sample data on the target population, the p value is examined. With the type I error set at 0.05 (5%), and the observed $p < 0.0001$, there is substantial evidence against the null hypothesis, implying a statistically significant association between DM and FMH. However, the observed association is unadjusted and may be due to the confounding effect of race or race may be an effect measure modifier.

```
. mhodds   DM FMH, by ( Race)
Maximum likelihood estimate of the odds ratio
Comparing FMH==1 vs. FMH==0
by Race


  Race | Odds Ratio    chi2 (1)    P>chi2    [95% Conf. Interval]

     1 |  7.222222       8.94      0.0028     1.58311   32.94820
     2 |  3.194444       2.29      0.1299     0.65199   15.65117
```

```
Mantel-Haenszel estimate controlling for Race
```

Odds Ratio	chi2(1)	P>chi2	[95% Conf. Interval]	
5.078158	10.78	0.0010	1.724242	14.955956

```
Test of homogeneity of ORs (approx): chi2(1) =   0.54
                                      Pr>chi2 = 0.4617
```

The previous stata output assesses race for the potential for confounding and/or effect measure modifier in the association between DM and FMH. The comparison of the crude and adjusted OR is indicative of race as a confounding (5.50 versus 5.07) as well as an effect measure modifier given the substantial difference in stratum-specific odds ratio for race (7.22 versus 3.19).

9.1.3   Measure of Effect/Association

As observed earlier, CSD reflects the prevalence of the disease. The risk period resulting in the prevalence may be either extended or restricted. When there is an extended risk period, noncases remain still at risk of developing the outcome after the study (instant cohort without a follow-up). In this context, one can consider the measure of effect to be incidence density ratio (IRD) or average incidence rate ratio expressed as $ID_{exposed}/ID_{unexposed}$. This measure is comparable to prevalence odds ratio (POR). In restricted risk period, the surviving cases are observed at the end of the risk period or end of the study. In this context, the measure of effect remains prevalence ratio (PR), and is assessed by $R_{exposed}/R_{unexposed}$, which is comparable to risk ratio (RR). In these two cases, if the disease prevalence is low, the effect measure of possible cause/etiology is the same, implying PR=POR (Figure 9.2).

9.2   Summary

Cross-sectional studies are used to examine the relationship between exposure and disease at the same point in time. These studies measure the prevalence of the exposure and disease or outcome of interest. One issue in this design is the difficulty in establishing temporal sequence as well as overestimation or underestimation of disease prevalence. In terms of the measure of effect or association in CSD, the prevalence of the disease is estimated by determining the proportion of the disease among the exposed and unexposed.

The proportion or prevalence of disease among the exposed is given by

$$\frac{\text{Cases who were exposed (a)}}{\text{Cases who were exposed plus control who were exposed (a + b)}}.$$

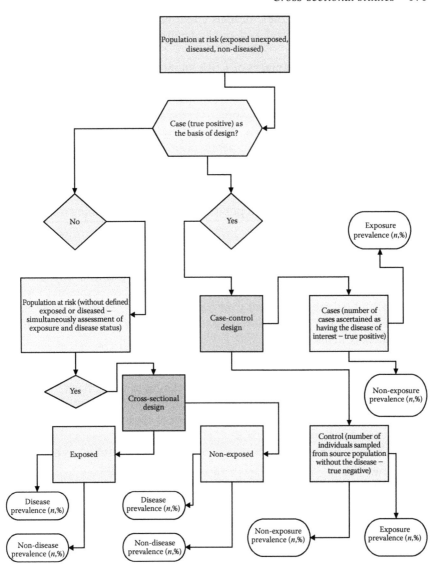

Figure 9.2 Cross-sectional and case-control comparison.

The proportion or prevalence of disease among the unexposed is given by

$$\frac{\text{Cases who were not exposed (c)}}{\text{Cases who were not exposed and control who were not exposed (c + d)}}.$$

The feasibility of the research question or issues and the available resources determine which of these designs is to be used in evidence discovery. Therefore, if appropriately applied, these designs could generate standard and reliable results in addressing clinical and public health issues, thus improving and maintaining health.

There are obvious advantages of CSD, mainly inexpensive, rapid, and easy to conduct. Remarkably, this design could generate reliable and generalizable findings given the large and random samples. However, the lack of temporal sequence tends to limit its application to association and hypothesis generating for causal or etiologic studies. A clear ambiguity on the causal pathway is the association between milk and peptic ulcer. Does milk cause peptic ulcer or are those with peptic ulcer more likely to consume milk in reducing the hyperacidity seen in this condition? Despite the observed limitations, a well-conceptualized and performed CSS could benefit clinical medicine and public health in terms of healthcare and public health program planning respectively.

Questions for discussion

1 Suppose you are a physician and have seen a few patients with prostate cancer, almost all of whom report that they have been exposed to whole milk and red meat. You and your colleagues hypothesized that the exposure to milk and red meat is related to the development of prostate cancer in these patients.
   a Which study design will be adequate in testing this hypothesis?
   b Do you need a control, and how will you select your control?
   c What would be the measure of association in your design?
   d What are the benefits and disadvantages of this design?
   e Comment on the measure of the effect of the exposure on the disease as a direct measure of risk.
2 A "healthy worker survivor effect" bias has been identified as one of the limitations of cross-sectional design. Comment on this.
3 If you were expected to examine the association between obesity and TV watching, would you consider CSD? What are the anticipated problems with sampling and response rate? Comment on the causal association in this relationship.
4 Cross-sectional studies are often criticized for lack of temporal sequence. Can this same criticism be applied to case-control design, and why?
5 Consider hypothetical study performed in an outpatient clinic on the association between vaccination and developmental disorders, autistic spectrum disorder (ASD), in children. If data were gathered on mothers with and without children with autism as outcome and history of vaccination before the diagnosis of autism was gathered simultaneously (survey questionnaire) as exposure, what is the design used in this study? Is it difficult or simple to establish causal relationship between exposure and outcome on the basis of this design? Suggest other alternative designs that may lead to causal association inference. Can we assess relative risk on the strength of this design? Finally, if among 300 of the children

vaccinated, ASD was ascertained on 15, and among 400 unvaccinated children, there were 30 children with ASD, what is the odds and the odds ratio?

6 Suppose among 200 children with cerebral palsy, 125 had feeding difficulties, and among 180 controls, 75 had feeding difficulties. Test the hypothesis that feeding difficulties are associated with cerebral palsy.

    a Compute the odds ratio relating cerebral palsy to feeding difficulties in children.

    b Provide a 95% CI for the estimate.

    c What can you conclude from these data?

References

1. K. A. Levin, "Study Design III: Cross-sectional studies," *Evid Based Dent* 7 (2006) 7: 24–25.
2. K. J. Rothman, *Modern Epidemiology*, 3rd ed. (Philadelphia: Lippincott, Williams & Wilkins, 2008).
3. L. Holmes, Jr., *Basics of Public Health Core Competencies* (Sudbury, MA: Jones and Bartlett, 2009).
4. R. S. Greenberg, *Medical Epidemiology*, 4th ed. (New York: Lange, 2005).
5. E. J. Essien et al., "Emerging Sociodemographic and Lifestyle Predictors of Intention to Use Condom in Human Immunodeficiency Virus Intervention among Uniformed Services Personnel," *Mil Med* 171 (2006): 1027–1034.
6. L. Gordis, *Epidemiology*, 3rd ed. (Philadelphia: Elsevier Saunders, 2004).
7. K. J. Rothman, *Epidemiology: An Introduction* (New York: Oxford University Press, 2002).
8. A. Aschengrau and G. R. Seage III, *Essentials of Epidemiology* (Sudbury, MA: Jones & Bartlett, 2003).
9. R. H. Friis and T. A. Sellers, *Epidemiology for Public Health Practice* (Frederick, MD: Aspen Publications, 1996).

10 Cohort studies

Design, conduct, and interpretation

10.1 Introduction

While epidemiologic studies do not primarily aim to establish causality but association, prospective cohort studies (also termed *longitudinal, concurrent, follow-up*, and *incidence* studies) are more likely to demonstrate cause and effect or temporal sequence, relative to other nonexperimental or observational designs. A cohort design in epidemiology simply refers to a nonexperimental study that involves follow-up of subjects with common characteristics, namely, exposed and unexposed. This design may involve an open or dynamic cohort, a fixed cohort, or a closed cohort. In these examples, loss to follow-up is not uncommon, except in the closed cohort, where no losses occur. Whereas the measure of effect or association in the open and closed cohort design is the relative risk (RR) or rate, the measure of effect in the closed cohort is the cumulative incidence or average risk since no losses occur because of the short observation or follow-up period.

To illustrate a cohort study, let us consider a hypothetical study to determine the effect of soccer on the development of the anterior cruciate ligament (ACL) injury among adolescent females. This study will involve

a A well-defined cohort of high school girls in a particular school who play soccer twice weekly and two hours per session (exposure/index group).
b A well-defined cohort of high school girls who do not play (unexposed/control/comparison/referent).
c Ascertainment of outcome (ACL) injury—investigators must determine that both the girls who play soccer and those who not have not developed ACL injury at the beginning of the study.
d The gathering of information on potential confounders from the two groups, which will allow the investigators to balance baseline differences (assuming that these factors, such as weight, nutritional status, other sports involvement, time spent on video games daily, etc., do not change during the follow-up period) at the analysis phase of the study.

e A defined follow-up period in which the girls who play soccer and those who do not are equally monitored for the development of an ACL injury (outcome ascertainment).

f Determination of whether or not an ACL injury occurs more among girls who play soccer by assessing the chance of developing an ACL injury through RR/rate analysis. For example, if the RR is 3.0, then girls who play soccer are three times as likely to develop an ACL injury relative to those girls who do not. However, if the RR is 0.30 (below 1.0), this means that girls who play soccer are 70% less likely to develop an ACL injury.

By way of recapitulation, nonexperimental studies are designs in which investigators do not assign study subjects to the study groups but passively observe events and determine the measures of association or effect. The goal is generally to draw inferences about a possible causal relationship between exposure and some health outcome, condition, or disease.[1] These studies (cohort) are broadly characterized as analytic. The analytic designs are traditionally identified as cross-sectional, case-control, and cohort and several hybrids of these designs (nest case-control, case-cohort, case-crossover, etc.), but such characterization remains inappropriate since every analytic study has a descriptive component.

Prospective cohort studies (where the investigator collects information about the exposed and unexposed at the commencement of the study and follows both groups for the occurrence of the outcome/s), relative to other nonexperimental epidemiologic studies, can be relatively expensive and time-consuming. However, these designs can provide information on a wide range of outcomes and can be used appropriately to assess the time sequence of events. In a *retrospective cohort*, the investigator collects information on exposure (for example, operative and nonoperative patients) and outcomes (for example, nosocomial infection) that were recorded at some time in the past and then determines whether or not the outcome (nosocomial infection) occurs more or less frequently in the operative (index) or nonoperative (referent) group. A retrospective cohort is less expensive and not time-consuming, but it is difficult to establish a clear temporal sequence and it can introduce measurement (selection and information) bias into the results of the study (Figure 10.1a and b).

As mentioned in previous chapters, a cohort study is one of the most employed nonexperimental epidemiologic designs, as it is most efficient in studying a rare exposure and reliable in establishing the temporal sequence (cause-and-effect relationship) and in assessing multiple disease/outcome/health-related event incidences. Therefore, cohort studies examine a single exposure in order to determine the outcome/s. Typically, study subjects are defined by exposure status and followed over a well-defined period of time to determine the occurrence or incidence of the outcome, disease, or health-related event. This chapter describes the types of cohort designs, namely, prospective, retrospective, and ambidirectional cohort design. Detailed discussion is provided on the

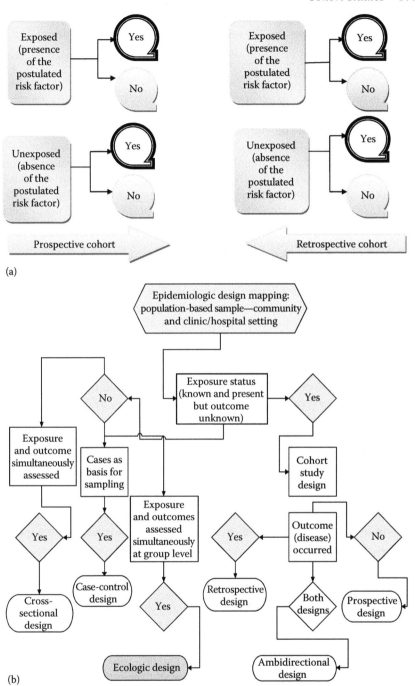

Figure 10.1 (a) Prospective versus retrospective cohort design. (b) Cohort studies: prospective versus retrospective.

design, conduct, and analysis of prospective and retrospective cohort studies. Finally, the advantages and limitations of the two main designs are presented.

10.2   Cohort designs

Cohort studies are nonexperimental designs that commence with the identification of the exposure status of each subject and involve following the groups over time to determine the outcome in both the exposed and unexposed. And like most epidemiologic studies, cohort designs are intended to allow inferences about whether exposure influences the occurrence of disease.[2] Whereas sampling (selection of study subjects) in case-control is based on the disease or health outcome, in cohort designs, sampling is performed without regard to the disease or health outcome but only exposure status.[1] In contrast to cohort study, cross-sectional design, which is an "instant cohort," involves sampling without regard to exposure or disease status.[1,3]

   Cohort design is basically classified into prospective cohort and retrospective cohort. Basically, prospective (concurrent events) and retrospective (historical events or nonconcurrent) denote the timing of the events under investigation in relation to the time the study begins or ends.[2,4] While this distinction is theoretically and conceptually useful, caution must be applied in the use of this dichotomy to describe designs, as it is not uncommon to have prospective cohort designs with a retrospective measurement of some variables and vice versa.[4]

   Prospective cohort design is that in which exposure and the subsequent outcome status of each participant are determined after the initiation or onset of the study.[1-4] This design involves selection of a sample from the population, measurement of the exposure or predictor variable (for example, exposed and unexposed gestational x-ray status or absence or presence of obesity) and measurement of the outcome that developed during the follow-up period (for example, a higher proportion of leukemia in offspring of mothers exposed to x-ray or a higher incidence of type II diabetes mellitus [DM] in the overweight and obese group). A retrospective cohort design, like a prospective design, is defined by exposure status and involves historical information on exposure and the subsequent outcome.[1,3-9] This design involves

a   Identification of a cohort that has been assembled in the past, such as through historical records or past medical records.
b   Collection of data on the predictor or exposure variable—for example, a retrospective cohort was designed to study risk of postoperative pancreatitis after spinal fusion in patients with neuromuscular scoliosis. The investigators used the medical records of all patients who underwent posterior spine fusion and ascertained gastro-esophageal reflux, reactive airway disease, and seizures as potential exposure variables to the outcome (postoperative pancreatitis).

c Collection of data on outcome, which was measured in the past according to the same medical records—for example, the outcome in the previous retrospective design was postoperative pancreatitis. This measure occurred prior to the onset of the study.

10.2.1 Measure of disease frequency and association/effect

The measure of association in cohort studies is the risk ratio or RR, which is quantified as the risk among the exposed divided by the risk among the unexposed.[2,4,9] A risk ratio greater than 1.0 is indicative that the exposure increases the risk of the disease; a risk ratio of 1.0 implies that there is no association between the exposure and the disease, while a risk ratio less than 1.0 implies that the exposure is protective of the disease.[2,7] Later in this chapter, the computation of the RR will be discussed and differs from the assessment of odds ratio from the probability of the exposure given case and comparison experience. However, it is important to note that the variability is sampling scheme between case-control and cohort studies influence the assessment of the relationship between exposure and outcome. Cohort risk assessment is A/A + B (risk in exposed) divided by C/C + D (risk in unexposed).

Other measures used in cohort designs include the attributable risk (AR) percentage,[2,4,7] number needed to harm, number needed to treat, etc.[9,10] The AR refers to the proportion of exposed cases that would not have gotten the disease if they had not been exposed.[5–7,10–13] For example, if investigators conducted a prospective cohort study to determine the incidence of oral cavity neoplasm associated with smokeless tobacco, the AR would be the proportion of those with oral cavity neoplasm who would not have had the disease (oral cavity neoplasm) if they were not exposed to smokeless tobacco. The AR is computed by subtracting the rate of disease in a population that does not have a risk factor from the rate of disease in a population with a risk factor.[5,12,13] This is mathematically presented in the following:

Attributable Risk (AR) = Rate of disease/exposed – Rate of disease/unexposed.

Also related to the AR is the AR fraction (ARF) as well as etiologic fraction (EF), which is a proportion of the rate among the exposed; it is attributable to the exposure. The ARF is mathematically given in the following:

Attributable Risk Fraction (ARF) = Re – Ru/Re,

where Re and Ru are the risk in the exposed and unexposed subjects, respectively. The AR percentage refers to the measure of the proportion of the total risk among the exposed subjects that is related to the exposure, if the exposure is associated with the disease or outcome.

The EF refers to the proportion of new cases in a specified or given period that occurred as a result of the risk factor of interest. Simply, EF is the chance or probability that a randomly selected case from the specific population developed the disease due to the risk factor of interest.

10.2.2   Prospective cohort (longitudinal/concurrent) study

10.2.2.1   Design

Cohort designs represent a nonexperimental study method for determining the incidence and natural history of a condition and may be prospective or retrospective; sometimes two cohorts are compared. In a prospective design, a group of subjects is chosen who do not have the outcome of interest (for example, DM). The investigator then measures a variety of variables that might be relevant to the development of DM. Over a period of time, the subjects in the sample are observed to see whether they will develop the outcome of interest, DM. In a single-cohort study, the participants who do not develop the outcome of interest are used as internal controls. Where two cohorts are used, one group has been exposed—for example, through obesity/being overweight or being treated with an antidiabetic/antihyperglycemic agent of interest like insulin while the others have not, thereby acting as a control (unexposed).

10.2.2.2   Prospective cohort study conduct

The first step in conducting a prospective study is defining the specific cohort or group based on the exposure status and not on the outcome of interest or the disease.[1-3] If the specific group definition is based on disease or outcome, then the design constitutes case-control or case-comparison study. In cohort investigation, each subject must have the potential to develop the outcome of interest (that is, both males and females should be included in a cohort designed to study, for example, the association between being overweight/obese and DM). Additionally, if a study is designed to examine the risk of cancer of the prostate (CaP), given exposure to fruits, vegetables, serum lipids, and red meat, all subjects recruited (men, older than 40 years of age) must have the potentials to develop CaP. Furthermore, the sampled cohort or population must be representative of the general population if the study is primarily designed to determine the incidence and natural history of the disease. However, as in a previous example with DM, a representative sample may involve studying females of a certain age only. In addition, if the investigators' aim is to examine the association between predictor variables and outcomes (analytical), then the sample should contain as many subjects or patients likely to develop the outcome (DM) as possible; otherwise, much time and money will be spent collecting information of little value (inability to detect the significant association because of small study size) (Figure 10.2).

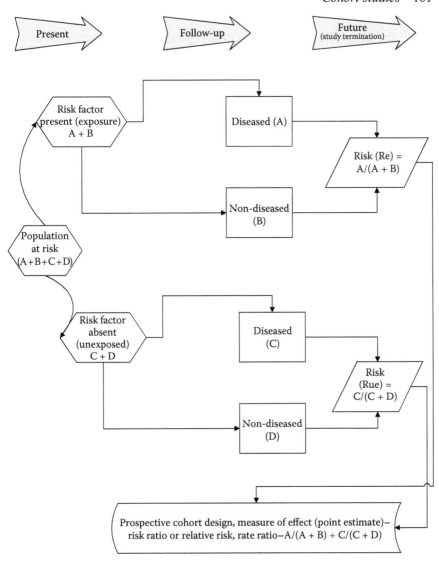

Figure 10.2 Prospective cohort study illustrating the design and estimation of the measure of effect or point estimate.

BOX 10.1   LONGITUDINAL (COHORT) STUDIES

- Cohort studies are based on exposure status for sampling of controls.
- Could be retrospective, prospective, or ambidirectional but must utilize more than one data point for assessment of effect unlike cross-sectional design (baseline and follow-up measures).
- The type of design depends on the temporal relationship between the initiation of the study and the occurrence of outcome.
- A design is considered a retrospective also termed historical or nonconcurrent, if the exposure and outcomes of interest have already occurred prior to the initiation of the study.
- In a prospective design, the exposure which defines the cohort has occurred in this exposed group prior to the initiation of the study but the outcome of interest has not occurred.
- Both groups (exposed and unexposed or controls) are followed to assess the incidence rate of the outcome or event of interest.
- Both retrospective and prospective designs compare the exposed to the unexposed groups in order to determine the measure of the effect of the exposure.
- The calendar time is the main distinction between the two designs.

10.2.2.3   Feasibility of prospective cohort design

While the randomized controlled clinical trial remains the gold standard among clinical research designs, its conduct may not be feasible because of ethical concerns on allocations of subjects to potential risk factors. For example, one cannot deliberately allocate or expose pregnant subjects to x-ray in order determine the risk of ionizing radiation on childhood thyroid cancer or leukemia. A prospective cohort becomes a feasible alternative design in determining such associations. As cohort studies measure potential etiology prior to the outcome, this design can demonstrate that these "causes" preceded the outcome, thereby avoiding the issue of temporal sequence—cause-and-effect nexus.

In addition, cohort designs have an advantage of allowing the examination of various outcome variables. For example, cohort studies of obesity as an exposure can simultaneously look at deaths from cancer and cardiovascular and cerebrovascular disease as end points or outcomes. A prospective cohort design allows the computation of the effect of each variable on the probability of developing the outcome of interest, measured by the RR.[5,12,13] However, since the design of the prospective cohort study is based on exposure, if the outcome is rare, this design is rendered inefficient. For example, a design to study the natural history of benign unicameral bone cysts with osteosarcoma as an outcome of interest may be inefficient because of the rare occurrence of osteosarcoma. The efficiency of a prospective cohort study increases as the incidence of any particular outcome increases. Therefore, a study of union after cervical spine fusion in patients with cervical instability of C1 through C2 will be efficiently investigated with a prospective cohort design if most patients who receive surgery experience union. Another problem with prospective cohort studies is the loss of some subjects to follow-up, which can significantly affect the outcome, thus resulting in biased estimate of effect.

10.2.2.4 Measure of effect

The measure of association or effect in cohort studies is the risk ratio or RR, which is quantified as the risk among the exposed divided by the risk among the unexposed. Primarily, this design describes incidence or natural history; analyzes predictors or risk factors or variables, thereby enabling calculation of the RR; and measures events in temporal sequence thereby distinguishing causes from effects. Mathematically, the RR is computed by using a 2×2 table:

Relative risk (or Risk ratio) = $(a/(a + b))/(c/(c + d))$.

Vignette 10.1 A prospective study conducted by Boice and Monson[14] on the exposure to x-ray fluoroscopy and breast cancer reported 41 cases among the exposed with a 28,010 person-time (PT) (year) observation and 15 cases among the unexposed with 19,017 PT observation. What is the incidence rate?

```
. iri 41 15 28010 19017
```

	Exposed	Unexposed	Total
Cases	41	15	56
Person-time	28010	19017	47027
Incidence Rate	.0014638	.0007888	.0011908

	Point estimate	[95% Conf. interval]	
Inc. rate diff.	.000675	.0000749	.0012751
Inc. rate ratio	1.855759	1.005684	3.6093 (exact)
Attr. frac. ex.	.4611368	.0056519	.722938 (exact)
Attr. frac. pop	.337618		

(midp)	Pr(k>=41) =	0.0177 (exact)
(midp)	2*Prk>=41) =	0.0355 (exact)

Note: iri represents incidence rate command when data are aggregate (summary data). Using the 2×2 table, a = 41, b = 15, c = 28,010 (person-years for the exposed) and d = 19,108 (person-years for the unexposed). The 95% CIs for the measures of disease association support the rejection of the null hypothesis of no association between x-ray fluoroscopy and the development of breast cancer. The incidence rate ratio = 1.85,

95% CI, 1.00–3.61 indicates a significant (85%) increased incidence of breast cancer among those exposed to fluoroscopy.

Vignette 10.2 Risk ratio estimation Glass et al. (1983) conducted a prospective cohort,[15] with a 10-day follow-up among 30 breast-fed infants colonized with vibrio cholera measured by antilipopolysaccharide antibody titers in the mother's breast milk. The high antibody was found in 7 children with diarrhea out of 19 children with diarrhea; 9 children without diarrhea out of 11 without diarrhea had high antibody. Construct a 2 × 2 table of this cumulative incidence study and calculate the risk ratio (Table 10.1).

Table 10.1 2 × 2 Table of the association between diarrhea and antibody level

Disease	Exposure–antibody level		Total
	High antibody (exposed)	*Low antibody (unexposed)*	*Total*
Diarrhea	7 (a)	12 (b)	19 (a + b)
Nondiarrhea	9 (c)	2 (d)	11 (c + d)

Using STATA syntax: iri 7 12 9 2.

```
. csi 7 12 9 2

                 |   Exposed   Unexposed  |      Total
-----------------+------------------------+------------
           Cases |      7          12     |       19
        Noncases |      9           2     |       11
-----------------+------------------------+------------
           Total |     16          14     |       30
                 |                        |
            Risk |   .4375     .8571429   |    .6333333
                 |                        |
                 |    Point estimate      |   [95% Conf. interval]
                 |------------------------+------------------------
 Risk difference |      -.4196429         |   -.7240828    -.1152029
      Risk ratio |       .5104167         |    .2814332     .9257086
 Prev. frac. ex. |       .4895833         |    .0742914     .7185668
 Prev. frac. pop |       .2611111         |
                 |------------------------+------------------------
                       chi2(1) =      5.66    Pr>chi2 = 0.0173
```

The STATA output indicates the protective effect of high antilipopolysaccharide antibody titers in the mother's breast milk with respect to childhood diarrhea, RR, 0.51, 95% CI, −0.028 to 0.93, $p = 0.02$.

```
. cs DM SMK
```

	SMK Exposed	Unexposed	Total
Cases	59	27	86
Noncases	14	11	25
Total	73	38	111
Risk	.8082192	.7105263	.7747748

	Point estimate	[95% Conf. Interval]	
Risk difference	.0976929	-.07240828	.2678364
Risk ratio	1.137494	.902267	1.434045
Attr. frac. ex.	.1208742	-.1083194	.302672
Attr. frac. pop	.0829253		

```
                         chi2(1) =        1.37   Pr>chi2 = 0.2424
```

The previous stata output above illustrates the association between diabetes (DM) and smoking (SMK) in a hypothetical sample of patients. Compared to nonsmokers, smokers are 14% more likely to develop DM. Despite a clinically meaningful effect of the exposure on the disease, there is no evidence against the null hypothesis, implying the inability to generalize the finding from this sample data to the target population ($p = 0.24$), with 0.05 as type I error tolerance level. Because this association could be confounded or explained by an effect modifier, namely race, sex and family history of hypertension, these variables are addressed for confounding and effect measure modification.

```
. cc DM SMK
```

	Exposed	Unexposed	Total	Proportion Exposed
Cases	59	27	86	0.6860
Controls	14	11	25	0.5600
Total	73	38	111	0.6577

	Point estimate	[95% Conf. interval]	
Odds ratio	1.716931	.6150071	4.678976 (exact)
Attr. frac. ex.	.4175655	-.6259974	.786278 (exact)
Attr. frac. pop	.2864693		

```
                         chi2(1) =        1.37   Pr>chi2 = 0.2424
```

```
. mhodds    DM   SMK, by ( Race)

Maximum likelihood estimate of the odds ratio
Comparing SMK==11 vs. SMK==0
by Race
```

Race	Odds Ratio	chi2(1)	P>chi2	[95% Conf.	Interval]
1	1.395000	0.37	0.5410	0.47746	4.07575
2	2.000000	0.52	0.4715	0.09185	13.70545

```
Mantel-Haenszel estimate controlling for Race
```

Odds Ratio	chi2(1)	P>chi2	[95% Conf.	Interval]
1.511713	0.76	0.3827	0.593751	3.848877

```
Test of homogeneity of ORs (approx): chi2(1) =    0.10
                                      Pr>chi2 =  0.7478
```

The stata output indicates race as a confounding in the relationship between DM and SMK (OR = 1.72 crude versus aOR = 1.52).

```
mhodds    DM    SMK, by ( Sex)

Maximum likelihood estimate of the odds ratio
Comparing SMK==1 vs. SMK==0
by Sex
```

Sex	Odds Ratio	chi2(1)	P>chi2	[95% Conf.	Interval]
1	1.777778	0.75	0.3880	0.47283	6.68417
2	1.905882	0.90	0.3431	0.49084	7.40034

```
Mantel-Haenszel estimate controlling for Sex
```

Odds Ratio	chi2(1)	P>chi2	[95% Conf.	Interval]
1.840577	1.64	0.2001	0.713437	4.748452

```
Test of homogeneity of ORs (approx): chi2(1)   =    0.01
                                     Pr>chi2   =  0.9426
```

The previous stata output above indicates sex as a confounding in the association between DM and SMK, (crude, RR = 1.72, versus adjusted, RR = 1.84).

```
. mhodds     DM  SMK, by (    FMH)

Maximum likelihood estimate of the odds ratio
Comparing SMK==1 vs. SMK==0
by FMH
```

FMH	Odds Ratio	chi2(1)	P>chi2	[95% Conf. Interval]	
0	0.638889	0.50	0.4805	0.18213	2.24109
1	6.000000	6.48	0.0109	1.24622	28.88742

```
Mantel-Haenszel estimate controlling for FMH
```

Odds Ratio	chi2(1)	P>chi2	[95% Conf. Interval]	
1.545905	1.02	0.3117	0.660275	3.619434

```
Test of homogeneity of ORs (approx): chi2(1)   =    5.36
                                      Pr>chi2   =  0.0206
```

The above stata output illustrate family history of hypertension (FMH) as a confounding (RR = 1.72 and aRR = 1.54) and effect measure modifier (non-FMH, 0.64 vs -FMH, 6.00) in the association between smoking and diabetes.

Vignette 10.3 Population attributable fraction Fleiss et al.[16] reported infant mortality by birth weight for 72,730 live births among the whites in 1974 in New York. There were 1,040 deaths during this period, and 618 deaths were reported among the low birth weights (≤2,500 grams), while 422 deaths were reported among those with normal birth weight (>2,500 grams). Of the 71,690 who were alive, 5,215 were born with prematurity. Construct a 2 × 2 table, and estimate the population attributable fraction and the attributable fraction for the exposed (Table 10.2).

Table 10.2 Association between diarrhea and birth weight

| Disease | Exposure–birth weight | | Total |
	≤2,500 g (exposed)	>2,500 g (unexposed)	
Diarrhea	618 (a)	422 (b)	1040 (a + b)
Nondiarrhea	4597 (c)	67093 (d)	71690 (c + d)

Examples of cohort studies include the following:

a   Lerner and Kannel[17]
b   Doll and Peto[18]
c   Smith et al.[19]

10.2.2.5   *Comparison of prospective cohort study with case-control*

Cohort studies, as compared to case-control studies, have outcome/s that are measured after exposure, yield accurate incidence rates and RRs, may uncover unanticipated associations with outcome, are best for common outcomes, are expensive, require large numbers, take a long time to complete, are prone to attrition bias (which can be compensated for by using PT methods), and are prone to the bias of change in methods over time. Unlike previously thought, case-control could be prospective, implying the ascertainment of the cases during the process of conducting the study.[4]

10.2.2.6   *Other measures of effect in prospective cohort designs*

10.2.2.6.1   ATTRIBUTABLE POPULATION FRACTION AND ATTRIBUTABLE FRACTION IN THE EXPOSED

Interpretation: prematurity, which is the exposure, characterized by birth weight less than or equal to 2,500 grams, accounts for 94.7% of the deaths among the premature children. This result represents the attributable population fraction. An estimated 56.3% of the mortality in this population could be prevented if prematurity (low birth weight) were eliminated (attributable exposure fraction).

STATA syntax: csi 618 422 4597 67093

The csi command is used to estimate risk ratio, attributable population fraction, and attributable fraction in the exposed in a cumulative incidence data.

```
STATA syntax

. csi 618 422 4597 67093
```

	Exposed	Unexposed	Total	
Cases	618	422	1040	
Noncases	4597	67093	71690	
Total	5215	67515	72730	
Risk	.1185043	.0062505	.0142995	
	Point estimate		[95% Conf. Interval]	
Risk difference	.1122539		.1034617	.121046
Risk ratio	18.95929		16.80661	21.38769
Attr. frac. ex.	.9472554		.9404996	.9532441
Attr. frac. pop	.5628883			

```
                       chi2(1) =   4327.92   Pr>chi2 = 0.0000
```

10.2.2.6.2 RISK RATIO IN CUMULATIVE INCIDENCE DATA

STATA syntax: csi 7 12 9 2

The csi command is used to estimate risk ratio in a cumulative incidence data.

```
. csi 7 12 9 2, exact
```

	Exposed	Unexposed	Total
Cases	7	12	19
Noncases	9	2	11
Total	16	14	30
Risk	.4375	.8571429	.6333333

	Point estimate	[95% Conf. Interval]	
Risk difference	-.4196429	-.7240828	-.1152029
Risk ratio	.5104167	.2814332	.9257086
Prev. frac. ex.	.4895833	.0742914	.7185668
Prev. frac. pop	.2611111		

```
                         1-sided Fisher's exact P = 0.0212
                         2-sided Fisher's exact P = 0.0259
```

Note: The risk ratio of 0.51 indicates a significant (49%) decreased risk of diarrhea among children with high antibody compared to those with low antibody, risk ratio (RR) = 0.51, 95% CI, 0.28–0.93, $p = 0.02$.

BOX 10.2 BASIC DISTINCTIONS OF EPIDEMIOLOGIC STUDY DESIGN

- A design that begins with exposure/s of interest and disease-free subjects and aims to assess the outcome in the future by following the subjects represents a *prospective cohort study.*
- The time relation in prospective cohort study is present and future (continuing).
- A *case-crossover design* uses the previous experience of the cases as a substitute for a control series, to estimate the person–time distribution in the source population.
- *Ambidirectional cohort* is a design that is both retrospective and prospective in its observation of the outcome.
- *Retrospective cohort* (historical cohort study) is a design in which the cohorts are identified from recorded information and the time during which they are at risk for disease occurred before the beginning of the study.
  - Simply, a retrospective study is conducted by defining the cohort and collecting information which applies to past time.
- *Case-control* is a design in which the groups of individuals are defined in terms of whether they have or have not already experienced the outcome under consideration and the exposure is then measured.

10.2.3 *Retrospective (historical/nonconcurrent) cohort study*

Retrospective cohort design involves the use of data already collected for other purposes. The methodology is the same, but the study is performed historically or post hoc and the cohort is "followed up" retrospectively. The study period may be many years, but the time to complete the study is only as long as it takes to collect and analyze the data. Depending on the time when the cohort study is initiated relative to occurrence of the disease(s) to be studied, a distinction could be made between historical (retrospective) and current (prospective) cohort studies. In a current cohort study, as described previously, the data concerning exposure are assembled prior to the occurrence of disease. In a historical cohort study, data on exposure and occurrence of disease are collected after the events have taken place, implying that the cohorts of exposed and nonexposed subjects are assembled from existing records or medical or healthcare registries. The methodological principle of historical cohort studies is, however, the same as those of prospective studies.

10.2.3.1 *Retrospective design*

An observational or nonexperimental design in which the medical records/registries of groups of individuals who are alike in many ways but differ by a certain characteristic (for example, androgen-deprivation therapy [ADT] and non-ADT) are compared for a particular outcome (such as locoregional CaP survival). This design is also termed a *historical cohort study.*[20]

10.2.3.2 *Retrospective study conduct*

This design is essentially the same as that of prospective, but it involves the investigator collecting data from past records and does not involve prospective follow-up of subjects/patients.[3] The starting point of this study is the same as for all cohort studies, with the first objective being to establish two groups—exposed versus nonexposed. The groups are then followed up in the ensuing time period (past). Compared to concurrent cohort design, this design is relatively less expensive and less time-consuming. For example, to assess the effectiveness of ADT in the prolongation of survival of older males with locoregional CaP, the investigator utilized the National Cancer Institute (NCI), Surveillance, Epidemiology, and End Results (SEER) data for a period of time, retrospectively followed these men (ADT and non-ADT), and captured the mortality events in the two cohorts (an outcome that had occurred prior to the onset of the study). We illustrate the design and conduct of a retrospective cohort study in the association between radiation exposure and TC in Figure 10.3.

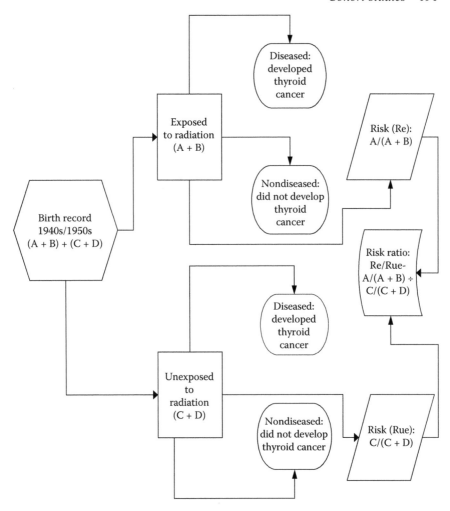

Figure 10.3 **Retrospective cohort design.** Thyroid cancer (TC) had occurred prior to the initiation of the study; both the exposed and unexposed are screened for thyroid cancer and compared with respect to the risk of thyroid cancer in the exposed (radiation) versus the nonexposed for the outcome (TC).

10.2.3.3   *Feasibility of retrospective cohort study*

The term *retrospective* in a clinical research environment often portrays an inherently less reliable design and lower level of evidence compared to a prospective cohort. But this is an incorrect claim. However, a retrospective cohort study could be as reliable as a prospective one if the methods of variable measurement preclude the possibility that exposure information could have been influenced by the disease. Therefore, high-standard and valid results could be obtained from retrospective designs if selection and information biases are substantially minimized.[4]

Where data are available (preexisting information on exposure and disease/outcomes), such as with medical records and disease registry, a retrospective design is a feasible epidemiologic design. However, the preexisting data may affect study validity if selection bias and missing-data bias significantly influence this historical ascertainment.

10.2.3.4   The measure of effect or association in a retrospective cohort design

The measure of effect or association in this design is similar to that of prospective, but since temporality is questionable in some instances, care is required in using risk and rate ratio in the interpretation of retrospective cohort data. Mathematically, rate ratio (data are based on the rate of the outcome-disease or event) is given in the following:

$$\text{Rate ratio (RR)} = \text{rate of outcome among the exposed/rate of the outcome among the unexposed,}$$

where rate is described as the number of the outcome (disease/event) divided by the PT. With this, rate ratio = A/PT (exposed)/B/PT (unexposed), where A is the number or count of the exposed subjects with the outcome of interest and B is the number or count of the unexposed subjects with the outcome of interest (2 × 2 table).

The risk ratio is often used as an appropriate measure of effect or association in a retrospective cohort study. Mathematically, the risk ratio (RR) is given as follows:

$$\text{RR} = \text{Risk (exposed)/Risk (unexposed),}$$

where risk in the exposed is measured by A/A + C and risk in the unexposed is measured by B/B + D (2 × 2 table). For example, in the retrospective study conducted to examine how developmental motor delay, sex of patients, and age at walking were related to thoraco-lumbar kyphosis (TLK) progression, the risk ratio was used as the measure of effect or association. To illustrate the use of this measure, the investigators used the binomial regression model to present the risk ratio as the measure of the association between sex and TLK progression. Using the data from this study, a (male with TLK progression) = 11, b (male without TLK progression) = 10, c (female with TLK progression) = 9, and d (female without TLK progression) = 18. The risk ratio is 11/(11 + 9)/10/(10 + 18) = (11/20)/(10/28) = 0.55/0.36 = 1.53. This means that males were 53% more likely to have TLK progression. However this association may be due to factual association, chance, confounding, or bias. To assess the possibility of chance in this effect measure or point estimate, STATA statistical software was used to compute the risk ratio, significance, and the 95% CI.

```
. csi 11 10 9 18

                  | Exposed  Unexposed |       Total
------------------+--------------------+---------------
           Cases  |    11         10   |        21
        Noncases  |     9         18   |        27
------------------+--------------------+---------------
           Total  |    20         28   |        48

            Risk  |   .55    .3571429  |      .4375

                  |   Point estimate   |  [95% Conf. Interval]
------------------+--------------------+---------------------------
 Risk difference  |     .1928571       |  -.0882779      .4739922
      Risk ratio  |       1.54         |   .8155379      2.908019
  Attr. frac. ex. |     .3506494       |  -.2261846      .6561233
  Attr. frac. pop |     .1836735       |
------------------+--------------------+---------------------------
                         chi2(1) =     1.76   Pr>chi2 = 0.1842
```

The STATA syntax csi is used to fit the estimate for aggregate data that simultaneously assesses the association between exposure and outcome (pre-existing data) or cross-sectional design.

Using binomial regression to assess the risk ratio associated with sex and TLK progression: The STATA syntax binreg is used to estimate risk in binomial regression involving failure and success (outcome) given the exposure such as sex.

```
STATA syntax: binreg varlist (dependent/response) varlist (independent)
binreg TLK sex, rr

Generalized linear models              No. of obs   =      48
Optimization   : MQL Fisher scoring    Residual df  =      46
               (IRLS EIM)              Scale parameter =     1
Deviance      = 63.43630961            (1/df) Deviance = 1.37905
Pearson       = 47.99777213            (1/df) Pearson = 1.04343

Variance function: V(u) = u*(1-u)      [Bernoulli]
Link function : g(u) = ln(u)              [Log]

                                       BIC= -114.6389

                           EIM
      TLK | Risk Ratio   Std. Err.     z    P>|z|      [95% CI]

      sex |.6363636      .2179903    -1.32   0.187   .3251779   1.245345
```

This result (using a regression model, binomial) indicates that girls were 36% less likely to have TLK progression: RR = 0.64, 95% CI, 0.32–1.24. However, this finding is not statistically significant, implying that one should fail to reject the null hypothesis of no association between TLK progression and sex in children with achondroplasia, but not that there is no clinical relationship between sex and TLK progression, given the magnitude of protective effect of sex on TLK progression.

BOX 10.3 CONFOUNDING AS AN ASPECT OF INTERNAL VALIDITY OF A STUDY

- *Confounding is derived from the Latin "confondere,"* meaning "to pour together," and indicates the confusion of two supposedly causal variables, so that part or all of the estimated effect of one variable (exposure) is actually due to the other (confounder).
- A confounding variable is considered an extraneous variable since it competes with the independent variable (exposure of interest) in explaining the outcome.
- In a study conducted to assess whether exposure (A) causes disease (B), C is a confounder if:
  - (1) C (smoking) is associated with A (coffee drinking) in the population that produced the cases of B (pancreatic cancer).
  - (2) C is an independent cause or predictor of B.
  - (3) C is not an intermediate step in the causal pathway between A and B.

10.2.3.5 Assessment of confounding in cohort design

Like other nonexperimental studies, confounding affects the internal validity of the study and should be assessed and controlled for prior to the interpretation of the results of an epidemiologic investigation. It is worth observing that confounding, while it is not a bias, can lead to a biased estimate of effect unless adjusted for in the association. There are ways to determine if a variable is a confounder or not. One approach is to examine the association between the suspected confounding variable and both the exposure and outcome. The first step is to examine the association between the confounder and the outcome among the exposed and unexposed. If there is an association, then the variable may be a confounding (suspect possible confounding effect of the variable). The next step is to examine the association between the confounder and the exposure. Therefore, if there is an association, then the variable is a confounding (Figure 10.4).

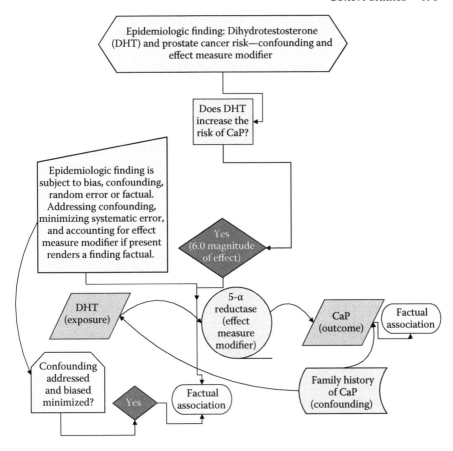

Figure 10.4 Confounding on the risk of DHT on prostate carcinogenesis.

10.2.3.6 Controlling for confounding

A confounding effect may be addressed at the analysis phase of the study by stratified analysis and multivariable analysis. At the design phase, matching is recommended in a nonexperimental design while the randomization process is required in an experimental design. The primary intent of these two strategies is to balance the baseline factors, thus achieving group comparability prior to exposure to treatment or placebo in experimental design or follow-up in nonexperimental cohort and case-control designs.

Specifically, we can examine whether or not there is a distortion in the anticipated association, given a potential confounding as the third external variable. First, the estimated measure of the association (odds ratio) will be compared before (crude) and after adjustment for the potential confounder (stratified) with Cochran–Mantel–Haensel Stratification Analysis. Second, if the difference between the crude and adjusted odds ratio is 10% or more, then the potential confounder is an actual confounder. Mathematically, the magnitude of confounder is determined by Crude odds ratio − Adjusted odds ratio/ Adjusted odds ratio. Third, if age is clinically related to second thyroid cancer, regardless of statistical significance ($p > 0.05$), then age will be considered a confounder. Finally, if age is a confounder only, the stratum-specific odds ratio will be similar to one another but will be different from the crude OR estimate by 10% or more. In effect, age will be adjusted for in the multivariable model.

In a hypothetical retrospective cohort study to determine the effect of extra virgin olive oil on the risk of female risk cancer, investigators assessed the potential confounding effect of family history of female breast cancer on the association. Using a stratified analysis, family history of female breast cancer was assessed. Examine these outputs to determine whether or not family history of female breast cancer is a confounder.

Also, the M-H stratification analysis could be used after examining the crude odds ratio.

```
STATA syntax: cc fbc evoo, by ( fh)
```

FH	OR	[95% Conf. Interval]		M-H Weight
0	3.5	.2433801	196.5367	.4 (exact)
1	1.666667	.1792658	15.0668	.9 (exact)
Crude	1.4	.3469866	5.453572	(exact)
M-H combined	2.230769	.5406183	9.204888	

```
Test of homogeneity (M-H)      chi2(1) =    0.23  Pr>chi2 = 0.6284

              Test that combined OR = 1:
                      Mantel-Haenszel chi2(1) =     1.20
                                      Pr>chi2 =    0.2740
STATA syntax: tabodds  fbc evoo, or
```

evoo	Odds Ratio	chi2	P>chi2	[95% Conf. Interval]	
0	1.000000	.	.	.	.
1	1.400000	0.29	0.5879	0.412131	4.755769

```
Test of homogeneity (equal odds): chi2(1)  =     0.29
                                  Pr>chi2  =    0.5879

Score test for trend of odds:     chi2(1)  =     0.29
                                  Pr>chi2  =    0.5879
```

```
STATA syntax: mhodds fbc evoo, by( fh)

Maximum likelihood estimate of the odds ratio
Comparing evoo==1 vs. evoo==0 by fh
```

fh	Odds Ratio	chi2(1)	P>chi2	[95% Conf. Interval]	
0	3.500000	1.06	0.3042	0.27349	44.79155
1	1.666667	0.30	0.5826	0.26430	10.50987

```
Mantel-Haenszel estimate controlling for fh
```

Odds Ratio	chi2(1)	P>chi2	[95% Conf. Interval]	
2.230769	1.20	0.2740	0.509659	9.764040

```
Test of homogeneity of ORs (approx): chi2(1)   =   0.22
                                      Pr>chi2   =  0.6399
```

The above stratification analysis is indicative of family history of breast cancer (fh) as both a confounding and effect/association measure modifier. With crude OR of 1.40 relative to aOR of 1.20, fh is a confounding in the association between female breast cancer and extra-virgin olive oil. The observation of the OR by the family history level or strata also indicates OR modification. With respect to application and findings interpretation, fh should be treated as effect or association measure modifier and not as a confounding, implying the presentation of such findings by the fh stratum.

10.2.3.7   Further example of cohort designs

• Meirik and Bergstrom[21]

This study of the outcome of delivery subsequent to induced abortion provides an example of a historical cohort study. This study aimed to examine if an induced abortion increases the risk of preterm birth or low birth weight in pregnancies following the abortion. From 1970 to 1975, the investigators assembled information on the date and type of abortion and the personal identification number of women having had an induced abortion in one hospital in Sweden. Sources of information were a computerized hospital discharge registries and ledgers kept in the surgical unit of the department of obstetrics and gynecology of the hospital. Information was obtained on 95% of the 5,292 induced abortions performed during the period studied. The computerized data on women having had a previous abortion were linked by means of the personal identification number to a national medical birth registry, which contains information on the outcome of all births in Sweden, including gestational duration and infant birth weight. Through this procedure, the investigators could identify women who gave birth after having had an induced abortion and were provided with information on the outcome from the medical birth registry. A control group was selected from the medical birth registry. The abortion history of women in the control group was checked from their antenatal care records. In this cohort study, the data collection was carried out from 1978 through 1981, whereas the abortions (exposure) had taken place from 1970 to 1975 and the deliveries (outcomes), from 1970 to 1978.

10.2.4 Hybrids of cohort designs

10.2.4.1 Ambidirectional cohort design

In clinical research, we sometimes need to collect data on certain measures after the studies have begun. This leads to a design that combines prospective measurement of some variables with retrospective measurement of some variables. A study that involves the mixture of prospective and retrospective measurements is sometimes called ambidirectional cohort design.[3] If presented with a mixed design, some epidemiologists have suggested the description of the study as prospective if the exposure measurement could not be influenced by the disease and retrospective if influenced by the disease. In addition, the measured variables could be described differently for different analyses.[4,13] A different analysis is required since a study with retrospective data is subject to concern that disease occurrence, diagnosis, or treatment outcomes (following medication or surgery) affect exposure evaluation (observers, information, misclassification, selection biases), thus influencing the internal validity of the study and making generalization questionable (external validity).

10.3 Rate ratio estimation in cohort study

Rate ratio may be estimated by rate in the exposed (Re)/rate in the unexposed (Ru). The Re is estimated by A/PT (exposed), while Ru is expressed by B/PT (unexposed). Rate ratio is A/PT(exposed)/B/PT (unexposed) (Table 10.3).

Table 10.3 Rate ratio estimation in cohort study (person-time denominator)

	Exposed	Unexposed	Total
Number of outcomes	A	B	A + B
Person-time	PT (exposed)	PT (unexposed)	PT (total)

Vignette 10.4 Rate ratio estimation A CaP study on the effect of selenium and vitamin D in reducing the risk of CaP was conducted (hypothetical) (Table 10.4). The study involved 12,000 older men on selenium and vitamin D and 8,000 controls, enrolled between 2000 and 2002 and followed for 10 years. At the end of the study, 136 men developed CaP among those on selenium and vitamin D, while 66 developed CaP among the unexposed (no selenium/vitamin D). Is selenium associated with decreased risk of CaP?

Table 10.4 Rate ratio estimation using a 2 × 2 table

	Selenium/VitD	*Nonselenium/VitD*	*Total*
Number of outcomes	136	80	202
Person-time	118,640	79,340	197,980

Rate ratio = 136/118,640 ÷ 80/79,340 = 0.0011/0.0010 = 1.1. The obtained rate ratio indicates no benefit of selenium/vitamin D in reducing the risk of CaP (Figure 10.5).[22]

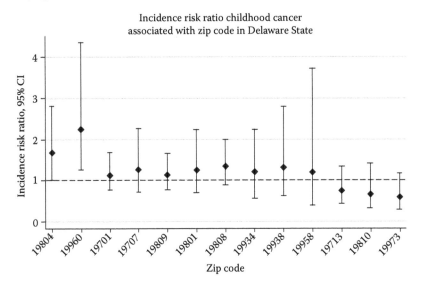

Figure 10.5 Incidence risk ratio (RR) estimation with point estimates and error bars in illustrating the result of a recent study on pediatric cancer and healthography. (From L. Holmes, J. Vandenberg, L. McClarin, and K. Dabney, *Int J Environ Res Public Health*, 13:ijerph13010049, 2015. doi: 10.3390 /ijerph13010049.)

10.4 Summary

Cohort studies are nonexperimental epidemiologic designs that are feasible for examining the outcomes or effects of an exposure. In terms of timing, this design could be prospective, retrospective, or ambidirectional (Figure 10.6). These studies, namely, prospective cohort, can provide valid and reliable scientific evidence in support of the effectiveness of surgical, medical, and behavioral intervention. Additionally, these studies have

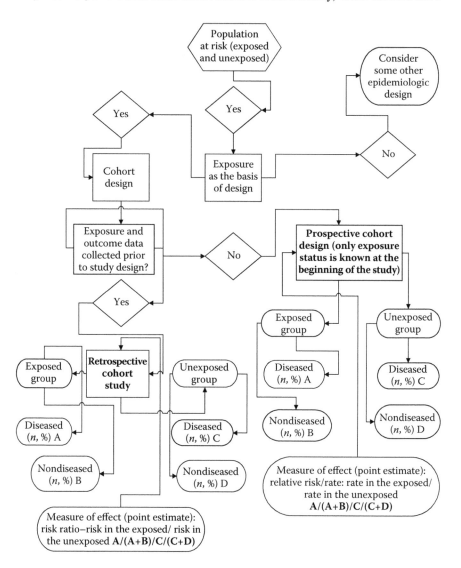

Figure 10.6 The design and measure of effect in retrospective and prospective cohort studies.

potentials in generating incidence and, hence, temporality in terms of cause and effect. Prospective cohort design, also termed *incidence, longitudinal,* and *follow-up,* involves

a Ascertainment of exposure,
b Identification or selection of the exposed group,
c Selection of the comparable group or groups, and
d Follow-up of the cohort (exposed and unexposed) for the occurrence or incidence of the outcome (disease or health-related event). Practical considerations in the design of cohort studies are definition of research question and hypothesis, selection of appropriate comparison group, confirmation of outcome-free status, determining the method of measuring the outcome, reducing the effect of confounders, and limiting the attrition rate or the loss to follow-up.[23]

The advantages of this design are

• Reliable data on incidence
• Efficiency in the examination of the effect of rare exposure on outcome,
• Less prone to bias
• Ability to establish a clear temporal sequence on the effect of exposure on the outcome

The limitations or weaknesses of prospective cohort designs are

• Inefficiency in studying rare outcomes or diseases (case-control remains a preferable design in this context)
• Inefficiency in studying a disease with a long induction and latent period[24]

Retrospective cohort studies could be conducted if there are preexisting data and if exposure status information does not suffer from misclassification bias, which may influence the result of the study toward the null. With this design, the advantage of prospective studies can be used without the need for the length of time required for prospective follow-up. The advantages of this design include the following:

• Efficiency for rare exposure
• Capability of assessing multiple effects of an exposure
• Efficiency for diseases with long induction and latent periods

The disadvantages of this design include the following:

• More vulnerable to bias relative to prospective cohort design or clinical trials
• Inefficiency for rare outcomes
• More prone to bias relative to prospective and RCTs

Questions for discussion

1 Historical and concurrent groups remain the two common types of comparison groups in classical cohort design.
  a Suppose you are conducting a cohort study in which you are expected to use a historical comparison group; explain how data will be collected for this comparison.
  b What are the possible sources of data for the historical comparison group?
  c What are the limitations of using a historical control group? Can changes in clinical factors, such as nursing practices, rehabilitation protocols, or adjunct medications, compromise the use of historical comparison?
2 Read the paper by Holmes et al.[20] and discuss the design and the analysis used to determine the effectiveness of ADT in prolonging the survival of older men treated for CaP. What are the potential biases in this design?
3 Suppose you are conducting a retrospective cohort study on the effect of spinal fusion on deep wound infection among children with neuromuscular scoliosis, where you looked back in time and examined exposure and outcomes that have already occurred by the time.
  a What are the advantages and disadvantages of this design?
  b Discuss the measure of effect or association.
4 Discuss how you will conduct a prospective cohort study to determine the incidence rate of CaP among men who are on a vitamin E supplement.
  a What would the expected limitations of this design be, and will they be addressed?
  b Comment on the consequence of nondifferential loss of participants due to follow-up.

References

1. D. A. Savitz, *Interpreting Epidemiologic Evidence* (New York: Oxford University Press, 2003).
2. H. Morgenstern and D. Thomas, "Principles of Study Design in Environmental Epidemiology," *Environ Health Perspect* 101 (Suppl 4) (1993): 23–28.
3. L. Holmes, Jr., *Basics of Public Health Core Competencies* (Sudbury, MA: Jones and Bartlett, 2009).
4. K. J. Rothman, *Modern Epidemiology*, 3rd ed. (Philadelphia: Lippincott, Williams & Wilkins, 2008).
5. C. H. Hennekens and J. E. Buring, *Epidemiology in Medicine* (Boston: Little, Brown, and Company, 1987).
6. M. Elwood, *Critical Appraisal of Epidemiological Studies in Clinical Trials*, 2nd ed. (New York: Oxford University Press, 2003).
7. A. Aschengrau and G. R. Seage III, *Essentials of Epidemiology* (Sudbury, MA: Jones & Bartlett, 2003).
8. R. H. Friis and T. A. Sellers, *Epidemiology for Public Health Practice* (Frederick, MD: Aspen Publications, 1996).

9. M. Szklo and J. Nieto, *Epidemiology: Beyond the Basics* (Sudbury, MA: Jones & Bartlett, 2003).
10. B. Dawson-Saunders and R. G. Trap, *Basic and Clinical Biostatistics*, 2nd ed. (Norwalk, CT: Appleton & Lange, 1994).
11. D. L. Katz, *Clinical Epidemiology and Evidence-Based Medicine: Fundamental Principles of Clinical Reasoning and Research* (Thousand Oaks, CA: Sage, 2001).
12. B. MacMahan and D. Trichopoulos, *Epidemiology: Principles and Methods*, 2nd ed. (Boston: Little, Brown, 1996).
13. K. J. Rothman, *Epidemiology: An Introduction* (New York: Oxford University Press, 2002).
14. J. D. Boise and R. R. Monson, "Breast Cancer in Women after Repeated Examinations of the Chest," *J Natl Cancer Inst* 59 (1977): 823–832.
15. R. I. Glass et al., "Protection against Cholera in Breast-Fed Children by Antibiotics in Breast Milk," *N Engl J Med* 308 (1983):1389–1392.
16. J. L. Fleiss, B. Levin, and M. C. Paik, *Statistical Methods for Rates and Proportions*, 3rd ed. (John Wiley & Sons, 2003).
17. D. J. Lerner and W. B. Kannel, "Patterns of Coronary Heart Disease Morbidity and Mortality in the Sexes: A 26 Year Follow-Up of the Framingham Population," *Am Heart J* 111 (1986): 383–390.
18. R. Doll and H. Peto, "Mortality in Relation to Smoking: 40 Years Observation on Female British Doctors," *BMJ* 208 (1989): 967–973.
19. G. D. Smith, C. Hart, D. Blane, and D. Hole, "Adverse Socioeconomic Conditions in Childhood and Cause Specific Adult Mortality: Prospective Observational Study," *BMJ* 316 (1998): 631–635.
20. L. Holmes, Jr., W. Chan, Z. Jiang, and X. L. Du, "Effectiveness of Androgen Deprivation Therapy in Prolonging Survival of Older Men Treated for Locoregional Prostate Cancer," *Prostate Cancer and Prostatic Diseases* 10(4) (2007): 388–395.
21. O. Meirik and R. Bergstrom, "Outcome of Delivery Subsequent to Vacuum Aspiration Abortion in Nulliparous Women," *Acta Obstet Gynecol Scand* 62 (1983): 499–509.
22. L. Holmes, J. Vandenberg, L. McClarin, and K. Dabney, "Epidemiologic, Racial and Healthographic Mapping of Delaware Pediatric Cancer: 2004–2014," *Int J Environ Res Public Health* 13 (2015):ijerph13010049. doi: 10.3390/ijerph13010049.
23. J. L. Kelsey, A. S. Whittermore, A. S. Evans, and W. D. Thompson, *Methods in Observational Epidemiology*, 2nd ed. (New York: Oxford University Press, 1996).
24. D. Jackowski and G. Guyatt, "A Guide to Health Measurement," *Clin Ortho Relat Res* 413 (2003): 80–89.

11 Clinical trials (human experimental designs)

11.1 Introduction

Clinical trials (CTs) translate results of basic scientific research into better ways to prevent, screen, diagnose, or treat diseases/clinical conditions. *Clinical trial* thus refers to a designed experiment involving human subjects in which investigators assign participants to treatment or control groups (randomized treatment allocation in a comparative CT).[1-4] CTs differ from nonexperimental or observational designs since active manipulation of the treatment by the investigator remains the basis of this design. Because this design involves a controlled environment that resembles a laboratory setting (chance assignment or unbiased treatment assignment, same physical environment), if conducted as designed and appropriately, a more scientifically rigorous result could be obtained, compared with observational epidemiologic designs. Randomized CTs (RCT) in comparative CTs balance the baseline prognostic factors and hence allow investigators to efficiently determine the effect of the treatment per se. However, despite the advantage of RCTs (more scientifically valid result due to minimized bias and confounding) over observational epidemiologic designs, there are ethical issues that will restrict this conduct in human research, and prospective cohort design becomes feasible (Table 11.1).

The objective of clinical practice is to modify the natural history of a disease so as to prevent or delay death or disability and to improve the patient's health and quality of life, and CTs provide the avenue for such assessment.[5]

11.1.1 Purpose of CT

A randomized trial is considered the ideal design for assessing the effectiveness and the side effects of new forms of intervention (treatment, procedure, behavior change, or modification).

This chapter describes and differentiates between CTs and observational epidemiologic studies, types of CTs, phases of CTs, designing and conducting RCTs, and analysis and interpretation of CTs. The measure of association in RCTs as well as the advantages and limitations of CTs are presented. Although not partitioned as one could have wanted them to be, given the

Table 11.1 Comparison of clinical trial and cohort studies

Design perspective	Clinical trials	Cohort studies
Comparison group	Two or more exposure groups	Two or more exposure groups
Follow-up	Participants followed for the development of the outcome/s	Participants followed for the development of the outcome/s
Outcome and outcome measure	Determines more than one outcome using incidence rates as the measure of effect	Determines more than one outcome, using incidence rates as the measure of effect
Subjects selection	Selection with randomization, thus balancing baseline prognostic factors	Selection to obtain comparability and efficiency without randomization
Subject allocation	Investigator allocates exposure to the treatment group	No active manipulation of exposure by investigators
Placebo assignment	Yes	No
Timing of study	Prospective	Prospective and retrospective

introductory nature of this chapter, the goal was to present three landscapes in the performance of CTs: conceptualization, design process, and statistical inference.

BOX 11.1   NOTION OF CLINICAL TRIAL

- A biomedical or behavioral research study of human subjects designed to answer specific questions about biomedical or behavioral interventions (drugs, treatments, devices, or new ways of using known drugs, treatments, or devices).
- Clinical trials are used to determine whether new biomedical or behavioral interventions are safe, efficacious, and effective.
- Clinical trials of an experimental drug, treatment, device, or intervention may proceed through four phases.

11.1.2   CT as experimental design

The core of the *experimental design* is the allocation. It denotes the assignment of individuals or subjects/participants by the investigator and may involve randomization.[1,3] The distinguishing feature from nonexperimental or observational designs is that the investigator controls the assignment of the exposure or treatment, but otherwise, the symmetry of potential unknown confounders is maintained through randomization.[1,3] Properly executed, experimental studies provide the strongest empirical evidence. The randomization of subjects to treatment or control arms also provides a better foundation for statistical procedures than observational studies do.

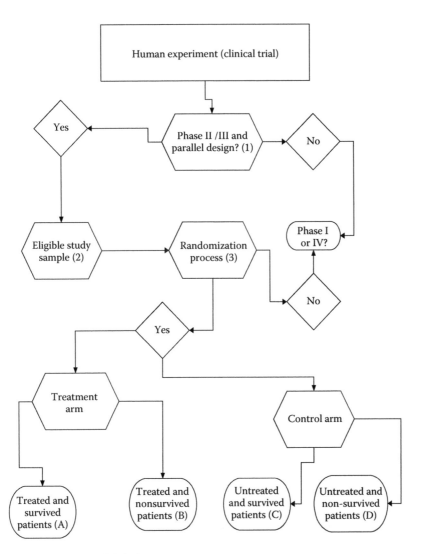

Figure 11.1 Clinical trial design.

A *randomized controlled CT (RCT)* is a prospective, analytical, experimental study using primary data generated in the clinical environment to draw statistical inference on the efficacy of the treatment, device, or procedure. Subjects similar at the baseline are randomly allocated to two or more treatment groups, and the outcomes from the groups are compared after a follow-up period.[1,3] This design, designated the gold standard, is the most valid and reliable evidence of the clinical efficacy of preventive and therapeutic procedures in the clinical setting. However, it may not always be feasible. The *randomized cross-over CT* represents a prospective, analytical, experimental design using primary data generated in the clinical environment to assess efficacy as in RCT. In this design, for example, subjects with a chronic condition, such as low back pain, are randomly allocated to one of two treatment groups and after a sufficient treatment period and often a washout period, are switched to the other treatment for the same period. This design is susceptible to bias if carried-over effects from the first treatment occur (sort of contamination) (Figure 11.1).[6]

BOX 11.2   RELIABLE CLINICAL TRIAL

A reliable clinical trial must employ a rigorous design and disciplined outcome ascertainment, involving:

- Complete and accurate specification of the study population at baseline
- Rigorous definitions of treatment
- Bias (systematic error) control
- Active ascertainment of end points

11.2   Phases of CTs

11.2.1   *What are the phases of a CT?*

Four stages are commonly identified in CTs (Figure 11.2). These phases are as follows:

Phase I. This phase involves testing in a small group of people (e.g., 20 to 80) to determine efficacy and evaluate safety (e.g., determine a safe dosage range and identify side effects). For example, in phase I cancer trials, small groups of people with cancer are treated with a certain dose of a new agent that has already been extensively studied in the laboratory. The dose is usually increased group by group in order to find the highest dose that does not cause harmful side

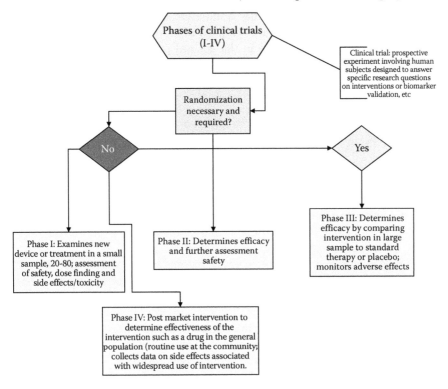

Figure 11.2 Phases of clinical trial.

effects. This process determines a safe and appropriate dose to use in a phase II trial.

Phase II. This is a study in a larger group of people (several hundred) to determine efficacy and further evaluate safety. For example, people with cancer who take part in phase II trials have been treated with chemotherapy, surgery, or radiation, but the treatment has not been effective. Participation in these trials is often restricted based on the previous treatment received. Phase II cancer trials usually have less than 100 participants.

Phase III. The phase III CT is conducted to determine efficacy in large groups of people (from several hundred to several thousand) by comparing the intervention to other standard or experimental interventions to monitor adverse effects and to collect information to allow safe use. The definition includes pharmacologic, nonpharmacologic, and behavioral interventions given for disease prevention, prophylaxis, diagnosis, or therapy. Community trials and other population-based intervention trials also are included.

Phase IV. This refers to studies done after the intervention has been marketed. These studies are designed to monitor the effectiveness of the approved intervention in the general population and to collect information about any adverse effects associated with widespread (routine real-world use).

BOX 11.3A   BASICS OF HUMAN EXPERIMENTAL DESIGN

- Experimental design, if feasible, is considered the gold standard compared with nonexperimental or "observational" studies.
- The active manipulation or assignment of the treatment by the investigator is the hallmark that differentiates experimental designs from nonexperiment studies.
- Whereas not all experimental designs utilize blindness to minimize bias, blindness is not a feature of nonexperimental designs.
- Neither in observational designs nor experimental ones are investigators required to manipulate the outcome.
  - Outcomes are observed as they occur. Hence, both designs apply observations and hence observational.
- Experimental designs, like nonexperimental or observational designs, are conducted in human as well as animal populations.

BOX 11.3B   GOALS OF CLINICAL TRIAL

- The art of designing trials is to provide a degree of error reduction that is efficient for the purpose of clinical objectives.
- Controls the effect of random error—sampling error due small sample size reflecting variability, and nonrepresentative sample.
- Controls the effect of bias (nonrandom error), including systematic error may occur as a result of measurement error and inaccuracy.
- Selection bias.
- Observer bias.
- Information bias.
- Misclassification bias.
- Confounding (not bias but may lead to bias estimate of effect)—The mixing effect of the third variable on the relationship between disease, for example, and the treatment drug.

11.2.2   Basic design in a CT

A sound scientific CT almost always demands that a control group be used, against which new intervention can be compared.[3] The process of randomization is the preferred way of assigning subjects to a control or treatment group.[3] Here are the basic designs of CT:

a   Randomized
b   Nonrandomized concurrent—assignment without randomization process
c   Historical—compare a group of participants on a new therapy or intervention with a previous group on a standard or control therapy
d   Cross-over—each participant is used twice
e   Factorial
f   Group allocation
g   Sequential—involves interim analysis

**BOX 11.4   STAGES (PRELIMINARY)
IN CLINICAL TRIAL CONDUCT**

- The concept development process assimilates observations from a variety of sources and frames a formal research question and testable hypothesis.
   a.   In clinical research, this process often results in a trial concept document.
   b.   The "what" and "why" questions raised in the previous section are particularly relevant to this process.
- Statement of research question.
- Translation of research question to testable hypothesis.

11.2.3   Feasible CT design

A good CT requires the following ingredients: it is randomized and controlled, able to ask a good question (testable research question), well designed and conducted, adequately powered (appropriate sample size), free from bias (measurement, selection, information), and generalizable to the target population; it has independent data collection and analysis and unbiased reporting of findings (report and publication).[1,3]

11.2.4   Blinding in CT

Blinding is ensuring that patients, healthcare providers, and researchers do not know to which group specific patients are assigned. Trials are said to be single, double, or triple blinded, depending upon how many of the relevant participants in the trial are unaware of patient assignment. The purpose of blinding is to minimize patients receiving different care or their data being interpreted differently, based upon the *intervention they are assigned.*[7–10]

An *open-label trial* or *open trial* is a type of CT in which both the researchers and participants know which treatment is being administered. This contrasts with single-blinded and double-blinded experimental designs, in which participants are not aware of what treatment they are receiving (researchers are also unaware in a double-blinded trial). Open-label trials may be appropriate for comparing two very similar treatments to determine which is more effective. An open-label trial may be unavoidable under some circumstances, such as comparing the effectiveness of a medication to intensive physical therapy sessions. An open-label trial may still be randomized. Open-label trials may also be uncontrolled, with all participants receiving the same treatment.[9–11]

11.2.5   Elements of an RCT

1   Comparative—two, three, or more arms, for example, a comparison of the standard versus a new treatment for asthma among children.
2   Minimizes bias—selection bias due to baseline study characteristic is balanced, making the control as similar as possible to the treatment arm.
3   Randomization—assigns patients to treatment arms by chance, avoiding any systematic imbalance in characteristics between patients who will receive the experimental versus the control intervention. Usually, patients are assigned equally to all arms, although this need not be the case. With a simple two-arm trial (one experimental and one control) randomization can be accomplished with a flip of a coin. When there are more than two arms or unequal numbers of patients are to be assigned to different arms, computer algorithms can be used to ensure random assignment.

11.3   Types of CT designs and statistical inference

11.3.1   Parallel design

This is a design in which subjects in each group simultaneously receive one study treatment. For example, if a study is conducted to determine the efficacy of drug A among men with advanced prostate cancer, a parallel design will involve men in the treatment group receiving drug A with men in the control arm receiving the standard drug (drug B) over the same calendar period. Elements of parallel designs are as follows:

• Efficiency—if randomized and controlled parallel design is considered effective.
• Treatment—each subject receives one treatment.
• Comparison—between-patient comparison and average difference between the treatment groups should be much larger than differences between subjects.

- Analysis—two groups, two independent-sample *t*-tests as a parametric test and the nonparametric alternative, which is the Mann–Whitney, also termed two-sample rank sum test, and if more than two groups are involved, the appropriate test is one-way analysis of variance (ANOVA) or its nonparametric alternative, the Kruskal–Wallis.

11.3.2 Series design

Comparison within subjects or patients: Differences between subjects or patients do not affect the treatments. Comparison within subjects reduces variability, giving a more precise comparison.

1 Statistical analysis: The analysis involving two groups utilizes a paired *t*-test and Wilcoxon signed-rank test for parametric data and nonparametric data, respectively, while for groups of greater than two, two-way ANOVA and Friedman's test are appropriate test statistics for parametric and nonparametric data respectively.
2 Disadvantages: It is not suitable for acute conditions where treatment is curative but is adequate for chronic conditions, and it is prone to analysis issues with loss to follow-up/withdrawals.
3 Design and conduct: Series design involves the assessment of results after each few subjects and deciding that one treatment is superior and then the trial stops or more subjects need to be tested. This design can detect large differences quickly.
4 Conduct: Conducting this type of study requires grouping subjects or patients; it is suitable for the evaluation of rapid outcomes and minimizes numbers of subjects when there are clear differences between subjects.

11.3.3 Cross-over design

Different groups have treatments in different orders. Basically, in this trial, all participants receive all of the treatments; what differs is the order of the treatments. Unlike parallel treatment trials, the groups usually switch treatments at the same time, and a washout period is normally expected. A washout period is the interval between the end of one treatment and the start of another treatment.

11.3.4 Factorial design

In factorial design, subjects receive a combination of treatments—for example, placebo, drug X, drug Y, drug X plus drug Y. This design involves the consideration of interactions. No interaction occurs if drug X increases the response in the same amount regardless of whether or not the subject takes drug Y.

11.4   Elements of a CT

CTs involve a huge amount of organization and coordination. Simply, the elements include the consideration of

- Study subjects—CTs involve human subjects.
- Design direction—prospective in design.
- A comparison group—new treatment versus placebo/standard care.
- Intervention measures—primary outcome (death, recovery, progression, reduction in SE, etc.).
- Effects of medication, surgery—relating to outcome.
- Timing of CT—conducted early in the development of therapies.[1]

Conducting the trial, which is the design and implementation, distinct from conceptualization, requires that the investigators to perform the following tasks:

1 Review existing scientific data and build on that knowledge.
2 Formulate testable hypotheses and the techniques to test these hypotheses.
3 Consider ethics.
4 Determine the scientific merits of the study through statistical inference.
5 Mitigate validity issues—biases and confounding.[1,3,6]

BOX 11.5   DESIGN AND STATISTICAL INFERENCE

- Study design is critical for inference—good trial design and conduct are considerably more important than analysis.
- No matter how sophisticated an analysis is, it cannot reliably fix selection and observer biases.
- Systematic errors, such as selection bias, must be minimized during the design and implementation phases of the study.
- Imprecision in the estimate of the treatment effect must be taken into consideration in the interpretation of the results.

11.5   Conceptualization and conduct of a CT

Essential to conceptualization of CTs are the following:

a *Primary question and response variable*: The question must be carefully selected, clearly defined, and stated in advance.[3] The primary research question is the one that the investigator is most interested in answering and one that is capable of being adequately answered. This could be framed in a form of hypothesis testing, for example, "The outcome in the treatment will be different from the outcome in the control."

b *Outcome*: The outcome in a CT could be survival prolongation, ameliorating an illness, reducing symptoms, improving quality of life, or modification of intermediate or surrogate characteristics (example, blood glucose, blood pressure). For example, a trial could be designed to determine whether or not drug X compared with nitroglycerin prolongs survival in patients with angina pectoris (AP).

c *Secondary objective*: This is related to the primary question and/or the subgroup hypothesis.[3]

d *Secondary question*: Survival differs by the ethnic/racial group of patients with AP treated with drug X.

e *Subgroup hypothesis*: Proposed to examine effect by sex, race, age, etc. In subgroup hypothesis testing, statistical power (SP) remains an issue. However, it is essential to conduct such an analysis even if it was not proposed at the beginning of the study, for example, in a factorial design trial of aspirin and streptokinase on vascular and total mortality in patients with myocardial infarction (MI) (subgroup—astrological birth signs, Gemini or Libra showed the worst outcome).

BOX 11.6   STAGE II OF CLINICAL TRIAL: EXPERIMENTAL DESIGN PROCESS

- Experimental design process translates the research question about a population of interest into a formal experiment or clinical trial protocol.
- The protocol includes patient eligibility requirements and detailed descriptions of the experimental and control interventions, as well as definitions of the objective and measurable outcomes.

BOX 11.7   CLINICAL TRIAL STAGE III: STATISTICAL INFERENCE

- Statistical inference is the process that allows researchers to draw conclusions about their hypotheses.
- There are two approaches to "Hypothesis Testing and Statistical Inference": (a) Bayesian Concepts, which provide two alternative approaches to statistical inference, and (b) Frequentist's approach.

In addition, adverse effects could be used to answer some questions in a trial. However, primary and secondary questions should be scientifically and medically relevant or have public health significance.

BOX 11.8　PARTICIPANT ENROLLMENT IN CLINICAL TRIALS

- Informed consent
- Eligibility assessment
- Baseline examination
- Intervention allocation—randomization

11.5.1　What is the study population in CT?

The study population is the subset of the population with the condition or characteristics of interest defined by the eligibility criteria.[3] This must be defined in advance, stating very clearly the inclusion and exclusion criteria (study eligibility). The selection of the study will involve the population at large, the population with the condition, entry criteria met, the study population, enrollment, and a study sample.[3] The participants with potential to benefit from the intervention are great candidates for enrollment if they met the inclusion criteria.

Adequate selection of study subjects requires that investigators select the subjects in whom the intervention may work, subjects in whom there is likelihood to detect the difference (hypothesized result of the intervention). There must be a reasonable number of participants, and it must be driven by a finite amount of funding, the effect size, and the scale of measurement of the response or outcome variable, such as continuous (fewer subjects) versus binary (increased number of subjects).[1,3,6]

11.5.2　Sample size for the study

In clinical trials where the parameter μ is the treatment-control difference, the probability of type I error (α) is usually set by investigators, while the probability that a statistically significant effect will be observed if a real difference exists between treatment and control ($1-\beta$) depends on the sample size, reflecting the power of the test/study. Simply, as the sample size increases, the spread of the distribution decreases and β decreases, implying increase in power ($1-\beta$). In effect, clinical trials with insufficient power (inadequate sample size) are less likely to observe a statistically significant difference even where there is a real difference ($\mu 1$) in outcome between treatment and control groups.

To address this question, the investigators need to set the SP of the study, which is the ability of a study to show a difference should one truly be present.[3,12-15] Beta (β), SP = $1 - \beta$ (tolerable type II error $- 0.2$). SP = $1 - 0.2 = 0.8$

(80% minimum SP to detect the difference if one really existed). They must determine effect size—difference in mean, considering the standard deviation (SD) or proportion between the treatment and controls, and the alpha or type I error (tolerable significance level − 0.05) and test statistic—proportion, mean, and survival estimate (hazard ratio). With these assumptions, the size of the study, which is always an estimation, is obtained.

BOX 11.9 ETHICAL CONSIDERATIONS IN A CLINICAL TRIAL

- Participants must give voluntary informed consent.
- Experiment must be for the good of society and results not obtainable by other means.
- Experiment should be based upon prior animal studies.
- Physical and mental suffering and injury should be avoided.
- There should be no expectation that death/disabling injury will occur from the experiment.
- Investigators must weight risk versus benefit.
- They must also protect subjects against injury, disability, or death.
- Only scientifically qualified persons are to be involved.
- Subject can terminate her/his involvement.

11.6 Example of a CT

Stephen Hulley, MD; Deborah Grady, MD; Trudy Bush, PhD; Curt Furberg, MD, PhD; David Herrington, MD; Betty Riggs, MD; Eric Vittinghoff, PhD; for the Heart and Estrogen/progestin Replacement Study (HERS) Research Group. Randomized Trial of Estrogen Plus Progestin for Secondary Prevention of Coronary Heart Disease in Postmenopausal Women.[16]

This is the Women's Health Initiative (WHI) randomized placebo-controlled trial of 16,608 healthy postmenopausal women assessing the effects of estrogen and progestin. Investigators assumed that the hormone replacement therapy (HRT) trial would find that HRT reduces coronary heart disease (CHD) and provides overall benefits to recipient.[17] After 5.2 years of average follow-up, an increase in breast cancer, CHD, and pulmonary embolism due to HT more than offset reductions in colorectal cancer and hip fracture. The trial ended early because of these findings.

>*Context.* Observational studies have found lower rates of CHD in postmenopausal women who take estrogen than in women who do not, but this potential benefit has not been confirmed in CTs.

Objective. To determine if estrogen plus progestin therapy alters the risk for CHD events in postmenopausal women with established coronary disease.

Design. Randomized, blinded, placebo-controlled secondary prevention trial

Setting. Outpatient and community settings at 20 US clinical centers.

Participants. A total of 2763 women with coronary disease, younger than 80 years, and postmenopausal with an intact uterus. Mean age was 66.7 years.

Intervention. Either 0.625 mg of conjugated equine estrogens plus 2.5 mg of medroxyprogesterone acetate in one tablet daily ($n = 1380$) or a placebo of identical appearance ($n = 1383$). Follow-up averaged 4.1 years; 82% of those assigned to hormone treatment were taking it at the end of one year and 75% at the end of three years.

Main outcome measures. The primary outcome was the occurrence of nonfatal MI or CHD death. Secondary cardiovascular outcomes included coronary revascularization, unstable angina, congestive heart failure, resuscitated cardiac arrest, stroke or transient ischemic attack, and peripheral arterial disease. All-cause mortality was also considered (Figure 11.3).

Results. Overall, there were no significant differences between groups in the primary outcome or in any of the secondary cardiovascular outcomes: 172 women in the hormone group and 176 women in the placebo group had MI or CHD death (relative hazard [RH], 0.99; 95% confidence interval [CI], 0.80–1.22). The lack of an overall effect occurred despite a net 11% lower low-density lipoprotein cholesterol level and 10% higher high-density lipoprotein cholesterol level in the hormone group compared with the placebo group (each $p > 0.01$). Within the overall null effect, there was a statistically significant time trend, with more CHD events in the hormone group than in the placebo group in year 1 and fewer in years 4 and 5. More women in the hormone group than in the placebo group experienced venous thromboembolic events (34 vs. 12; RH, 2.89; 95% CI, 1.50–5.58) and gallbladder disease (84 vs. 62; RH, 1.38; 95% CI, 1.00–1.92). There were no significant differences in several other end points for which power was limited, including fracture, cancer, and total mortality (131 vs. 123 deaths; RH, 1.08; 95% CI, 0.84–1.38).

Conclusions. During an average follow-up of 4.1 years, treatment with oral conjugated equine estrogen plus medroxyprogesterone acetate did not reduce the overall rate of CHD events in postmenopausal women with established coronary disease. The treatment did increase the rate of thromboembolic events and gallbladder disease. Based on the finding of no overall cardiovascular benefit and a pattern of early increase in risk of CHD events, we do not recommend starting this treatment for the purpose of secondary prevention of CHD.

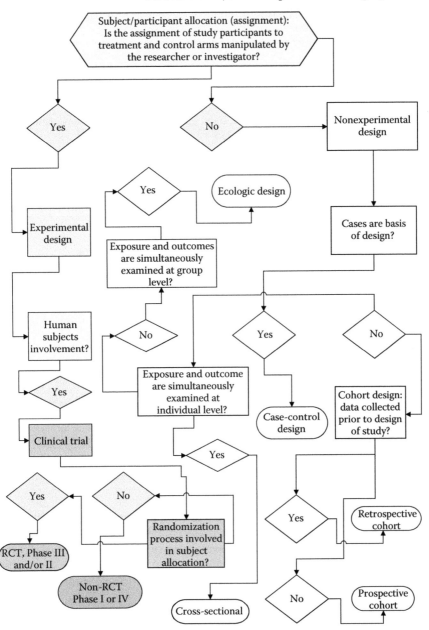

Figure 11.3 Clinical trial illustrating the hallmark of the design by investigator's allocation of subjects.

Table 11.2 Experimental designs: description, measure of association, strengths, and limitations

---

Description
- Experimental and involves random assignment of subjects to treatment and control groups.
- Best design of studying new interventions on individual or community basis.
- Prospective in time relationship.
- Gold standard of epidemiologic investigation when feasible; allows randomized double-blinded placebo-control assessment.

Measure of association
- Same as prospective cohort study (relative risk, odds ratio, hazard ratio).
- Unlike prospective cohort, the analysis to yield the point estimate could be *intent-to-treat analysis* (data on the effectiveness of treatment under everyday practice condition; all randomized subjects whether or not there is an assurance on treatment compliance) and *efficacy analysis* (data on treatment effects under ideal conditions).

Strengths and advantages
- Randomization—most appropriate way to control confounding.
- Double-blinded—most appropriate way to control bias.
- Provides direct measure of association for benefits or risk (relative risk, risk ratio, hazard ratio).

Limitations
- Loss to follow-up (prospective), especially in long-term trials involving many years of follow-up.
- Generalizability—efficacy treatment may not necessarily translate to effectiveness of the treatment in real-world situations (community settings).
- Ethical consideration—patients cannot be assigned to exposure with known adverse effects, such as tobacco ingestion.

However, given the favorable pattern of CHD events after several years of therapy, it could be appropriate for women already receiving this treatment to continue (Table 11.2).

11.6.1   *ERT and HR: Compliance Bias*

The benefit of ERT on heart disease had been associated in part with compliance bias, implying that those who take ERT are compliers, thus the possibility of compliance bias (CB) in explaining the observed benefits of ERT on HR. The possibility of CB in clinical trials and other nonexperimental studies requires caution in the application of epidemiologic studies in clinical guidelines development and in practice change.

11.6.2   *Types of trial*

We mentioned types of CTs earlier in this chapter:

a   Cross-over—each group receives all treatment but not simultaneously.
b   Parallel—each group receives one treatment but treatments are administered concurrently.

c Simple—each group receives only one treatment.
d Factorial—each group receives two or more treatments.
e Community.
f Individual.
g Preventive.
h Therapeutic.[18]

11.6.3 Blinding and placebo-control designs

CT can be *single-blinded* trials, in which the participants are not aware of which study arms they are being assigned to; *double-blinded* trials, in which neither the experimental nor the study subjects have knowledge of the intervention assignment; or *triple-blinded* trials, in which neither the study staff (investigators), study subjects, nor the committee monitoring the response or outcome have knowledge of the intervention assignment.

Placebo control refers to a design in which the control group is given an inactive treatment (water pill/nondrug), which resembles the intervention drug.

**BOX 11.10 ANALYSIS STRATEGIES
IN INTERVENTION TRIAL**

- Analysis strategies in intervention trial—intent to treat versus efficacy analysis.
- Two types of analytic approaches are often used in clinical trials (randomized), namely, efficacy and intent-to-treat.
- The latter is a method of analysis used in which all patients randomly assigned to one of the treatment arms are analyzed together, regardless of whether or not they completed or received that treatment.
- On the other hand, efficacy analysis is performed only on those who comply with the assigned treatment.

Vignette 11.1 Consider a CT of 2000 subjects (close cohort) with AP of whom half (1000, intervention/treatment) received nitroglycerin-G2 (new drug) and the other half (1000, control) received the standard therapy (nitroglycerin). After five years of follow-up, 200 deaths were reported in the intervention group and 350 from the control. If we assume nondifferential loss to follow-up or no loss in the two arms, what is the relative mortality associated with the new drug? What is your interpretation of the result?

Computation: Mortality rate in the intervention = Number of deaths/ Population at risk. Substituting $\rightarrow$ 200/1000 = 0.2 (20%). Mortality rate in the control = Number of deaths (control group)/Population at risk (control group). Substituting → 350/1000 = 0.35 (35%). Relative mortality associated with the new drug = Rate in the intervention group/Rate in the control group. Substituting → 0.2/0.35 = 0.57.

Interpretation: Relative risk less than 1.0 is indicative of the protective effect of the new drug with respect to mortality in the intervention population compared to the control.

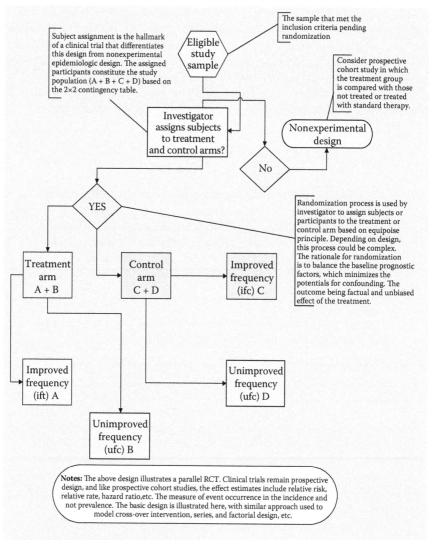

Figure 11.4 Randomized clinical trial.

Vignette 11.2 Consider a CT of a Bacillus Calmette–Guérin (BCG) vaccination in which 556 children were vaccinated and 8 died and 528 were not vaccinated (control) and 8 died. Assuming this was an RCT, what is the relative risk of dying? Is the vaccine protective against dying compared with the placebo (control)?

Computation: Mortality rate in the vaccinated = Number of deaths in the vaccinated group/Population at risk (vaccinated children). Substituting → 8/556 = 0.014 (1.44%). Mortality rate in the control group = Number of deaths in the control group/Population at risk (control). Substituting → 8/528 = 0.015 (1.51%). Relative risk = Rate in the vaccinated children/rate in the control. Substituting → 1.44/1.51 = 0.95.

Interpretation: The relative risk less than 1.0 (null—no association) is indicative of the benefit of the vaccine in decreasing mortality in the vaccinated group compared with the control (Figure 11.4).

11.7 Summary

Often considered as the father of physiology, Claude Bernard (1813–1878) observed that the first requirement in practicing experimental medicine is to be an observing physician and to start from pure and simple observations of patients made as completely as possible. The decision to provide a certain treatment to a patient may come from past experience, diagnosis, opinion, and natural observation, none of which is scientifically valid in determining the effect of treatment. The evaluation of therapeutic benefits or efficacy of treatment depends largely on CTs, especially RCTs. These designs are ethically suitable and necessary in several circumstances of medical and public health uncertainties.

CTs are designed experiments on human subjects that involve, as a hallmark, the allocation of participants to treatment and control group/s. Unlike observational epidemiologic studies, the exposure status in CTs is assigned by the investigator. However, like prospective cohort studies, it presents the opportunity to study more than one outcome. And because of its potentials in minimizing systematic errors (bias) and balancing baseline prognostic factors through randomization (allocation of study subjects by chance), it is considered the gold standard of epidemiologic designs. However, like other designs, care must be taken in the performance of RCTs by considering the impact of (a) size of the trial, (b) design, and (c) analyses in the determination of treatment effect.

There are four phases in CTs:

Phase I (20 to 25 subjects) is usually conducted to assess drug distribution and elimination (pharmacokinetics). The intent is to quantify the kinetic parameters, such as drug elimination rate and half-life. The result from this phase is used to provide information on dosing, without evidence on efficacy.

Phase II (25 to 50 subjects) focuses on side effects, thus assessing treatment feasibility and toxicity and, if feasible, providing simple estimates of clinical efficacy as success and failure rates. This phase estimates the success and failure rates based on the predetermined criteria (based on the hypothesis *t*-tested).

Phase III (formal sample size and power estimations depending on the hypothesis to be tested) determines the relative effects of treatment. The measure of effect may be the mean difference, ratio (risk, rate), or other measures of effects. This phase may involve information on repeated measurements as when all patients undergo surgery, when outcomes are correlated with one another, or when predictor variables change over time (time-dependent covariate).

Phase IV (large sample) is a nonrandomized widespread assessment of treatment effectiveness and adverse effect in the general population. This phase is termed postmarketing and is conducted after the drug's efficacy has been established.

There are several designs and design concepts involved in RCTs: parallel, series design, cross-over, factorial, noninferiority or equivalence design, superiority design, treatment masking or blinding, blocking, stratification, randomization, nesting, and replication. While the understanding of these concepts is necessary in the gaining of knowledge on the design of RCTs, some were not covered in detail in this chapter. However, detailed discussions on these design perspectives are covered in well-written texts on CTs and include some of those referenced in this chapter.

The analysis of CT data may involve simple analysis without statistical models. These techniques are covered in *Applied Biostatistical Principles and Concepts*, a companion volume to this text. Statistical techniques commonly used for time-to-event data analysis, such as Kaplan–Meier survival estimates, are useful to know, as are the log rank test used to examine the survival equality while comparing the treatment groups, Cox regression for the effects of covariates, ANOVA, and logistic regression, etc.

Questions for discussion

1 Suppose you are interested in determining the effect of vitamin C on the common cold, and your control group is to receive a placebo.
   a   What design would be adequate if all subjects are to receive the treatment but at different times? Discuss the advantages and how to address the potential limitations in the design that you select.
   b   How will the efficacy of vitamin C be measured?
   c   Would a repeated measure design be efficient in this context?

2 Discuss the advantages and limitations, if any, of the following design concepts in RCTs:

  a   Randomization
  b   Stratified randomization
  c   Double and triple blinding
  d   Drop-in nonadherence and sample size
  e   Noninferiority design
  f   Difference in response rate to be detected and sample size

3 Suppose you are to plan a safety and activity (SA) or phase II CT to study the efficacy and side effects of a new drug against hormonally refractory prostate cancer and the toxicity is likely to be low while the potential treatment effect is expected to be high based on animal studies. There is a constraint to complete the study as quickly as possible, because of cost and scientific priorities. Which design would you consider feasible in this study? Please discuss.

4 One could use a prospective cohort study or an RCT to study the effect of selenium on prostate cancer progression. Discuss the strengths and weaknesses of each, and recommend which design to use in yielding more scientific evidence.

References

1. S. Piantadosi, *Clinical Trials*, 2nd ed. (Hoboken, New Jersey: Wiley-Interscience, 2005).
2. J. L. Fleiss, *The Design of Clinical Experiments* (New York: Wiley, 1986).
3. L. M. Friedman et al., *Fundamentals of Clinical Trials*, 3rd ed. (New York: Springer-Verlag, 1998).
4. S. Yusuf et al., "Why Do We Need Some Large, Simple Randomized Trials?" *Stat Med* 3 (1984):409–420.
5. L. Gordis, *Epidemiology*, 3rd ed. (Philadelphia: Elsevier Saunders, 2004).
6. B. W. Brown, "The Cross-Over Experiment for Clinical Trials," *Biometrics* 36 (1980):69–79.
7. B. S. Everitt, *The Cambridge Dictionary of Statistics in the Medical Sciences* (Cambridge: Cambridge University Press, 1995).
8. R. S. Greenberg, *Medical Epidemiology*, 4th ed. (New York: Lange, 2005).
9. J. Howard et al., "How Blind Was the Patient Blind in Aspirin Myocardial Infarction Study (AMIS)?" *Clin Pharmacol Ther* 32(5) (1982):543–553.
10. L. Hansson et al. "Prospective Randomized Open-Blind End-Point (PROBE) Study: A Novel Design for Intervention Trials," *Blood Pressure* 1 (1992):113–119.
11. M. Moscucci et al., "Blinding, Unblinding, and the Placebo Effect: An Analysis of Patients' Guesses of Treatment Assignment in a Double-Blind Clinical Trial," *Clin Pharmacol Ther* 41 (1987):256–265.
12. A. Donner, "Approaches to Sample Size Estimation in the Design of Clinical Trials—A Review," *Stat Med* 3 (1984):199–214.
13. J. M. Lachin, "Introduction to Sample Size Determination and Power Analysis for Clinical Trials," *Cont Clin Trials* 2 (1981):93–113.
14. J. D. Dawson and S. W. Lagakos, "Size and Power of Two-Sample Tests of Repeated Measures Data," *Biometrics* 49 (1993):1022–1032.
15. W. J. Shih, "Sample Size Reestimation in Clinical Trials," in K. E. Peace, ed., *Bio Pharmaceutical Sequential Statistical Applications* (New York: Mercel Dekker, 1992).

16. S. Hulley et al. "Randomized Trial of Estrogen Plus Progestin for Secondary Prevention of Coronary Heart Disease in Postmenopausal Women." *JAMA* 280(7) (1998):605–613.

17. M.J. Stampfer, G.A. Colditz. "Estrogen Replacement Therapy and Heart Disease: A Quantitative Asseesement of the Epidemiologic Evidence." *Int J Epidemiol* 33(3) (2004): 445–453.

18. A. Aschengrau and G. R. Seage III, *Essentials of Epidemiology* (Sudbury, MA: Jones & Bartlett, 2003).

12 Causal inference in clinical research and quantitative evidence synthesis

12.1 Introduction

Epidemiologic evidence (nonexperimental and experimental) requires that investigations be carefully designed to minimize measurement errors and bias and control for the effect of confounders on the association between exposure and disease/or outcome, as well as account for effect measure modifier. The inability of studies to address these issues at the design phase (measurement errors/bias/confounding) or at the analysis phase (stratified and multivariable analysis to control for the effect of confounders) signals threats to the internal validity of the study. Since the internal validity cannot be ensured, given these methodological issues, the findings from such flawed studies cannot be generalized, hence the threat to external validity as well. However, despite the need to increase both the internal and external validity of studies, it is not feasible to use a single study to establish a causal inference in terms of epidemiologic evidence. Therefore, established epidemiologic evidence must come from mechanisms that involve the consideration of methods used to claim a cause-and-effect relationship, as well as the quantitative combination of valid and reliable individual studies. Meta-analysis or quantitative evidence synthesis (QES), which is the combination of results or scientific evidence on a specific relationship or effect of treatment after a heterogeneity of studies has been assessed, remains one of the methods of assessing epidemiologic evidence and determining causality.

The primary goal of epidemiologic investigation is not to establish causality but to demonstrate valid and reliable evidence of association between exposure and outcome. This evidence cannot be claimed with crude (unadjusted for the potential confounding effects) findings and in the midst of systemic and random errors clouding the studies. Meta-analysis, or QES, if based on accurate and valid individual studies, can shape the direction of evidence toward causal inference.

This chapter focuses on the design and conduct of quantitative systematic review, called quantitative evidence synthesis (QES). Quantitative systematic review is often conducted when there are conflicting results on a specific research question. The search methods for articles is described as well as the inclusion and exclusion criteria and the specific methods (random or fixed effect), and the use of forest plots to illustrate the combined effect is presented. The critique of scientific literature is illustrated with the intent to explain how internal and external validity of a scientific paper are assessed.

12.1.1   Causal inference

Causal association involves the assessment of a given study for evidence of causation (causal inference). Arriving at causality is a complex process, which involves a causal and non-causal explanation of association based on the evidence from the study. A balanced assessment of these explanations then presents the likelihood that the association is explained by causal and not by noncausal factors, such as confounding, bias, and error.[1–5]

The search for causal evidence involves the examination of evidence description, internal validity, external validity, and comparison of results with other evidence.[1] In assessing the description of evidence, the investigator or researcher is expected to determine or assess the exposure or intervention, outcome, study design, study population and study sample, and the main result.[1] The internal validity of the study involves the consideration of both noncausal and causal or positive features of association. With respect to noncausal explanations of the association, the study should be assessed for observation bias, confounding, and chance variation. The positive features of causation involve the assessment of temporality, which is the timing of the study on cause and effect; the strength or magnitude of an association; dose-response relationship; consistency with other studies; and specificity within the study.[1,4]

External validity is the generalization of the results of the present study to the target or populations beyond the target population. External validity or generalizability is possible if the study result can be appropriately applied to the eligible, source, or other relevant population. In terms of the comparison of the results with other evidence, it is essential to assess consistency with other studies, specificity, biologic plausibility, and coherency (exposure and outcome distribution).[1]

Association in clinical research may be due to observation bias, confounding, chance, or facts. The variation between the true value of a factor being

---

BOX 12.1   MINIMIZING ERRORS OF MEASUREMENT

How are measurement and recording errors minimized?

- Precision, reliability, and practicability must be combined.
- Study must be conducted by carefully planning and monitoring the phases or stages of the study.
- Methods used must be applied in the same way and with the same care to all the subjects in the study regardless of the groups compared.

assessed and the value of the variable chosen to represent that factor in the study simplifies error and its possible source. Consider a study to examine the association between electrocautary and deep wound infection after posterior spine fusion in children with neuromuscular scoliosis. How could electrocautary be best assessed? If a questionnaire was developed and used to extract information from medical records on whether a particular surgeon used electrocautary on each study subject, electrocautary as measured shows a considerable departure from the physio-electrical or biologic measure of this variable. Measurement of this sort does not appropriately reflect the causal hypothesis intended by the study. Therefore, a study designed to assess such an association must consider acceptability, reproducibility, and the relevance of the measures of electrocautary to the outcome: deep wound infection.

The appraisal of evidence depends on the design used in the study. Let us consider randomized clinical trials using a hypothetical study.

BOX 12.2   TYPES OF ERRORS IN OBSERVATIONS

What are the types and sources of errors in observations?

- Within-subject variation—random variation and biological variation, such as circadian or seasonal rhythms
- Measurement and recording methods—result from measurement techniques, the recording of the data (manually or electronically), and data transformation

---

12.2   Critique of randomized clinical trials

The critical appraisal of RCTs involves a brief summary of the study in an abstract form, introduction, materials and methods, patient recruitment and assessment, end-point assessment, randomization processes, and statistical analysis. The causal association follows the steps outlined earlier. Using a hypothetical RCT study on the efficacy of ADT in reducing PSA level (biochemical end-point) in men with locoregional prostate cancer, the appraisal of RCTs is illustrated below.

12.2.1   Evidence description

1 *Identification of exposure or intervention (treatment):* What was the treatment or intervention? ADT.
2 *Identification of outcome:* What was the outcome? PSA level (biochemical end-point) assessed with an intention-to-treat analysis.
3 *Identification of the study design:* What was the specific study design? Randomized controlled parallel design.

4 *Identification of the study population:* What was the study population? Eligible older men diagnosed with localized and regional prostate cancer and who were Medicare recipients.
5 *Identification of the main result:* What was the main result of the study? Describe the summary of the results indicating which results were statistically significant and which ones were not.

12.2.2 *Internal validity of RCTs*

Assess the study for noncausal explanations of the result. This assessment involves the following questions:

1 *Were the results of the study likely to be affected by observation bias?* Assessing level of PSA may be influenced by observation bias, but if the end point was assessing survival (dead or alive), this could be highly unlikely.
2 *Were the results likely to be affected by confounding?* Randomization might have balanced the differences in the baseline prognostic factors between the treatment group (ADT) and non-ADT group (control). Assess the study for multivariable analysis and stratification, which are both useful in controlling for confounding during the analysis stage of the study. Also, the intent-to-treat analysis may protect against confounding. Therefore, randomization as a measure of balancing the difference in the baseline prognostic factor or confounding is realized or effective if the intention-to-treat analysis is appropriately utilized in the analysis of clinical trials data.[1,3]
3 *Were the results likely to be affected by chance variation?* Assess whether appropriate statistical tests were used, such as the log rank test for equality of survival, which is a chi-square with n-1 degree of freedom. It is also essential to assess multiple testing. Figure 12.1 is the STATA syntax to graphically examine the equality of survival by race is on the next page.

BOX 12.3   EFFECTS OF ERRORS IN CLINICAL RESEARCH

What are the effects of errors in observations?

- Inability to show differences between groups if the measurement is grossly inaccurate (no relationship or recorded values with true values or hypothesized value)
- Tendency of moving the point estimate toward the null—a strong association is not produced by error in measurements used, but a weak or no association may be due to error in the observations
- Difficulty in detecting a true difference between the groups being compared

---

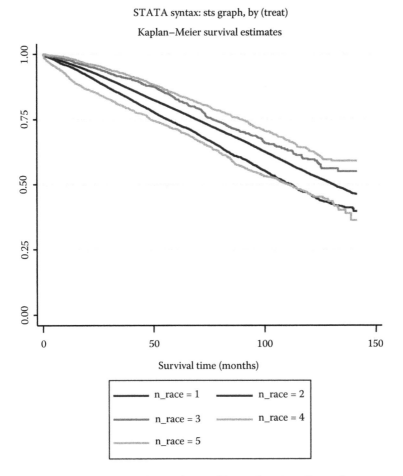

STATA syntax: sts graph, by (treat)

Kaplan–Meier survival estimates

Figure 12.1 **Kaplan–Meier survival estimates illustrating the effects of treatment on survival.** Because the lines do not cross, it is highly likely that the effect of treatment on survival is not due to chance.

The following is the test of the effect of race on survival. The STATA syntax following is used to test the equality of survival by race, which simply determines the statistical stability of the observed racial differences in survival.

```
STATA Syntax : sts test race
Log-rank test for equality of survivor functions
```

race	Events observed	Events expected
1	657	632.57
2	157	154.06

```
3                 26        39.00
4                 95       109.37
         _____
Total            935       935.00


         chi2(3)  =         7.23
         Pr>chi2  =         0.0649
```

The log rank test output above gives a chi-square value with three degrees of freedom of 7.23 (3) and a probability value, $p = 0.06$. So a difference as large or larger than that observed would be expected to occur in 6.0% of trials if the true situation were that the four races/ethnicities had the same mortality or survival. By applying this statistical test, the researcher is attempting to ask the question of how likely it is that the observed racial difference in survival occurred by chance. More technically, the log rank test estimates the probability of having obtained results as or more extremely divergent from the null as those observed, under the assumption that the null hypothesis is true (*p value interpretation*). Formally or traditionally, the significance level or p value is pre-established at 0.05; thus, when the observed p value is below 0.05, we declare that the results are unlikely to have arisen by chance only if the null hypothesis is true. In contrast, the log rank test of the equality of survival by race showed $p = 0.06$; therefore, we failed to reject the null hypothesis and observe that the results are likely to have arisen by chance alone, implying no statistically significant racial difference in survival.

```
STATA syntax: sts test treat

Log-rank test for equality of survivor functions


         Events      Events
Treat    observed    expected
        _____
0             94       44.42
1            591      381.41
2            109      144.99
3            141      364.18
        _____
Total        935      935.00


         chi2(3)  =       326.34
         Pr>chi2  =         0.0000
```

The log rank test output above gives a chi-square value with three degrees of freedom of 326.34 and a p value of < 0.0001. So a difference as large or larger than that observed would be expected to occur in $< 0.01\%$ of trials if the true situation were that the four treatment groups had the same survival. Therefore, we reject the null hypothesis and declare that the results are unlikely to have arisen by chance alone, implying a statistically significant treatment difference in survival.

In the following, we present the effect of a covariate on survival using the univariable Cox regression model. The STATA syntax *"xi"* allows for the utilization of the lowest group as the reference group.

BOX 12.4   CLINICAL TRIAL ASSESSMENT

- Determine the null hypothesis—What was it?
- Groups tested—Arms of study
- Study/sample size—Adequate, estimated a priori
- Experimental and control arms selection—How was the selection made?
- Treatment regimens—Were these adequately described?
- Blindness—Was it single, double, or triple blinded?
- Analysis and Results—Type of analysis, CI used, power assessed, inference drawn from data; were the findings biologically plausible, and were they consistent with previous studies?

```
STATA syntax: xi:stcox i.stage

No. of subjects =    1404              Number of obs  =        1404
No. of failures =   935
Time at risk = 63537.92533
                                       LR chi2(4)     =      450.28
Log likelihood = -6046.2402                 Prob > chi2    =      0.0000
```

_t	Haz. Ratio	Std. Err.	z	P>|z|	[95% Conf. Interval]	
_Istage_2	2.087446	.2128682	7.22	0.000	1.709281	2.549276
_Istage_3	2.978452	.3007237	10.81	0.000	2.4437	3.630224
_Istage_4	4.880411	.4956942	15.61	0.000	3.99946	5.955405
_Istage_9	8.308861	.8981957	19.59	0.000	6.722423	10.26969

The above output indicates a dose–response risk of dying, given tumor stage at diagnosis. The hazard ratio (HR) increases with advancing stage at tumor at diagnosis. While the Cox Proportional Hazard Model will be discussed in detail, it is good to note that this model assumes that the effects of a covariate do not change with time. This model is expressed by $h(t \mid x) = ho(t) \exp(x\beta_x)$ and is inherent to the linear predictor $(x\beta_x)$, which is the logarithm of the relative hazard $\exp(x\beta_x)$. The linear predictor is the log relative hazard (LRH), $x\beta_x = x\beta_{x1}, + x\beta_{x2}, + x\beta_{x3}$, for k covariates.

The STATA output above shows the results of treatment expressed here as hazard ratios (HR) and indicates a significant (27%) decreased risk of dying comparing treatment 0 (referent group) to treatment 1, (HR= 0.73, 95% CI, 0.59-0.91); there was a 66% decreased risk of dying among patients who received treatment 2 compared to treatment 0 (HR=0.34, 95% CI, 0.26-0.45), and an 82% decreased risk of dying among patients who received treatment 3 relative to treatment 0 (HR=0.18, 95% CI, 0.13-0.23).

```
STATA syntax: xi:stcox i.treat

No. of subjects  = 1404                     Number of obs  =    1404
No. of failures  = 935
Time at risk  = 63537.92533
                                            LR chi2(3)    =    338.75
Log likelihood = -6102.0067                   Prob > chi2  =    0.0000
```

_t	Haz. Ratio	Std. Err.	z	P>|z|	[95% Conf. Interval]	
_Itreat_1	.7344221	.0815979	-2.78	0.005	.5907083	.9131001
_Itreat_2	.3453433	.0487169	-7.54	0.000	.261923	.4553322
_Itreat_3	.1762317	.0235626	-12.98	0.000	.1356052	.2290296

12.2.2.1   Internal validity

Nonconfounding and factual attributes of RCTs—assess for temporality (cause-and-effect relationship), magnitude of association, dose–response relationship, consistency, and specificity.[1,2,4]

1 *Temporality:* Was there a correct time relationship? Assess whether or not the outcome follows randomization. Was there a clear timing between the cause (intervention or treatment) and the effect (outcome)?

2 *Magnitude of association:* Was the association strong? Assess whether the observed association is strong enough to be clinically important, if the results are valid.

3 *Dose–response relationship:* Was there a dose-response association? Assess whether the benefits are relative to the dose if a higher versus lower dose of the same agent was compared in the trial.

4 *Consistency:* Are the results of the current RCTs consistent within the study? Assess whether or not the treatment produces improvement in some groups of patients. This is feasible if the trial was designed to answer questions about subgroups of patients. The use of posthoc analysis to examine subgroup effects may be affected by multiple comparison issues as well as comparisons between nonrandomized groups. However, when feasible, subgroup analysis (though unplanned) is recommended since this could add more information to the study.

5 *Specificity:* Was there any specificity within the study? Assess whether or not the drug expected to reduce mortality in cervical cancer, for example is related to cervical cancer death reduction, and not other cancers or other conditions in the study population.

If internal validity from causal explanation is possible as in well-designed large RCTs, we can claim that it is very unlikely that the observed results are due to confounding or observation bias and errors. However, given the significance level, *p* value, chance variation may be a possible explanation if the *p* value is greater than 0.05 (assuming that this was the set significance level for the hypothesis testing).[6]

BOX 12.5   STUDY ACCURACY: VALIDITY—SYSTEMATIC ERROR (BIAS) AND RANDOM ERROR ACCURACY

The objective of a study, which is an exercise in measurement, is to obtain a valid and precise estimate of the effect size or measure of disease occurrence.

- Value of parameter is estimated with little error.
- Related to the handling of *systematic errors* or biases and *random error*.
- Involves the generalization of findings from the study to a relevant target or source population.
- Comprises *validity* and *precision*.
  - Validity refers to the estimate or effect size that has little systematic error (biases)
    - There are two components of validity: internal and external.
- *Internal validity* refers to the accuracy of the effect measure of the inferences drawn in relation to the source population.
  - Inference of the source population
  - A prerequisite for external validity*
  - Measures of internal validity are (a) confounding, (b) selection bias, and (c) information bias (measurement error)
- *External validity* refers to the accuracy of the effect measure of the inferences in relation to individuals outside the source population.
  - Involves representation of the study population to the general population
  - Do factors that differentiate the larger or general population from the study population modify the effect or the measure of the effect in the study?
  - Involves combination of epidemiologic and other sources, for example, pathophysiology
  - Related to criteria for causal inference
- *Precision* refers to estimates or measures of effect or disease occurrence with little random error.

* K. J. Rothman et al., *Modern Epidemiology*, 3rd ed. (Philadelphia: Lippincott, Williams & Wilkins, 2008).

12.2.3 External validity—study results generalization

- *Eligible population application:* Can the study results be applied to the eligible population? Assess what percentage of the subjects who met the inclusion criteria was randomized. Assess whether losses occurred after randomization. Assess whether the end-point PSA level was confirmed for every subject at the completion of the study, thus implying that the end-point data applied to all of the eligible population.

- *Source population application:* Can the result of the study be applied to the source population? The source population in this example is all older women with cervical cancer who were Medicare recipients in the cancer registries utilized for eligibility assessment. Assess whether the results could be applied to the source population based on the specific eligibility and exclusion criteria of the study population. For example, in the cervical cancer hypothetical study, the external validity excludes younger women and women who are not recipients of Medicare.

- *Relevant population application:* Can the study results be applied to other relevant populations or beyond the target population? Assess whether the diagnostic procedure or treatment used in this study is consistent with those used in normal clinical practice. If the results of the study show causal relationship with the treatment or intervention, it is likely that these results could be applied beyond the target population, for example, outside the cancer registries that the study populations represented in the cervical cancer hypothetical RCT. The application of the result to the relevant population should assess the difference in the natural history of the disease; for example, older women with cancer from other sites or concomitant disease affecting the cell or inflammatory disease may have a different natural history of cervical cancer. Further, since the natural history of the disease may vary by sex and age, care must be taken on the application of RCTs beyond the source or target population. This is an important consideration involving subgroup analysis, the absence of which does not necessarily imply that the results will be substantially different. Therefore, in the absence of a subgroup analysis, when the overall result is presented and is indicated to be efficacious, it is reasonable to expect no difference in treatment efficacy by sex or age group. Also consider the most generalizable measure of effect, which is relative risk, risk ratio, or hazard ratio. In the example with cervical cancer and the risk of dying, compared with women who received drug 0, those who received drug 1 had a significant (27%) decreased risk of dying, with HR, 0.73, which corresponds to a risk difference = treatment 1 – treatment 0. That is the absolute benefit, and 1/absolute benefit = number of older women offered treatment 1 for one death prevented (number needed to treat).

BOX 12.6   NUMBER NEEDED TO TREAT (NNT)

- Number of patients needed to be treated or exposed to a procedure in order to prevent or cure one individual
- Probability of a particular beneficial effect before, on average, one individual experiences the beneficial effect
- The reciprocal of the absolute risk reduction (ARR): 1/ARR
- ARR = Postintervention absolute risk − Preintervention absolute risk
- Absolute risk decreases in the rate of specific adverse events associated with intervention

---

BOX 12.7   NUMBER NEEDED TO HARM (NNH)

- Number of patients needed to be treated or exposed to a procedure in order to prevent or cure one individual
- Probability of a particular beneficial effect before, on average, one individual experiences the adverse effect
- The reciprocal of the absolute risk reduction (ARR): 1/ARR
- ARI = Preintervention absolute risk − Postintervention absolute risk
- Absolute risk increase is the rate of specific adverse events associated with intervention

---

12.2.4   Results comparison with other evidence: causal relationship

1 *Consistency of evidence:* Were the results consistent with other evidence? Assess whether or not the results of the RCTs are consistent with other evidence, especially evidence from studies of similar or more powerful design, such as randomized clinical trial meta-analysis or quantitative evidence synthesis.

2 *Specificity:* Does the evidence suggest specificity? Assess whether or not the end-point is specific to the treatment. For example, if the end point was reduction in prostate cancer mortality, are there similar reductions shown equally with other diseases, such as cardiovascular diseases?

3 *Biologic Plausibility:* Are the results of the RCTs plausible in terms of the biologic mechanism? Assess the biologic, pathophysiologic, and clinico-pathologic mechanism of the treatment.

4 *Coherency:* If there is a large or major effect, is it coherent with the distribution of the exposure and outcome? Assess whether the result shown is of clinical importance, including assessing the *number needed to treat*, side effects, and cost effectiveness. Assess the result of the current study with results obtained from alternative methods.

The appraisal of other designs follows a similar approach. Therefore, regardless of the design, the basic approach is

1 Evidence description, which involves the identification of exposure or intervention, outcome, study design, study population, and main result
2 Noncausal explanations, which involve other possible explanations beyond factual for the observed results, such as bias and error, confounding, and chance
3 Factual attributes or positive features of studies: temporality, magnitude, or strength of association, dose-response, consistency, and specificity
4 Generalizability as external validity: application of study findings to eligible, source, and other relevant populations
5 Results comparison with other evidence: consistency, specificity, plausibility, and coherence[1]

BOX 12.8 NONSTATISTICALLY SIGNIFICANT RESULT INTERPRETATION

- A test based on a null hypothesis may suffer from random error, rendering the observed result smaller than the true result as well as losing statistical significance.
- To what extent can it be accepted that there is no true difference between the groups being compared?
- A type II or beta error is committed if the result is nonsignificant when there is a true difference (truth in the universe).
- Relying on the significance level in interpreting such a result is not encouraged and requires the computation of the confidence limits (example, 95% confidence interval [CI]), which will show the range of values of the association with which the results are compatible.
- If the nonsignificant result is due to a small sample size or study, the CI will be wide.
- A wide CI is indicative that one cannot conclude that there is no appreciable difference between the groups being compared.
  - It is uncommon to find two studies with inconsistent findings, which raises the question of type II errors.

12.3 Special consideration: Critical appraisal of public health/epidemiologic research

The appraisal of public health research utilizes a similar process as that discussed earlier. This section details the practical application of the outlines
indicated here. Specific critical appraisals of observational studies include
prospective cohort study, retrospective cohort study, case-control and
matched case-control study, and cross-sectional study and large-population-
based study.

Study Designs: Determine the study design to address the research questions: experimental (clinical trial, therapeutic, parallel, preventive, community,
individual, etc) and observational (cross-sectional, case-control, cohort, etc).

12.3.1 Scale of measurement and distribution

The scale of measurement and the shape of the data are essential in the selection of the test statistic. This aspect was covered in Section I of this book but
needs to be reemphasized:

1 Determine the scale of measurement of the variables (nominal, categorical, discrete, ratio, interval) for the dependent and independent variables.
2 Determine if the data presented are assumed to follow normal distribution or not, parametric or nonparametric.
3 If data are assumed to be normally distributed, are the descriptive statistics appropriate (mean, standard deviation, standard error, etc)?
4 If data are assumed to be nonparametric, are the descriptive statistics
  presented in terms of proportions or percentages?

Internal validity (random error, bias, and confounding) refers to accurate
measurement of study effects without bias—bias presents threats to the internal validity of the study. The precision and accuracy of measurement are
essential to studying validity. Whereas precision refers to the degree to which a
variable has nearly the same value when measured several times, accuracy per-
tains to the degree to which a variable actually represents what it is supposed
to represent or measure. Precision may be enhanced by repetition; refine-
ment; observer's training and performance verification; standardization; and
automation, which minimizes variability due to observers. Accuracy may be
improved by specific markers and better instruments, unobtrusive measurement, blinding, and instrument calibration.

12.3.2 Role of random error

Assuming a random sample was taken from the population studied, is this
sample representative of the population? Is the observed result influenced by
sampling variability? Is there a recognizable source of error, such as quality of

questions, faulty instruments, etc.? Is the error due to chance, given no connection to a recognizable source of error? Random error can be minimized by improving design, enlarging sample size, and increasing precision, as well as by using good quality control during study implementation. It is important to note here that the sample studied is a random sample and that it is meaningless to apply statistical significance to the result designs that do not utilize random samples.

12.3.3   Null hypothesis and types of errors

The null hypothesis states that there is no association between the exposure and the disease variables, which in most instances translates to the statement that the ratio measure of association = 1.0 (null), with the alternate hypothesis stated to contradict the null (one-tail or two-tail)—that the measure of association is not equal to 1.0. The null hypothesis implies that the statistics (mean, odds ratio, relative risk) being compared are the results of random sampling from the same population and that any difference in OR, RR, or the mean between them is due to chance. There are two types of errors that are associated with hypothesis testing: type I (rejecting the null hypothesis when it is in fact true) and type II (failing to reject the null hypothesis when it is in fact false) (Table 12.1).[7,8]

12.3.4   Significance level (alpha)

The test statistics that depend on the design as well as the measure of the outcome and independent variables yield a *p* value. The significance level or alpha (α) is traditionally set at 5% (0.05), which means that if the null hypothesis is true, we are willing to limit type I error to this set value.[6] The *p* value (significance level) is the probability of obtaining the observed result and more extreme results by chance alone, given that the null hypothesis is true. The significance level is arbitrarily cutoff at 5% (0.05). A *p* less than 0.05 is considered statistically significant, implying that the null hypothesis of no association should be rejected in favor of the alternate hypothesis. Simply,

Table 12.1 Hypothesis testing and type I error

	No Association	Association
No association	Correct	Type II error
Association	Type I error*	Correct

* The *p* value is the probability of a type I error. Because samples come from the population, the *p* value plays a role in inferential statistics by allowing a conclusion to be drawn regarding the population or the universe of subjects. Since population parameters remain unknown but could be estimated from the sample, *p* value reflects the size of the study, implying how representative the sample is with respect to the universe or population of subjects upon which the sample was drawn.

this is indicative of the fact that random error is an unlikely explanation of the observed result or point estimate (statistically significant). With p greater than 0.05, the null hypothesis should not be rejected, which implies that the observed result may be explained by random error or sampling variability (statistically insignificant).[6–8]

> *Vignette 12.1 Study interpretation* Consider a study to examine the association between physical inactivity and body mass index (BMI) among school-age children. Assume that the investigators found the risk of obesity (BMI > 30 kg/m²) was four times higher among children with low levels of physical activity, and the p associated with the relative risk is 0.03. What is the possible explanation of this result, and is this result statistically significant?
>
> *Solution*: This simply means that if the null hypothesis is true, there is a 3% probability of obtaining the observed result or one more extreme (RR = 4.0 or greater) by chance alone. Because $p < 0.05$, the observed result is statistically significant.

BOX 12.9   TYPES OF ERRORS IN HYPOTHESIS TESTING

- Type I or alpha error refers to an incorrect rejection of the null hypothesis, implying the rejection of the null hypothesis when indeed the null hypothesis is true.
- When the null hypothesis is true and the investigator rejects the null hypothesis, a type I error is committed (false-positive).
- Type II or beta error refers to erroneously failing to reject the null hypothesis when indeed it is false.

12.3.5   Confidence interval and confidence limit

The confidence interval (CI) is determined by quantification of precision or random error around the point estimate, with the width of the CI determined by random error arising from measurement error or imprecise measurement and sampling variability, and some cutoff value (95%). The CI simply implies that if a study were repeated 100 times and 100 point estimates and 100 confidence intervals were estimated, 95 out of 100 confidence intervals would contain the true point estimate (measure of association). It is used to determine statistical significance of an association. If the 95% fails to include 1.0 (null), then the association is considered to be statistically significant.

The confidence interval (CI) reflects the degree of precision around the point estimate (OR/RR/HR). If the range of RR or OR (point estimate) values consistent with the observed data fall within the lower and upper CI, the data is consistent with the inference, implying the rejection of the null hypothesis. Therefore, when the null value (1.0), implying no association, is excluded from the 95% CI, one can conclude that the findings are statistically significant. Consequently, such data are not consistent with the null hypothesis of no association, implying that such association cannot be explained solely by chance.

12.3.5.1 Application of CI in assessing evidence

While large studies may not necessarily convey clinical importance, small studies are often labeled "nonsignificant" because of the significance level being greater than 0.05. This is due to the low power of these studies, which precludes a detection of a statistically significant difference. The magnitude of effect (quantification of the association) and 95% CI, which may appear to be wide, indicating considerable uncertainty, are reliable interpretations of small and negative findings. The p value interpretations of such studies are misleading, clearly wrong, and foolhardy.[3]

> *Vignette 12.2* Consider a study conducted to examine the role of passive smoking on lung carcinoma. If the OR – 1.56 and 95% CI = 1.4 – 1.9, can we claim that there is a statistically significant association between passive smoking and lung carcinoma?
>
> *Solution*: Because the point estimate for the association lies within the upper and lower confidence limits, and 1.0 is not included, the observed result is statistically significant.

12.3.6 Bias (systematic error) and sources of bias

One has to determine if bias, which is systematic error, contributes to the observed results. *What are the types of bias? In critical apparoasal of clinical and biomedical research findings*, creating a laundry list of biases is not a useful practice, but one should assess what systematic errors may possibly influence the result. Examples of bias are selection bias, prevalence or incidence bias (admission rate bias—Berkson's fallacy studying hospitalized patients as cases), nonresponse, and volunteer bias. Measurement validity may introduce recall bias, detection bias, information bias, and compliance bias. Systematic error is likely to occur because of observer bias, subject bias, or instrument bias. However, systematic errors are minimized by improving design and increasing accuracy.

12.3.7 Randomization and blinding (experimental and clinical trial)

We have to determine whether or not randomization was properly achieved. Also, was double blinding utilized?

12.3.8 Power (rejecting a false alternative hypothesis) and sample size

Power measures the ability of the test to correctly reject the null hypothesis when the alternative hypothesis is true. This is presented mathematically as

Statistical power $= (1-\beta)$, where false negative applies.

Both alpha (type I) and beta (type II) errors are involved in sample size computation of a study. Lowering alpha decreases power because it makes it less likely to reject the null hypothesis, even where true differences exist. A small number is unlikely to show the difference between the two groups. Smaller sample sizes reduce power because the translation of sigma (σ) into standard error (SE) of the mean produces a larger SE for smaller samples. Sample size varies with the magnitude of the outcome effect expected. *Thus, when variance is large, the outcome effect, even if robust, will be obscured by the underlying variation.* Conversely, when the variation is modest, even modest effect may be perceived clearly with a small sample size (Table 12.2).

Table 12.2 Choice of statistical test for selected data types

Data distribution	Groups (number)	Test statistic— independent	Test statistic—paired
Continuous (nonnormal)	2	Mann–Whitney U test	Wilcoxon signed-ranked test
Continuous (normal)	2 ($n > 30$)	t-test	Paired t-test
Normal (nonnormal)	≥ 3	Kruskal–Wallis test	Friedman test
Normal (normal)	≥ 3	ANOVA	Repeated-measures ANOVA
Ordinal	2	Mann–Whitney U test	Wilcoxon signed-ranked test
	≥ 3	Kruskal–Wallis test	Friedman test
Nominal	2	Fisher exact test, chi-square	McNemar test
	≥ 3	Pearson chi-square test	Cochran Q test
Binary outcome	–	Unconditional logistic regression	Conditional logistic regression
Continuous outcome	–	Linear regression	

A simplified guide to the selection of statistical test is presented by the author in the text: *Applied Biostatistical Principles and Concepts.*

12.4   Quantitative evidence synthesis (QES) applied meta-analysis

The purposes of QES are (I), one, to minimize random error, and (II) two, to marginalize measurement errors, which have a huge effect on the point estimate by down drifting away from the null. Small samples in epidemiological research studies have increased random errors. All studies have measurement errors and some studies have more measurement errors than others. Therefore, QES is useful in assessing the differences between studies that are due to measurement errors. QES is a method of summarizing the observed effect across studies., It increases the study or sample size and thus, minimizing random error and enhancing the generalization of findings. Further, QES integrates results across studies to identify the patterns and, to some extent, it establishes causation. As a result of the accumulating literature in medicine and public health, and given the confounding and contradicting claims, QES is an attempt to utilize study integration practices for public health and clinical decision making.

A unique feature of QES is temporality, in which findings in QES accumulate with time. For example, if QES is performed on the impact of culturally competent care on pediatric care improvement, this finding must identify time of conduct and continue to add studies and reanalyze the data for contrasting or negative findings with time. Subsequently, the emergence of new knowledge has impact in changing the results of QES and move evidence toward the factual association.

Despite the fluidity of QES in enhancing knowledge as well as informing intervention, science and scientific endeavors cannot be static, but rather dynamic. The scientific community cannot wait until evidence accumulates to such a point that no further addition is required with respect to evidence discovery in order to start intervention. QES can inform and provide at any point in time the knowledge required in order to improve care of our patients, as well as control and prevent disease at the population level. Because scientific knowledge is cumulative, as new data become available, QES data are subject to change in line with scientific innovation (Figure 12.2).

12.4.1   Quantitative systematic review

This is a method of combining the results from a number of studies of similar design to produce an overall estimate of effect, which incorporates the information provided by all the studies.[3,9,10] The quantitative evidence synthesis (QES) is comparable to traditional meta-analysis since both methods aim at quantifying the summary effect of the individual studies. However, the two methods differ since the QES applies biologic and clinical relevance in the interpretation of the pool estimates as well. It is a popular method of critically assessing the value of evidence used to support health interventions—evidence-based medicine, quantitative evidence synthesis (QES). It is useful

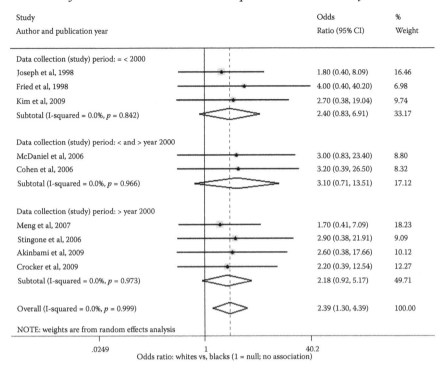

Figure 12.2 Forest plot of childhood asthma mortality stratified by time to illustrates temporal trends by race (white versus black).

in answering research questions whenever an investigation of a particular research subject presents with conflicting or contradictory results.[11–13] For example, some research groups may report a statistically significant difference in the use of anti-androgen in prolonging the survival of men treated for locoregional prostate cancer while other groups report no statistically significant difference. Additionally, unlike traditional meta-analysis, the random effect method of summarizing the result, termed pool estimate is used. The only exception to this technique or analytic tool involves the QES of studies from multicenter trial with the assumption of similar study protocol, and hence very marginal difference in protocol adherence and protocol or methodologic variability.[14]

12.4.2   *Meta-analysis and pool analysis*

Meta-analysis is a method of summarizing, integrating, and interpreting research studies that produces quantitative findings.[11–13] It is a technique of encoding and analyzing the statistics that summarize research findings. If full data sets of studies of interest are available, a pool analysis is the preferred method. Because meta-analysis focuses on the aggregation and comparison of findings of different research studies, meaningful comparability is required. For example, studies assessing the association between selenium intake and prostate cancer can be compared with meta-analytic design using prospective cohort or case-control studies but not mixed, given the differences in the point estimates generated by these two designs. Likewise, observational and experimental cannot be mixed in meta-analytic designs but can be compared separately.[10]

Meta-analysis represents each study's findings in the form of effect sizes or point estimates.[3] An effect size encodes the quantitative information from each relevant study's findings. Studies that produce bivariate correlations cannot be combined with those that compared groups of subjects on the mean values of the dependent variables.

12.4.3   Methodology in meta-analysis and QES

Meta-analytic and QES methods involve

1 Defining the research question
2 Defining the criteria for studies to be included
3 Identifying and retrieving the studies that meet the inclusion criteria
4 Abstracting information
5 Analyzing statistics (fixed effect or random-effect analysis)
6 Reporting results

12.5   Statistical/analytic methods

Common analytic methods used in QES include fixed and random effect models.

12.5.1   Heterogeneity test

The heterogeneity or homogeneity statistic tests whether the overall summary estimate is an adequate representation of the data set; compares each of the individual study results with the summary estimate; and examines the differences between the studies. The meta-analytic method is based on a weighted average of the differences of the results of each study and the summary estimate of the effect. If there is significant heterogeneity, the analysis may be repeated after excluding the studies that are particularly divergent. The heterogeneity statistics produce a χ^2 value for each individual study, based on the comparison of that study's result to the summary result.

12.6   Fixed effects model: Mantel–Haenszel and Peto

There are two commonly used fixed effects methods: *Mantel–Haenszel and Peto*. The Mantel–Haenszel method attempts to derive the most useful summary estimate of effect from the data given in all the studies included in the analysis. This test is similar to the analysis of stratified data, where the stratification variable is the individual study. The *Peto method* utilizes a 2 × 2 table for the observed and expected, the chi-square value is obtained by (O_i - E_i), and the variance of the expected (V_i) calculated.[1,11]

12.7 Random effects models: DerSimonian–Laird

The random effect model assumes that the studies that have been included are a representative sample of a hypothetical larger population of studies. Where there is no heterogeneity between studies, the fixed effect and random effects model yield the same result. But where there is heterogeneity, the random effects model may give a substantially different result (Figures 12.3 and 12.4). The most widely used random effects model is the DerSimonian–Laird method. This method weighs the inverse of a combination of within-study variation and between-study variation; as this variance will be larger, the confidence interval of summary measure of effect will be wider. With substantial

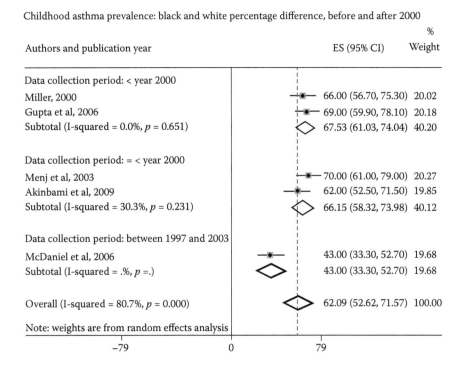

Figure 12.3 Forest plot of random effect of combined or pool estimate of childhood asthma prevalence by temporal trends and race.

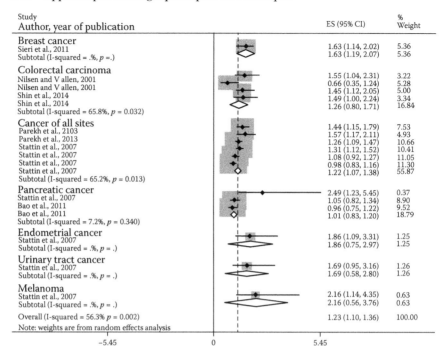

Study Author, year of publication		ES (95% CI)	% Weight
Breast cancer			
Sieri et al., 2011		1.63 (1.14, 2.02)	5.36
Subtotal (I-squared = .%, p =.)		1.63 (1.19, 2.07)	5.36
Colorectal carcinoma			
Nilsen and V allen, 2001		1.55 (1.04, 2.31)	3.22
Nilsen and V allen, 2001		0.66 (0.35, 1.24)	5.28
Shin et al., 2014		1.45 (1.12, 2.05)	5.00
Shin et al., 2014		1.49 (1.00, 2.24)	3.34
Subtotal (I-squared = 65.8%, p = 0.032)		1.26 (0.80, 1.71)	16.84
Cancer of all sites			
Parekh et al., 2103		1.44 (1.15, 1.79)	7.53
Parekh et al., 2013		1.57 (1.17, 2.11)	4.93
Stattin et al., 2007		1.26 (1.09, 1.47)	10.66
Stattin et al., 2007		1.31 (1.12, 1.52)	10.41
Stattin et al., 2007		1.08 (0.92, 1.27)	11.05
Stattin et al., 2007		0.98 (0.83, 1.16)	11.30
Subtotal (I-squared = 65.2%, p = 0.013)		1.22 (1.07, 1.38)	55.87
Pancreatic cancer			
Stattin et al., 2007		2.49 (1.23, 5.45)	0.37
Bao et al., 2011		1.05 (0.82, 1.34)	8.90
Bao et al., 2011		0.96 (0.75, 1.22)	9.52
Subtotal (I-squared = 7.2%, p = 0.340)		1.01 (0.83, 1.20)	18.79
Endometrial cancer			
Stattin et al., 2007		1.86 (1.09, 3.31)	1.25
Subtotal (I-squared = .%, p = .)		1.86 (0.75, 2.97)	1.25
Urinary tract cancer			
Stattin et al., 2007		1.69 (0.95, 3.16)	1.26
Subtotal (I-squared = .%, p = .)		1.69 (0.58, 2.80)	1.26
Melanoma			
Stattin et al., 2007		2.16 (1.14, 4.35)	0.63
Subtotal (I-squared = .%, p = .)		2.16 (0.56, 3.76)	0.63
Overall (I-squared = 56.3% p = 0.002)		1.23 (1.10, 1.36)	100.00
Note: weights are from random effects analysis			

-5.45   0   5.45

Figure 12.4 **Hyperglycemia and carcinogenesis.** The random effect method used in this pool estimate indicated a 23% increased risk of cancer in those with high glycemic index carbohydrates.

between-study variance (heterogeneity), the DerSimonian–Laird method gives relatively more weight to the smaller studies (Table 12.3).[1,3,11–13]

BOX 12.10   STUDY VALIDITY

- Validity (internal validity) refers to the lack of bias and confounding in the design of an epidemiologic study.
- External validity refers to the generalization of the findings from a study to a larger population different from the population that was sampled.
  - External validity cannot be established without internal validity.

12.7.1   Bias

Bias was mentioned earlier. Please remember that bias is a type of error. It is a systematic error that occurs as a result of the investigator's design or conduct of the study that eventually causes inaccurate assessment of the association between the exposure and the outcome of interest.

Table 12.3 Advantages and disadvantages of QES

Advantages
  • Utilizes structured research techniques to summarize and analyze a body of research studies.
  • Represents key study findings (i.e., more differentiated from the conventional review process) that rely on qualitative summaries.
  • Capable of finding effects or associations that are obscured in qualitative reviews.
  • Provides an organized and structured way of handling information from a large number of study findings under review.
  • Homogeneity test, which indicates if a grouping of effect sizes are from different studies, shows more variation than would be expected from sampling error alone.
  • Capable of performing meta-regression that is not feasible from other types of review.
  • Utilizes random effect pool summary estimates method to minimize between studies methodologic variabilities.
  • Examines heterogeneity post hoc and not a priori as in traditional meta-analysis.
Disadvantages
  • Time-consuming and requires specialized skills.
  • Methodological issues—study mixing, different effect sizes or measure of effect.
  • Publication bias.
  • Cannot overcome limitations of the individual studies that make up the sample size (k).

12.7.1.1 Types of bias

While the laundry list of errors is not what we advocate for a critical appraisal of scientific literature, the following are examples of bias that are commonly encountered in clinical research: recall bias (commonly encountered in case-control study) refers to the inability to remember information regarding exposure, especially among the control resulting in misclassification bias; misclassification bias (errors or mistakes in data acquisition that result in the wrong grouping of study subjects; information bias (record abstraction, interviewing, surrogate interviews, recall bias, surveillance, reporting; and selection bias.

12.7.1.1.1 SURVEILLANCE BIAS

Because populations with disease are more closely monitored compared with those who do not have the disease, disease ascertainment may be better in the monitored population and may introduce surveillance bias (monitoring of one population [diseased] more than the other [disease-free]). This bias may lead to erroneous estimations of the effect of the disease in the monitored population, thus inflating the point estimate (RR, OR).

12.7.1.1.2 CONTROLLING AND MINIMIZING BIAS

Biases can be controlled or minimized by accurate definition of items, methods of measurement, standardization of procedures, and quality control of data collection and processing.

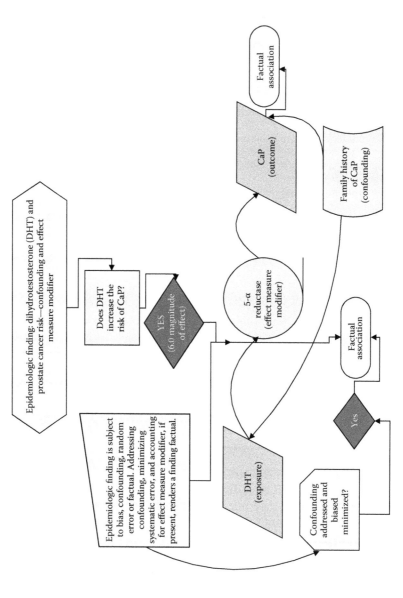

Figure 12.5 **Confounding.** Confounding, although not a bias, may lead to a biased estimate in the relationship between the exposure (DHT) and outcome (CaP development).

12.7.2 *Confounding*

Confounding has been addressed previously, in Chapter 3. One of the issues in the validation of epidemiological research is to assess whether associations between exposure and disease derived from observational epidemiological studies are of a causal nature or not (because of systematic error, random error, or confounding). Confounding refers to the influence or effect of an extraneous factor(s) on the relationship or associations between the exposure and the outcome of interest. Observational studies are potentially subject to the effect of extraneous factors, which may distort the findings of these studies. To be a confounding, the extraneous variable must be a risk factor for the disease being studied and associated with the exposure being studied but is not a consequence of exposure.

Note that confounding occurs when the effects of the exposure are mixed together with the effect of another variable, leading to a bias, and if exposure X causes disease Y, Z is a confounder if Z is a known risk factor for disease Y, and Z is associated with X, but Z is not a result of exposure X (Figure 12.5).

Vignette 12.3 Consider a study to assess the association between coffee drinking (X) and pancreatic cancer risk (Y). The exposure variable is coffee drinking, and coffee drinking is known to be associated with cigarette smoking (Z). Likewise, cigarette smoking is a known risk factor for pancreatic cancer. If causal association is observed between coffee drinking and pancreatic cancer, this might be due to the confounding effect of smoking. Therefore, to be confounding, smoking must be a risk factor for pancreatic cancer and be associated with coffee drinking.

If a causal association, such as X → Y occurs, then this causal relationship may be due to Z (confounder).

Controlling for confounding is a method of producing an unconfounded effect (point) estimate: (1) During the design phase of the study → (a) restriction, (b) matching, (c) randomization. (2) During the analysis phase of the study→ (a) restriction, (b) stratification (stratified analysis), (c) multivariable method (analysis).[5,15]

BOX 12.11 ELEMENTS AND CHARACTERISTICS OF CONFOUNDING

A confounder is an agent or extraneous factor that accounts for differences in disease occurrence or frequency or the measure of effect between the exposed and unexposed.

- Predicts disease frequency in the unexposed or referent population. For example, in the association between oral cancer and alcohol consumption, smoking is considered confounding if it is associated with both oral cancer and alcohol consumption.
  - A confounder is not qualified by this association only.
  - To qualify as a confounder, smoking must be associated with the occurrence of oral cancer in the unexposed or referent group, apart from its association with alcohol consumption.
  - Also, smoking must be associated with oral cancer among nonconsumers of alcohol.
- If the effect of alcohol consumption is mediated through the effect of smoking, then it is not a confounder, regardless of whether there is an effect of exposure (alcohol consumption) on oral cancer (outcome or disease).
- Any variate that represents a step on the pathway between the exposure and disease does not represent a confounder but could be termed an intermediate variate.

    Alcohol consumption → Smoking → Oral cancer

- Surrogate confounders refer to factors associated with confounders. For example, in chronologic age and aging, chronologic age is a surrogate confounder[16]
- Features of confounder—it must be
  - An extraneous risk factor for disease
  - Associated with the exposure in the source population or the population at risk from which the case is derived
  - Not be affected by the exposure or disease, implying that it cannot be an intermediate in the causal pathway between the disease and exposure.

12.8   Random error and precision

12.8.1   *Random error*

Basically random error remains an unaccountable error that needs to be quantified. Random error refers to unsystematic error that arises from an unforeseeable and unpredictable process, such as a mistake in assessing the exposure and disease and sampling variability (unrepresentative sample or chance).

12.8.2   *Precision*

This is the lack of random error. Precision, and hence reduction in random error, may be induced by increasing the sample size, repeating measurement within a study, and utilizing an efficient study design in order to maximize the amount of information obtained.

Precision (lack of random error) may be influenced by sampling, hypothesis testing and *p*-values, confidence intervals estimation, random variable probability distribution, and sample size and power estimation.[17,18]

Systematic error may be present in a study despite the absence or reduction of random error (study may be precise but findings are inaccurate). It is important to note that no matter the degree of random error in minimization, random error exist implying some element of uncertainties in all studies no matter the sampling technique utilized, study size and the magnitude of effect.

12.8.3 *Interaction*

As used in epidemiology, interaction is a biologic phenomenon indicating biologic interaction. Interaction is said to occur when the incidence rate of a disease or outcome in the presence of two or more risk factors differs from the incidence rate expected to result from their individual effect. This rate may be greater than what is expected (synergism) or less than what is expected (antagonism).[17,18] Like effect measure modifier, interaction is said to occur if there is a difference in the strata-specific risk point estimate (RR, OR) on the basis of the third variable.

12.8.4 *Additive model*

This occurs in association with effect if the effect of one exposure is added to the effect of the other (e.g., if those with neither exposure have an incidence of 2.0, while for those with a smoking history, the incidence is 8.0 and in those with smoking history and heavy alcohol consumption, 16.0).[17,18] The additive model assumes that the incidence will be X in those with both types of risk. What is X? X is 22. Because smoking adds 6.0 to those with no risk, it will be expected to add 6.0 to those with a history of alcohol drinking. The additive model is not accurate in describing the effect of exposure to two independent factors in disease causation.

12.8.5 *Multiplicative model*

This is the appropriate model for describing the effects of two independent factors or exposures in disease causation (e.g., if absence of neither exposure has an incidence of 2.0 and those exposed to cigarette smoking have an incidence of 8.0, while those exposed to heavy alcohol consumption have an incidence of 16.0). The multiplicative model assumes that the incidence will be Y in those with both risks. What is Y? Y is 64. Because smoking multiplies the risk by four times in the absence of alcohol, we also expect it to multiply the risk in alcohol users by four (16×4). If so, the effect of exposure to both smoking and alcohol will be $16 \times 4 = 64$.

12.8.6   *Effect/Association measure modifier*

Effect measure modification remains an appropriate epidemiologic concept in assessing heterogeneity of a third variable on the pathway of association. Suppose we wish to examine the data on the association between second primary thyroid cancer and radiation therapy for the first primary cancer in children, and to determine whether or not the effect of radiation on second primary thyroid cancer differs by the level of age or age group, with age as the third variable. Does age modify the OR of the association between radiation and second primary thyroid cancer? If it does, then the result of the association based on the overall estimate without stratum-specific result is invalid, flawed and misleading. Specifically to examine the OR effect modification, one has to examine the OR by separate level of age or age groups namely <0, 1–4, 5–9, 10–14 and 15–18 in the association between radiation and second primary thyroid cancer. Practically, if there is no association between radiation and second primary thyroid cancer in the pool analysis (age grouped lumped), the consideration of the stratified analysis by age group may lead to reliable and meaningful result and interpretation. The following steps should be taken in assessing the OR effect modification of age: (1) Estimate the overall or crude OR, (2) use C-M-H method to stratify the data by age, and (3) observe the effect of age on the OR of the association between radiation and second primary thyroid cancer. If effect measure modification is observed, the pool estimate should not be reported but the stratum specific OR in order to address this as a biologic phenomenon. Additionally, if there is only effect measure modification, the stratum-specific estimates differ from one another significantly and should be tested with the chi square test of homogeneity.

12.8.7   *Consider another example of effect measure modifier*

Is age a modifier in the association between ethnicity and hypertension? Differences are not observed between black and white men under the age of 35 with respect to hypertension incidence. After age 35, incidence tends to be two to three times higher in blacks relative to whites of the same age. Biologically, an effect measure modifier is the third variable that is not a confounder but enters into a causal pathway between the exposure and the disease of interest.[12] For example, the relationship between lung cancer and cigarette smoking is modified by asbestos, because asbestos exposure has been known to increase the risk of dying by 92 times among smokers, whereas the risk of dying from lung cancer among those exposed to asbestos only is tenfold. Another example is the modifying effect of cigarette smoking and obesity on the association between oral contraceptives and myocardial infarction in women. Effect measure modifier and confounding have similarities. Both confounding and effect measure modifier involve a third variable and are assessed or evaluated by performing stratified analysis.[1,5] Effect measure modifier also differs from confounding. In confounding, one is interested in knowing whether the crude measure of association (unadjusted point estimate) changes (distorted) and whether the stratum-specific and adjusted summary estimate differs from the crude or unadjusted estimate. In effect measure modification, one is interested in finding out if the association differs according to the third variable (the difference in stratum-specific estimates from one another).

Vignette 12.4 Consider a case-control study of the effect of lycopene on prostate cancer stratified by body mass index (BMI) (normal versus overweight). The stratum-specific odds ratio for men with a BMI of greater than or equal to 24.99 kg/m² = 2.2, and the stratum-specific odds ratio for men with normal BMI (<24.99 kg/m²) is 1.0. Does this illustration indicate the presence of effect modifier or confounding by BMI?

Solution: Because the stratum-specific odds ratio differs between men with normal and abnormal BMI, BMI is an effect measure modifier between lycopene and prostate cancer in men. In this example, the BMI needs to be described or explained in the causal pathway of prostate cancer and does not need to be adjusted for since it is not a confounder.

Question: Can the same variable (gender) be an effect measure modifier and confounder in the same setting (simultaneously)? Explore this possibility using the combined odds ratio and stratum specific odds ratio illustration.

12.8.8   Epidemiologic causal inference

Epidemiologic investigation is concerned with association as well as causal association. Simply, *cause* refers to whatever produces an effect (result, outcome, response variable). Cause may be understood as a factor if its operation increases the frequency of an event (outcome, result). Cause is also described as an event, condition, or characteristic that preceded a health-related event and without which the event would not have occurred at all or would not have occurred until some later time. Causal inference in epidemiology involves two steps:

1   Valid result—internal validity of the study (association that is not as a result of bias, confounding, and random error)
2   Assessment of whether the exposure actually caused the effect (outcome, result)

Causal relationships may be

- Necessary and sufficient (*necessary* if the outcome occurs only if the causal factor operated and *sufficient* if the operation of the causal factor *always* results in the outcome)

Table 12.4 Bradford Austin Hill's criteria for causal inference

Criteria	Explanation
Temporality	• The cause must precede the outcome (disease). • Complete consensus among investigators and most relevant criterion. • Easily established in prospective studies.
Strength of association	• Measured by relative risk or odds ratio. • Larger relative risk or odds ratio is more indicative of a stronger association.
Dose-response	• Effect increases as the exposure level increases.
Consistency of association	• Association is most likely to be causal if observed repeatedly by different persons, in different places, circumstances, and times.
Plausibility	• Coherency with the current body of knowledge (existence of biologic or social model to explain the association).
Coherence	• Cause-and-effect interpretation of the data should not seriously conflict with generally known facts of the natural history and the biology of the disease.
Experiment	• If exposure causes a disease, the disease is expected to decline when the exposure is reduced or eliminated.
Analogy	• Similarities between the observed association and other associations.
Specificity	• A cause should lead to a single effect, and vice versa. • An association is specific when a certain exposure is associated with only one disease.

- Necessary but not sufficient
- Sufficient but not necessary
- Neither sufficient nor necessary, implying that the operation of the causal factor increases the frequency of the causal factor, but the outcome does not always result and the outcome can occur without the operation of the causal factor[1,5]

The criteria commonly used to assesses causal inference in epidemiologic studies follows that used by Bradford Hill (Table 12.4).[19]

12.9 Rothman's component cause model (causal pies)

1 *Sufficient cause:* complete causal mechanisms that inevitably produce disease
2 *Component cause:* each participating factor in a sufficient cause
3 *Necessary cause:* a causal component that is a member of every sufficient cause

The causal pies model indicates that a sufficient cause is not a single factor but rather a minimal set of factors that unavoidably produce disease, implying that the termination of the action of a single causal component, blocks the completion of a sufficient cause, thus preventing disease occurrence by that pathway.[14,16]

Vignette 12.5 Consider an epidemiologic investigation conducted to assess the association between exposure to sulfur and brain tumors in children. If the investigator wishes to compare the findings in this study with other evidence, which criteria according to Bradford Hill, might be worth considering, and what sort of study design may provide a more valid and reliable comparison?

Solution: Evidence from one study may be compared with another in terms of Hill's criteria of consistency, plausibility, coherence, and specificity. The most appropriate design would be prospective studies.

Vignette 12.6 Consider an investigator who wishes to examine published studies on the evidence of estrogen replacement therapy in postmenopausal breast cancer. If s/he wishes to examine the features consistent with causation using the Bradford Hill criteria, which features should be taken into consideration?

Solution: Bradford Hill's features consistent with causation are (a) temporal sequence, (b) strength of association, (c) dose response-biologic gradient (d) consistency, and (e) specificity.

Vignette 12.7 Consider an investigation of epidemiologic causal inference that attempts to examine the study validity prior to assessing whether the exposure actually led to the disease. Which aspects of the study must the investigator consider in order to determine if the observed result was valid?

Solution: The first step in epidemiologic causal inference is to illustrate that the result was not due to (a) systematic error (bias), (b) confounding, or (c) random error (Figure 12.6).

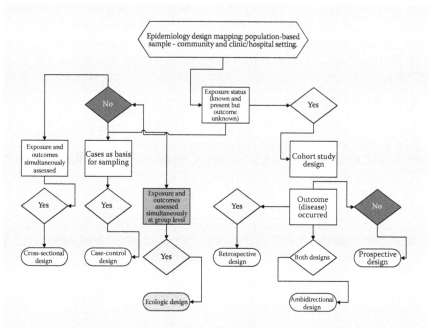

Figure 12.6 **Ecologic Study.** An ecologic fallacy is illustrated by group level inference to individual inference.

BOX 12.12   TYPES OF BIASES (SYSTEMATIC ERROR)

Bias is a systematic error in the design, conduct, or analysis of a study that results in a mistaken estimate of exposure's effect on the risk of disease.*

- Can be considered a systematic error or nonrandom error in a study that leads to a distorted result.**
  Selection bias refers to distortion of the effect size or association measure due to the procedure of subject selection and other factors that influence participation in the study.
- Estimates of effects or point estimates are based on participation.
- Association represents the mixture of forces that determine participation and forces that drive disease occurrence.
- Types of selection bias:
  - Self-selection bias refers to the self-referral of subjects; it may threaten the validity of the study since the reason for self-referral may be linked with the outcome of interest.***

- Systematic error in selection of subjects (exposed and non-exposed or cases and controls) within the study can distort the internal validity of the study as well as the conclusion or generalization of findings to a population outside the source population.
- Exclusion bias is a type of selection bias that occurs if investigators apply different eligibility criteria to cases and controls regarding which previous clinical conditions permit eligibility.
- Berksonian bias is a selection bias that is said to occur when both exposure and disease affect selection. It occurs because of the different probabilities of admission to the hospital for those with the disease, without the disease, and with the characteristics of interest.****

Information bias—refers to errors in estimating effect and may result from measurement errors.

- These errors include (a) classification error—misclassification (further classified as differential (errors depending on actual values of other variables) and nondifferential (does not depend on actual values of other variables).
- Misclassification also occurs when as in case-control those with the disease are classified a control, and some without the disease (control) may be classified as cases.
- Differential misclassification occurs when the rate of misclassification differs in different group (cases versus control).
- Nondifferential misclassification occurs when the rate of misclassification does not differ in different group (cases versus control).

Others: Dependent error (depends on error in measuring), independent or nondependent error (depends not on measuring error) and correlated error (dependent errors that have a nonzero correlation coefficient)

* J. J. Schlessman, *Case-Control Studies: Design, Conduct, and Analysis* (New York: Oxford University Press, 1982).

** R. S. Greenberg et al. *Medical Epidemiology*, 4th ed. (New York: Lange Medical Books/McGraw-Hill, 2005).

*** M. H. Criqui, M. Austin, E. Barrett-Connor, "The Effect of Non-Response on Risk Ratios in a Cardiovascular Disease Study," *J Chronic Dis* 32 (1979): 633–638.

**** J. Berkson, "Limitations of the Application of Fourfold Table Analysis to Hospital Data," *Biometrics* 2 (1946): 47–53.

12.10   Summary

Epidemiologic and clinical research evidence requires the disentangling of bias, random errors, and confounding prior to sustaining internal and external validity of the study. A single study, no matter how scientifically valid, rarely establishes causal inference. The claim of causality or causal inference involves the combination of criteria, one of which is the combination of studies for the summary effect termed meta-analysis, quantitative systematic review, or quantitative evidence synthesis (Table 12.5).

QES is contingent on the validity of the individual studies that form the basis of the summary point estimate. The more homogeneous the studies are, the more likely that the summary point estimates will reflect the effect of the intervention studied. There are two commonly used methods of summary effect in meta-analysis: the fixed effect and random effect models. The fixed effect model is used when the test of heterogeneity indicates homogeneity of the studies combined, while the random effect model is appropriate if heterogeneity of studies is assumed.

The search for causal inference in epidemiologic studies relies primarily on the assessment of the internal and external validity of studies. The external validity process involves the assessment of the statistical stability or significance level in order to determine whether or not the result is representative of the population from which the sample arose. The test of significance (statistical stability), simply asserts that a random sample represents the population, and hence the result from the sample can then be generalized to the

Table 12.5 Critical appraisal of scientific literature

A Research question: Assess the clarity and relevance of the question.

B Design process: Examine the appropriateness of the design to the proposed study question.

C Outcome measure/variable: Is the outcome or response variable well determined and is the measure clinically relevant?

D Predictor/independent variable: Assess how the exposures were determined and the appropriateness of the exposures in influencing the response.

E Analysis: Is the analytic method appropriate with respect to the scales of measurement of the outcome and predictor variables as well as the design of the study? What are the assumptions behind the test? Sample size and power estimation? Errors?

F Systematic error (bias): Assessment and minimization: Were biases recognized and addressed?

G Results and interpretation: Are the findings clinically relevant (effect size)? If negative findings were reported, did the authors document the power of the study?

H Study implications: Will the findings impact medicine, public health, and clinical practice?

target population. Traditionally, this level of significance is set at 5% error tolerance should one reject the null hypothesis if indeed the null hypothesis is true. Once the obtained probability value is less than 0.05, the null hypothesis is rejected since the obtained result is unlikely to be explained by chance only. With this claim (statistical significance establishment), researchers are required to examine the significant association in the data in the light of bias and confounding, since significance does not rule out the possibility of bias and confounding. Therefore, a result can be statistically significant but clinically and biologically irrelevant, as the finding may be driven by measurement or observation bias and confounding.

The internal validity of the studies involves the assessment of studies for temporality cause and effect relationship, magnitude of association, dose-response relationship, consistency, and specificity. The external validity should be assessed but not unless the internal validity is achieved, implying the deemphasis of the *p* value.

Questions for discussion

1 Suppose you are appointed as the director of a clinical taskforce to establish the guidelines for the assessment and treatment of avascular necrosis associated with sickle cell disease, and you intend to base this guideline on the meta-analysis or systematic quantitative review.
   a   What will your inclusion and exclusion criteria be?
   b   What method of meta-analysis will you employ if the studies indicate heterogeneity, and why?
   c   What are the limitations of this approach in establishing clinical guidelines?
2 A study was conducted to examine the role of paternal exposure to cigarette smoking and asthma in children. The result was found to be consistent with a causal relationship.
   a   If genetic predisposition was also a likely explanation, can we affirm a conclusion regarding a causal relationship?
   b   In terms of internal validity and causation, comment on the
      i   consistency of this study with other evidence,
      ii   specificity,
      iii biologic plausibility, and
      iv   coherency of the effect with the distribution of the exposure and the outcome.
3 Discuss the role of QES in epidemiologic causal inference.
4 Differentiate between effect measure modifier, biologic interaction, statistical interaction and confounding. Discuss of to assess for effect measure modifier and confounding, Can a variable be both effect measure modifier and a confounding? If that is th case, how will you handle the inference and report the findings?

5 Comment on the assessment of random error, bias, and confounding in the establishment of study validity.

   a   How relevant is the assessment of bias and confounding if the result of a study is statistically insignificant?

   b   What is the significance of probability value in the interpretation of study finding if the sample studied was not a random sample?

References

1. M. Elwood, *Critical Appraisal of Epidemiological Studies in Clinical Trials*, 2nd ed. (New York: Oxford University Press, 2003)
2. A. Aschengrau and G. R. Seage III, *Essentials of Epidemiology* (Sudbury, MA: Jones & Bartlett, 2003).
3. M. W. Lipsey and D. Wilson, *Practical Meta-Analysis* (Thousand Oaks, CA: Sage Publications, 2001).
4. K. J. Rothman, *Epidemiology: An Introduction* (New York: Oxford University Press, 2002).
5. M. Szklo and J. Nieto, *Epidemiology: Beyond the Basics* (Sudbury, MA: Jones & Bartlett, 2003).
6. E. L. Lehmann, *Testing Statistical Hypothesis*, 2nd ed. (New York: Wiley, 1989).
7. G. D. Murray, "Statistical Guidelines for *British Journal of Surgery*," *Br J Surg* 78 (1991): 782–784.
8. S. M. Gore et al., "*The Lancet's* Statistical Review Process: Areas for Improvement by Authors," *Lancet* 340 (1992): 100–102.
9. R. DerSimonian and N. Laird, "Meta-Analysis in Clinical Trials," *Control Clin Trials* 7 (1986): 177–188.
10. D. R. Jones, "Meta-Analysis: Weighing the Evidence," *Stat Med* 14 (1995): 137–139.
11. J. Lau et al., "Quantitative Synthesis in Systematic Reviews," *An Intern Med* 127 (1997): 820–826.
12. I. Olkin, "Meta-Analysis: Reconciling the Results of Independent Studies," *Stat Med* 14 (1995): 457–472.
13. I. Olkin, "Statistical and Theoretical Considerations in Meta-Analysis," *J Clin Epidemiol* 48 (1995): 133–146.
14. M. Kadhim, L. Holmes Jr, M. G. Gesheff, and J. D. Conway, "Treatment Options for Nonunion with Segmental Bone Defects: Systematic Review and Quantitative Evidence Synthesis," *J Orthop Trauma* 31 (2017): 111–119. doi: 10.1097/BOT .0000000000000700. Review. PMID: 27611666
15. C. H. Hennekens and J. E. Buring, *Epidemiology in Medicine* (Boston: Little, Brown, & Company, 1987).
16. K. J. Rothman et al., *Modern Epidemiology*, 3rd ed. (Philadelphia: Lippincott, Williams & Wilkins, 2008).
17. L. Gordis, *Epidemiology*, 3rd ed. (Philadelphia: Elsevier Saunders, 2004).
18. D. A. Savitz, *Interpreting Epidemiologic Evidence* (New York: Oxford University Press, 2003).
19. A. B. Hill, "The Environment and Disease: Association or Causation?" *Proc R Soc Med.* 58 (1965): 295–300.
20. K. Muayad, L. Holmes, M. G. Gesheff, and J. D. Conway. "Treatment Options for Nonunion With Segmental Bone Defects: Systematic Review and Quantitative Evidence Synthesis," *J Orthop Trauma* 31 (2017): 111–119.

Section III

Perspectives, challenges, and future of epidemiology

Over the past five decades, scientific knowledge and evidence discovery had become very complex as technology evolves and human environment mutates, requiring team and collaborative effort in an attempt to improve patient and population health through scientific effort. The era of epidemiology as an independent discipline or profession is over. Epidemiology is required to exert its role of leadership in scientific research geared at population health improvement.

This section explores the various perspectives in epidemiologic investigation and identifies epidemiology not as a discipline but as a profession. The role of epidemiology in health and healthcare policy is discussed with the need to engage epidemiologic findings as the basis for evidence in policy development. Further, as epidemiology remains to be purposive and accountable, consequentialist epidemiology becomes necessary in meeting the goal of public health, which is to control disease and promote health. Most importantly today is the obligation of epidemiology to transfer its findings to public health intervention in the areas of aging, disabilities, opium and obesity epidemics (translational epidemiology).

13 Perspectives, challenges, and future of epidemiology

13.1 Introduction

Epidemiologic dimensions or aspects have evolved with advances in the bio-medical sciences and clinical medicine. During the 1900s, the driving forces for mortality were infectious diseases. In the late 1960s, we experienced an epidemiologic transition, where chronic diseases (CDs) became the leading cause of mortality in the United States. With the advances in the genome, a new focus became inevitable: the stress on the genetic determinants of disease and disease outcomes. Since epidemiology follows transitions in the human population, epidemiologic focus shifted from infectious diseases and infant mortality to CDs and chronic disabilities as well as competing risk of dying, given the demographic transition in the United States' elderly population. The advent of genetic and molecular determinants of diseases and disease progressions over the past few decades transformed epidemiology from traditional association of external or exogenous exposure to the assessment of the cellular and molecular level events in the disease association. The recognition of the "internal dose" and the ability to identify biomarkers of disease initiation and progression resulted in more emphasis on molecular and genetic epidemiology. Medicine being molecular, any attempt to understand disease risk and etiology at the population level requires a careful attempt at examining the molecular (physiologic, cellular, biochemical, and microstructural, etc.) alteration at the population level that may serve as predisposing or risk factor as well as play a causal or etiologic role. Further, the effort to examine treatment outcomes, namely, drug benefits and adverse effects, enabled the development of pharmaco-epidemiology and health outcomes research as unique fields of epidemiology.

Since epidemiology remains on the frontline of science, it must follow new technologies, and learn from these advances in order to stay in this leadership position.[1] Epidemiology is faced with the challenges of applying innovative approach to "big data" and complex data modeling.[2] Specifically, innovative approach is required in addressing data from electronic medical records and the healthcare system linkage data, mHealth and social media data. This challenge involves collaboration with other disciplines such as computational biology, genetics, bioinformatics, social and behavioral sciences and systems science in managing, processing and analyzing data.[1] In meeting these challenges, epidemiology stands to benefit from collaboration with other disciplines in making sense of hyperdense data for reliable inference that is often impossible with small samples (sparse data bias). This collaboration requires epidemiologists to be informed on biological processes as components of disease etiology, in order to apply the mechanism disease in mapping the etiologic pathways in morbidities and mortalities. Epidemiologic research now and in future will require team science, translational and transdisciplinary approach. Therefore, scientific creativity needed in meaningful evidence recovery requires transdisciplinary innovation, and epidemiology has the opportunity, given its very broad scope, to provide innovative designs and statistical models to the utilization of these complex biologic, biotechnologic, behavioral, and genetics data in disease etiology and intervention mapping.

BOX 13.1   SOCIAL EPIDEMIOLOGY (SE)

- Emerged during the 1960s as a field of epidemiology that studies the relationship between social attributes or factors and disease, injuries, disabilities, and health-related events at the population level.
- With social factors contributing to mortality, social epidemiology has demonstrated the role of culture, social class, and education in disease initiation, progression, and prognosis.
- Characterized by inclusion of social, economic, and cultural exposure in the explanation of the outcome.
- These factors include race/ethnicity, sex/gender, socioeconomic status/class/position, education, income.
- Surveillance and etiologic influence are addressed in an attempt to examine social variation in disease and mortality.
- Data are assessed at individual as well as aggregate levels.
- Individual-level variables include marital status, material deprivation, social support, family support, status incongruity.
- Aggregate-level exposure in SE includes social network, economic inequality, social capital, and neighborhood deprivation.

In environmental epidemiology, time-related disease patterns are common and include time-clustering (occurs with the introduction of new exposure in an environment that is not commonly encountered on a large scale), cyclic patterns (increase in respiratory disease in the winter), and longitudinal trends (period effect, cross-generation changes, and birth-cohort effect).

This chapter focuses on the evolution of fields of epidemiology as hybrids of biologic, medical, economic (health outcomes epidemiology), or behavioral sciences. The attempt is to introduce the reader to a brief or introductory notion of these hybrids, namely, molecular/genetic epidemiology, cancer epidemiology, and cardiovascular, environmental, and nutritional epidemiology. In spite of the special subjects and the methodology involved in evidence discovery in these fields of epidemiology, the designs and the measures of effect or association remain the same as in the traditional epidemiology. These fields are unique, given that the research conducted therein follows fundamental epidemiologic research design and statistical inference. There are introductory books written during the past decade on these fields, and readers are encouraged to explore further if they wish to focus on some specialized areas of epidemiology. A detailed discussion of the principles and methodologies of each is beyond the scope of this book.

13.2   Clinical epidemiology

The most unspecific aspect of epidemiology tends to be "clinical epidemiology," which renders this subdiscipline so broad and unnecessary, it had be described as an oxymoron.[3] Basically, the distinction between epidemiology and clinical epidemiology is not the sample or study population but the subject matter or variables studied. We can understand clinical epidemiology as an attempt to study the natural history of a disease, disease risk factors, or the effect of treatment within the clinic setting. When epidemiologic principles are focused on disease screening, diagnosis, treatment, and prognosis,[4] this tends to be described as clinical epidemiology.

13.2.1   What then is clinical epidemiology?

Using practical experience to describe clinical epidemiology seems more appealing, in spite of the lack of specificity in the application of this concept as a unique field of epidemiology. Historically, epidemiology characterizes human beings at a population level, which partly qualifies the application of epidemiologic principles in the understanding of disease distributions and determinants of such distribution and treatment variability among groups of patients. However, clinical epidemiology includes not only patients but also agents (pathogenic microbes) in its investigative approach to improve health-care outcomes.

a   The subject matter of investigation in clinical epidemiology includes, but is not limited to, the natural history of the disease—assesses health outcomes in patients who received treatment relative to those who did not.
b   Diagnostic and screening tests (discussed in Chapter 4).
c   Treatment effectiveness (randomized and nonrandomized)—discussed in Chapter 10.

The design and analytic approach used in this field of epidemiology is similar to the methods and principles of general epidemiology. However, recently, healthcare outcomes within clinical or hospital settings have dominated the subject matter of clinical epidemiology. For example, if investigators examined the natural history of hip dysplasia in children with cerebral palsy with the intent to compare the outcomes (adverse events/complications) of untreated hips relative to the treated ones, this approach could be classified as a clinical epidemiologic study. Another example of a clinical epidemiology subject is the use of a prospective cohort design to study the natural history of unicameral bone cysts (UBCs) in a pediatric population. In this hypothetical example, the investigators may follow patients with UBCs who are treated with bone marrow injection (arm I), prednisone (arm II), and untreated or watchful waiting, also called observational management (arm III), to determine the healing of the cysts at the end of the study.

BOX 13.2   NUTRITIONAL EPIDEMIOLOGY (NE)

- Examines the relationship between dietary (micronutrients and macronutrients) exposure and disease- and health-related events.
- Provides validity in the assessment of the effect of diet on major disease and the modalities for prevention.
- Exposures are an aspect of diet, including though not limited to essential nutrients, natural constituents of food, chemicals coated in food, food preservatives, and noninfectious food contaminants.
- The classic and modern epidemiologic designs and analytic techniques used in general epidemiology are also used in NE.
- Migrant studies and secular trends are important in examining the correlation observed in ecologic studies.
- The measurement of diets involves the assessment of nutrients, food, and dietary patterns.
- Specifics of NE include the understanding of dietary assessment methods (short- and long-term dietary recalls, food frequency questionnaire, and biochemical indicators—serum or plasma, RBCs, subcutaneous fat, hair, and nails).

13.3   Infectious disease epidemiology

Infectious disease refers to diseases caused by pathogenic microbes, implying that for infectivity to occur, there is a minimum requirement of contact between the host (human) and agent (pathogenic microbe) as well as the environment that promotes pathogenicity and infectivity. However, when an infection is transmitted from host to host, a population pattern is established that reflects an infectious disease epidemiology. Koch's postulates in terms of causal influence are most applicable in infectious disease epidemiology, which implies the presence of the organism in every case and isolation in pure culture. Infectious disease epidemiology could be viewed as the interaction between the host, agent, and environment that resulted in disease transmission and infectivity in a human population. A definition of infectious disease epidemiology is that aspect of epidemiology that deals with illness due to a specific infectious agent or its toxic products that arises through transmission of that agent or its products from an infected person, animal, or reservoir to a susceptible host, either directly or indirectly, through an intermediate plant or animal host, vector, or the inanimate environment.[5]

Since contact with the agent, which may be an animal/insect or human (vector), is necessary as is the environment, infectious disease epidemiology involves other populations besides humans. Infection (outcome) is unlikely to occur without the contact between the host and the agent (exposure), and infectivity or disease manifestation is not possible without the pathogenic ability to compromise the immune system response (inert and adaptive). As a result of this pathway, infectious disease epidemiology aims at identifying the pathogen in those with clinical manifestations of the disease (signs and symptoms) or other end points (death), while excluding the pathogen from those without disease manifestation. Infectious disease epidemiology also aims to identify the risk factors that resulted in the transmission of the disease. The factors resulting in disease progression and survival remain the focus of infectious disease epidemiology. The factors affecting the transmission of disease have been described by epidemiologists as the forces that result in infectivity, namely, host (age, sex, genotype, and nutritional status), agent (virulence, pathogenicity, and antigenicity), and environment (weather, geography, air quality, and occupational setting).

While the measure of disease frequency and association in infectious disease epidemiology is comparable with methods used in general epidemiology, a certain measure of disease frequency, such as attack and fatality rates, is common between the two. These measures are discussed in Chapter 4 and in most textbooks on epidemiology.

Infectious disease epidemiology is used to examine factors influencing the occurrence of infection once the exposure or infection is determined and assess the determinants of recovery (resolution of infection), death, and persistent and recurrent infection. Further, this field of epidemiology explores the factors associated with infectivity or infectiveness and transmission. For example, if investigators wish to study retrospectively the factors associated with recurrent infection by chlamydia (host-to-host transmission) among undergraduate college students, such assessment could be performed as infectious disease epidemiology.

13.4 Molecular and genetic epidemiology

For years, traditional epidemiology has focused on exposure and disease association—exposure including such factors as behavior, diet, lifestyle, environment, and air and water pollutants implicated in disease outcome (cancer, diabetes mellitus, cardiovascular disease, etc.). In the past decade, following the stress on the genetic and molecular nature of human diseases, there has been a shift in the use of molecular biology and biochemistry tools in the understanding of disease causation and progression. Similar to traditional epidemiology, molecular epidemiology is concerned with population-based events, not separate individuals. In this example, molecular epidemiology seems to be comparable to population genetics.

Molecular epidemiology has been defined by several authors[6–10] as the analysis of nucleic acids and proteins in the study of health and disease determinants in human populations.[6] This definition emphasizes the biochemical bases of disease at the population level. Molecular epidemiology studies are sometimes performed to determine genetic polymorphism and association with disease risk or predisposition. Traditional epidemiologic designs, such as cross-sectional and case-control, are often used. Molecular biomarkers[7] have been used to characterize molecular epidemiology as the application of molecular biology to the study of infectious disease epidemiology.[8] The traditional approach in epidemiology has been to relate exposure to an environmental agent, such as a drug or infective agent, but with molecular epidemiology, genetic susceptibility is used to define risk, amplifying risk identification without necessarily adjusting for demographic variables and other confounders.[9]

Molecular epidemiology is the use of biologic markers or biologic measurements in epidemiologic research.[10]

What distinguishes molecular epidemiology is both the "molecular," the use of the techniques of molecular biology to characterize nucleic-acid- or amino-acid-based content, and the "epidemiology," the study of the distribution and determinants of disease occurrence in human populations. Molecular techniques may be applied to the measurement of host or agent factors and exposures. When applied to studies of disease, the resulting enhanced measurement increases our ability to more reliably detect associations. Molecular techniques help to stratify and to refine data by providing more sensitive and specific measurements, which facilitate epidemiologic activities, including doing disease surveillance, investigating outbreaks, identifying transmission patterns and risk factors among apparently disparate cases, characterizing host–pathogen interactions, detecting unculturable organisms, providing clues for possible infectious causes of cancer and other CDs, and providing better understanding of disease pathogenesis at the molecular level.

The application of molecular techniques to the study of heterogeneous organisms enhances epidemiologic studies by improving our ability to subclassify these organisms into meaningful groups. This facilitates the detection of disease outbreaks that may otherwise be undetected and allows the epidemiologist to identify risk factors of outbreaks, sporadic cases, or both.

The ongoing emphasis on the social determinants of individual and population health is indicative of how income, education, neighborhood factors, social support network, and other related socioeconomic factors predispose to health and disease. While these factors are recognized today by clinical medicine and public health to be relevant to patient and community health per se, they do not completely explain outcomes or disease incidence variability across diverse populations. This observation has resulted in the emergence of socio-epigenomics and sociogenonomics. The emergences of these perspectives open the window for health disparities and social epidemiologists to work within team science environment to determine the genomic or epigenomic basis of health disparities.

BOX 13.3   MEDICAL CARE/HEALTHCARE OUTCOMES EPIDEMIOLOGY

- Evolved over the past two decades as an approach to understanding health outcome determinants among treated and untreated patients at the population level
- Examines the predictors (exposure) of outcomes of treatment
- Determines treatment effectiveness and safety (complications and adverse events) in the healthcare delivery system
- Studies the benefit of treatment, including behavioral intervention in routine use in the community
- Utilizes traditional and modern epidemiologic designs, including survival (time to event) design and analysis in longitudinal assessment of care effectiveness and life prolongation
- Confounding is germane to this field of epidemiology
- Valid and reliable findings in this field involve a careful assessment of intermediates, effect measure modifiers, bias, and random error quantification
- Important in examining health equity and factors associated with health disparities in health care utilization, access, and outcome of treatment

---

13.5   Cancer epidemiology

The study of cancer and cancer precursor distribution and determinants at the population level that utilizes the traditional and molecular epidemiology techniques may be described as cancer epidemiology. Cancer epidemiology thus seeks to identify cancer risk factors in susceptible groups and populations at risk and determine treatment effectiveness and measures to prevent cancer risk and predisposing factors. The contribution of this field to the understanding, treatment, and prevention of human malignancies is undisputable in current thinking. Therefore, it is unimaginable to conceive a cancer research and treatment program without cancer epidemiologists as members of the team. This science is required in the cancer elimination effort of human society. In addition, as the caner genome project increases our knowledge of carcinogenesis, treatment will be genetically directed and will result in improved therapy. Anatomic site isolation of malignancies, although useful in terms of tumor classification, remains inadequate in informing cancer therapeutics. Cancer epidemiology will require clinical trials and prospective designs to demonstrate efficacy and effectiveness, respectively, in the future struggle against cancer.

The term *carcinoma* originated from the Greek word *karkinos*, as used by Hippocrates (fourth century BC); it literally means "crab." Hippocrates, despite his writings on the environmental determinants of human diseases, attributed cancer to the excess of black bile. Ramazzini, in his book *De Morbis Artificum* (1713), attributed excessive rates of breast cancer in Catholic nuns to their celibate life. Arabic and Chinese medical literatures both described symptoms that may be malignancy, implying the "aging of malignancy." The occupational (chimney sweeps and soot) implication in scrotal cancer was observed by Percival Pott (1775). This observation by Pott provided the opportunity for the prevention of scrotal sac cancer among chimney workers in England. However, the systematic study of cancer began in the eighteenth century with Bichat (1771–1802), who described tumors as an "accidental formation" of tissue built up in the same manner as any other part of the organism.

The patterns of cancer occurrence in specific populations were described by William Farr (1807–1883) in London. Doll and Hill (1954), in a prospective study, investigated the relationship between tobacco smoking and lung cancer. The relation between bladder cancer and British chemical industries was investigated in an occupational epidemiologic setting (1954). Epidemiologic cohort studies on industrial workers, patients treated with radiation and cytotoxic chemotherapy, and so on, have provided reliable evidence of exposure to specific carcinogens and the risk of developing cancer. The relationship between pipe smoking and squamous cell epithelioma was uncovered using a case-control design by Broders in 1920. The understanding of the association between late first birth and breast cancer was illustrated by a case-control design (MacMahon et al., 1970). Similarly, case-control design was used by Herbst et al. to observe the association between diethylstilbesterol and vaginal clear-cell adenocarcinoma in young women (1971).

Retrospective cohort design has been used to study the outcomes of cancer and survival. These studies represented the extended use of healthcare outcomes data in cancer epidemiology. Holmes et al. investigated the effectiveness of androgen-deprivation therapy (ADT) in prolonging the survival of older men with loco-regional prostate cancer (2007), the impact of ADT on racial/ethnic variance in prostate cancer survival (2009), and the association between dental care utilization and oral cavity neoplasm (2009).

While substantial advances have been made in cancer epidemiology, this field remains challenging. First, the long induction period of cancer following exposure requires many years of follow-up prior to the observation of outcome. Second, since some cancers are rare, many years of follow-up of many exposed individuals are necessary for the observation of outcome (cancer). Third, in pediatric cancer, the risk factors are often surrogate (parental exposure), limiting the assessment of the direct exposure in the development of malignancy.

Survival from most malignancies has improved not only because of medical care only but also the use of epidemiologic methods to identify and prevent the social, genetic, environmental, and occupational risk factors. While epidemiologic evidence resulted in an interdisciplinary effort to prevent cancer occurrence, advances in molecular biology and biochemistry and the application of epidemiologic tools in the understanding of cancer at the population level remain the direction to follow in an attempt to eliminate cancer in human populations.

13.6   CD and cardiovascular epidemiology

A CD can be described as a condition that is treatable but not curable and has a tendency to deteriorate. Because CD is most prevalent in the older or aging population, *aging epidemiology*, although not interchangeably used, focuses on the web of causality including decline in bodily functions that predisposes a person to CD and disabilities. For example, hypertension and diabetes mellitus are both treatable by controlling blood pressure and sugar level, respectively, but once diagnosed, these conditions progress unless managed. Classic examples of CDs are asthma and arthritis.

A CD may be defined as an illness that is prolonged in duration, does not often resolve spontaneously, and is rarely cured completely. CDs are complex and varied in terms of their nature, how they are caused, and the extent of their impact on the community. While some CDs make large contributions to premature death, others contribute more to disability. Features common to most CDs include

a   Complex causality, with multiple factors leading to their onset
b   A long development period, for which there may be no symptoms
c   A prolonged course of illness, perhaps leading to other health complications
d   Associated functional impairment or disability[11]

CD epidemiology (CDE) refers to the branch of epidemiology that focuses on the distribution and determinants of CDs and chronic disabilities at the population level. Studies in CDE following the principles and methods used in both traditional and CDE became instrumental in the 1960s in assessing cardiovascular risk factors. Classic examples are the large-scale studies, such as the Framingham Heart Study, the Seven Countries Study, and the British Physicians Study. These studies demonstrated the contributions of cigarette smoking, diet, physical inactivity, and high blood pressure to cardiovascular and cerebrovascular disease and malignancies. These and other studies have facilitated the establishment of the behavioral causes of many CDs. CDE continues to study the relationship between risk factors and major CDs. CDE shifted the focus from CDs to the behavioral risk factors preceding the diseases. CDE continues to demonstrate the contributions to health by factors beyond the physical environment, medical care, and health behaviors, including although not limited to socioeconomic position, race/ethnicity, social networks and support, work conditions, economic inequality, and social capital.[12]

BOX 13.4   ENVIRONMENTAL AND OCCUPATIONAL EPIDEMIOLOGY (EOE)

- Environmental factors are considered in epidemiology as those that are nonendogenous to and nonessential for the normal development and functioning of humans.
- Environment so considered has the potential to influence human health and disease process.
- So characterized, environment includes but is not limited to physical, chemical, biologic, social, political, cultural, and physical structure (architectural/civil engineering) factors.
- The distribution and determinants of these factors and the interaction of the physical, biologic, and physical factors with social, political, and cultural ones in disease predisposition and precipitation remain the subject of environmental and occupational epidemiology.
- Environmental epidemiology has been instrumental to the assessment of several exposures, including volatile organic substances, metals, particulate matter, pesticides, and radiation and historical issues like water contamination, air pollution, and organic pollutants.
- Natural disasters, such as war, floods, hurricanes, earthquakes, tsunamis, and global warming, are subjects of environmental epidemiology. Current challenges include climate/global warming.
- Designs and analytic issues are similar to those used in general epidemiologic research, but emphasis is placed on clusters, ecologic design, mapping, time-series analysis, analysis of clusters around point sources, and social class as a confounder.
- Specific to this field of epidemiology is risk assessment and the utilization of the steps in such assessment: hazard identification, exposure assessment, dose-response, and risk characterization.

13.7   Epidemiology and health policy formulation

The core functions of public health, namely, assessment, policy formulation, and assurance, reflect the role of epidemiology in the assessment of health issues across populations. Although the goal of epidemiology is not disease control and health promotion, the findings from epidemiology are essential for data-driven decision making regarding prioritization of intervention, intervention development, and implementation in promoting population health.

13.7.1 *Health disparities epidemiology*

Health disparities epidemiology examines the relationship between an independent variable (treatment/health service) and a dependent variable (outcome) to determine the effectiveness of treatment across diverse population. This approach considers the influence of other factors such as environment (possible confounding) in the relationship between health services and outcomes across subgroups (sex, race/ethnicity, disability), given that health inequity remains an exposure effect of health disparities. While confounding is not bias per se, inability to assess for and address confounding may introduce bias into the findings of health disparities research. Choosing a particular measure of health disparity reflects, implicitly or explicitly, different perspectives about what quantities or characteristics of health disparity are thought to be important to capture. To better monitor the population health burden of disparities over time, disparity indicators should be sensitive to two sources of change: (1) change in the size of the population subgroups involved and (2) change in the level of health within each subgroup. The first step is to provide an assessment of health disparity with a simple tabular and graphical presentation of the underlying "raw" data (rate, proportion, etc., and subgroup population size). Such presentation addresses the question of whether the particular disparity has increased or decreased over time—trends.

The challenges for health disparities epidemiology are inherent in the core understanding of unequal outcomes and how to measure such outcomes with accuracies as well as the feasible application of team science environment in an attempt to understand the "bioneuro-social" determinants of outcomes and morbidity variabilities. The measures of health disparities offer challenges in the context of a measure that could lead to intervention mapping in narrowing and eventually eliminating such gaps. When and how the absolute and relative measures of health disparities are used in assessing the differences in health and health outcomes across diverse populations or within a health disparity subpopulation depend on several factors, including the purpose of the measurement. For example, determining the racial/ethnic differences in hypertension may require the absolute measure (risk/proportion/prevalence difference) if the intent is to develop programs to target the population at most risk (Figure 13.1). In contrast, if the intent is to examine differences in association and/or causation of the outcome with the diverse populations, then the relative measure (relative odds/risk) remains appropriate (Figure 13.2).

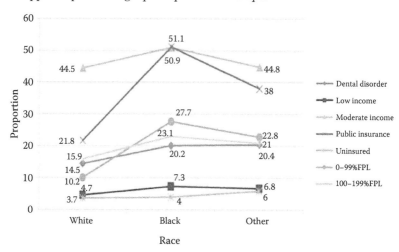

Figure 13.1 Absolute measure of health disparities. Figure illustrates variances in health disparities indicator, which is assessed by observing the difference in prevalence or proportion between subgroups.

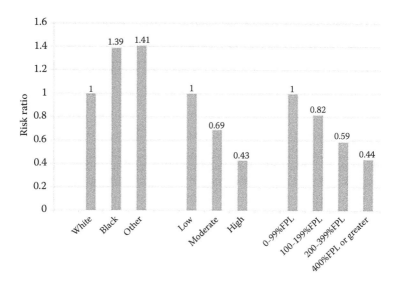

Figure 13.2 Relative measure of health disparities. The relative measure involves the preselection of the reference group based on the best or worst outcome and sample size (strata-specific estimate stability).

**BOX 13.5   PROCESS AND OUTCOMES MEASURES
OF HEALTH AND HEALTHCARE**

- *Health process*—What constitutes the components of good and standard of care? The answer to this reflects health process investigation/evaluation This can be studied by assessing the hospital by departments/clinics or healthcare providers to determine whether or not the care provided to children with ACL for example meets the established criteria by ASCO.
- This measure remains inadequate since we are unable to determine if the children with ACL are better off based on simply adhering to the established treatment criteria. In addition, since process measure is based on expert opinion, criteria used in process measure may change over time.
- *Health outcomes*—reflects whether or not a pediatric patient with asthma for example benefits from the medical/health care provided.
- *Health disparities epidemiology focuses on outcomes*—morbidity such as disease severity/prognosis, mortality, patient satisfaction, quality of life, degree of dependence, disability, complications, functional status, health status perception (symptom recognition, etc).
- Terms used to assess outcomes: (a) efficacy, (b) effectiveness, (c) efficiency–cost–benefit ratio.
- *Outcomes measures*—criteria: (a) clear quantification, (b) easy definition, ascertainment/diagnosis, (c) standardization, (d) comparability of the population at risk (treatment population vs. control population), (e) reflection of outcome endpoint with the specific research question.

Epidemiology, the science of disease detection, has evolved from exposure–disease association to the application of molecular biologic tools to the understanding of early changes in the course of exposure and disease. This transition presents better opportunities for our understanding of disease at the population level, thus allowing the social phenomena used to describe disease to have a biologic basis as well. A very interesting opportunity in using this tool is our ability to determine subpopulations' predisposition to disease. For example, if IgE concentration, on average, is higher among African Americans, this subpopulation may be more predisposed to asthma or type-I hypersensitivity reaction (Figure 13.3).

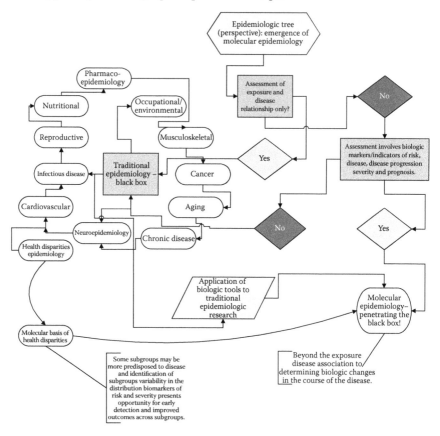

Figure 13.3 Perspectives in epidemiology (epidemiologic tree/taxonomy).

13.7.2   *Epidemiology: Future challenges and opportunities*

Of all disciplines involved in research initiatives and scientific evidence discovery, epidemiology has the broadest scope and expanded focus. This position in research taxonomy places epidemiology in a leadership position. While epidemiology assesses the distribution and determinants of events of interest, including disease, disabilities, injuries, and natural disasters, at a population level, this role has become complex due to exponential technological advances in data sources and gathering system. Because of these hyperdense data, implying complex modeling of causation, epidemiology is challenged with meaningful collaboration with other disciplines. Among other fields, epidemiology needs to collaborate with clinical and biomedical researchers using innovative approach to data processing and analysis for reliable evidence discovery. Within this framework of collaboration is the "3Ts" concept, namely, Team Science, Translational Research, and Transdisciplinary Research.[1]

There is, in this complex model initiative for causation, an inherent opportunity for epidemiology to lead in design, data collection, and processing as well as proper statistical modeling of these hyperdense data. Clinical and biomedical research by involving epidemiology in screening, diagnostic, and therapeutic research stand to benefit from reliable evidence discovery that will ultimately result in patient care improvement. Systems science creates another opportunity for epidemiologist to collaborate and go beyond the simple models of disease- or health-related events causation to complex ecologic explanatory models.[2] Such models result in understanding of biologic, genetic, social, and behavioral determinants of disease at the population level.

The epidemiologic challenge in team science environment creation is obvious. To create an effective team science environment, epidemiology must redefine its leadership in peer mentoring. This approach requires the collective achievement of the team's goals and objectives. Without such approach, the performance of the team remains to be compromised, resulting in impaired outcomes. Such an impaired outcome reflects poor/invalid and unreliable research findings, flawed methodology, and inability to translate or apply the research findings in improve patient and population health. Specifically, epidemiologic leadership in team science must involve the development and maintenance of team climate, team cohesion, team composition, and professional team development.

BOX 13.6   CHALLENGES OF EPIDEMIOLOGY AND RESEARCH DESIGN INNOVATION

- *Big data, hyperdense data, legacy data*—Large population data with genetics, biotechnology, population-based data with novel variables need to be handled with innovative design and analytic method.[13]
- *mHealth data source*—Use of mobile devise to gather data on health issues from specific populations. While exciting approach to rapid data collection, sampling remains a main concern to inference and causation.
- *Social media data source*: Data from Facebook and other social media are in current use and provide the opportunity for "real time" data processing and rapid analysis. However, sampling issues limits the inference from these data, requiring caution.
- *Transdisciplinary research*—Epidemiologic collaboration with social/behavioral scientists, computational biologists, biotechnologists, geneticists, bioinformatics, and clinical medicine remains a meaningful and useful approach to the understanding of the complex etiology of disease and causal inference.

- *Team research*—Epidemiology remains in the frontline of research sciences but given the advances in technology requires a team effort to reliable evidence discovery.
- *Translational research*—Addressing diagnostics, therapeutics and prevention requires the flow of information from the laboratory to the clinic and community/population.[1,2]
- *Systems science*—Collaboration among disciplines to solve a complex health issues require approaching disease etiology from a complex ecologic model. Systems science provides the opportunity for the development of complex explanatory as well as descriptive model.[14]
- *Health disparities*—The complex interplay of health disparities indicators, namely, race, ethnicity, sex, disability, substance abuse, obesity/overweight in incidence, prevalence, and mortality, requires the development and application of health disparities measures in understanding the etio-pathogenesis of the persisting differences in sub-population health.
- *Research design, data collection, and analytic methods*: Innovation in data collection, processing and analysis, as well as complex and ecologic modeling of causation.
- *Health and healthcare policy*: Data-driven policy is necessary in improving population health and narrowing health disparities. Epidemiology needs to influence policy formulation and implementation with reliable evidence on health (incidence, prevalence) and health outcomes assessments.

13.8 Summary

Epidemiology can be viewed as the basic science of public health concerned with disease detection (distribution and determinants) at the population level and the use of the findings from such detection initiatives for the control and prevention of diseases and health-related events at the population level. Epidemiologic research must continue to elucidate the causes of diseases and "mortagenics" (factors predisposing to mortality). While success in medicine has been attributed to advances in diagnostics and therapeutics, much of the gains during the past decades in life expectancy have been brought about by the contributions of epidemiology and public health. However, cases of CDs remain largely unknown, and we need large, prospective population-based studies to determine the influence of genetic, behavioral, social, economic, and environmental exposures on health outcomes over the lifespan. Further, more research is needed to identify the specific social, socioeconomic, cultural, or environmental factors that influence health behaviors, such as exercise and healthy diets.

Epidemiologic research, since it involves humans, remains complex. Epidemiologic investigations begin with an attempt to assess the association between exposure (risk factor) and outcome (disease). This effort or exercise in measurement requires a feasible design and appropriate analytic process for evidence discovery. Therefore, standard and reliable epidemiologic evidence is possible in all aspects of epidemiology provided the attempt is made to identify, assess, and control for confounding; interpret the influence of effect measure modifiers and intermediates; minimize bias; and quantify random error.

Epidemiology as a discipline is challenged with "big data" research that requires innovation in research design and statistical modeling beyond the traditional individual researcher's strategy to discovery. In addressing these complex data, thanks to advances in technology, epidemiology requires systems science approach to evidence discovery as well as transdisciplinary, team science, and translational research collaboration. There is an opportunity, given the brood scope of epidemiology, to assume leadership in design process as well as statistical modeling of these large data for meaningful evidence discovery in improving screening, diagnostics, therapeutics, and preventive health modalities (Figure 13.4).

Questions for discussion

1 Discuss the importance of epidemiology in the control and prevention of CD.
2 What would you consider to be the contributions of molecular epidemiology to our understanding of disease determinants?
3 Differentiate between social and biologic risk factors in cardiovascular diseases.
4 Does epidemiology play a role in health policy formulation and implication?
5 Epidemiologists are essentially concerned with disease-factor determination for disease prevention, while a clinician's role is to treat disease. Discuss the role of a clinician in the prevention of health complications and in health maintenance.
6 Risk assessment is important in estimating risk factors in situations in which they cannot be measured or observed directly, either because the risks are too low, population size is fairly small, or exposure does not occur in isolation from other hazardous materials or exposure. As an environmental epidemiologist, which design could be used to quantify the risks for environmentally induced acute lymphocytic leukemia in children? In this design, utilize the steps in risk assessment.
7 Discuss team science and the potential application of this approach in improving research findings and translation to improve patient and population health.
8 Socio-epigenomics requires an effective team science climate. Discuss the role of health disparities and social epidemiologist in developing and nurturing such climate.

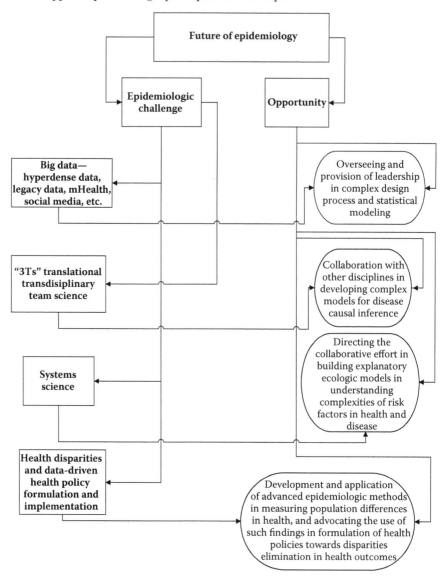

Figure 13.4 Challenges and opportunity of epidemiology.

References

1. B. C. Drolet and N. M. Lorenzi, "Translational Research: Understanding the Continuum from Bench to Bedside," *Transl Res* 157 (2011): 1–5. doi: 10.1016/j .trsl.2010.10.002.
2. R. A. Hiatt, "The Social Determinants of Cancer: A Challenge of Transdisciplinary Science," *Am J Prev Med* 35 (2) 2008: S141–S150.
3. J. M. Last, "Clinical Epidemiology," *J Public Health Policy* 9 (1988): 159–163.
4. K. J. Rothman, *Epidemiology: An Introduction* (New York, Oxford University Press, 2002).
5. J. M. Last, *A Dictionary of Epidemiology* (New York: Oxford University Press, 1995).
6. A. Hall, "What Is Molecular Epidemiology?" (Editorial) *Trop Med Int Health* 1 (1996): 407–408.
7. A. J. McMichael, Invited Commentary—"Molecular Epidemiology": New Pathway or New Travelling Companion?" *Am J Epidemiol* 140 (1994): 1–11.
8. L. S. Tompkins, "Molecular Epidemiology: Development and Application of Molecular Methods to Solve Infectious Disease Mysteries," in V. L. Miller, J. B. Kaper, D. A. Portnoy et al., eds., *Molecular Genetics of Bacterial Pathogenesis: A Tribute to Stanley Falkow, Part 1, Retrospective Look at Early Advances* (Washington DC: American Society for Microbiology, 1994): 63–73.
9. O. Shpilberg, J. S. Dorman, R. E. Ferrell et al., "The Next Stage: Molecular Epidemiology?" *J Clin Epidemiol* 50 (1997): 633–638.
10. P. A. Schulte and F. P. Perera, eds., *Molecular Epidemiology: Principles and Practices* (San Diego, CA: Academic Press, 1993).
11. Australian Institute of Health and Welfare (2012). Risk Factors Contributing to Chronic Disease. Available at: http://www.health.gov.au/internet/main/publishing .nsf/content/chronic (accessed 10/3/2016).
12. S. H. Woolf, R. E. Johnson, R. L. Phillips, Jr., and M. Philipsen, "Giving Everyone the Health of the Educated: An Examination of Whether Social Change Would Save More Lives than Medical Advances," *Am J Public Health* 97 (2007): 679–683.
13. American College of Epidemiology (2012). Promoting Innovation. Available at: http://acepidemiology.org/sites/default/files/Promoting%20Innovation%20in%20 Epidemiology%20August%203%202012%20REPORT.pdf (accessed 6/12/2013).
14. NIH, Office of Behavioral and Social Sciences Research. Methodology: Sytems Science. Available at: http://obssr.od.nih.gov/scientific_areas/methodology/systems _science/index.aspx (accessed: 9/12/2013).

14 Health and healthcare policies
Role of epidemiology

14.1 Introduction

The implication of science or scientific findings in decision-making involving the overall operations in the human society remains vital to the success and growth of civilized societies. By using the data from science as cumulative knowledge and evidence, policy formulation can benefit greatly in enhancing the success of policies in improving human life and health. Specifically, policies to improve human health must be contingent on scientific evidence derived from epidemiologic investigations with translational research focus (bench-bedside-population).

Epidemiology is not a mere scientific discipline but a professional practice area, and like biostatistics, it is an information science that operates within a complex system, given human complexities and biodiversity. As a purposive science, epidemiology generates data through investigation, analysis, and interpretation in order to improve population health. Since human population is not a mere integration of molecules and cells but beings of intent and spiritual dimension, epidemiologic investigations and the data generated therein are used in decision-making in improving healthcare, individual health, and population health. We can conceptualize the role of epidemiology in policy making by considering hypothetical public health issues, for example, e-cigarettes and lung carcinoma among youths. Basically, epidemiologic investigation on the association and causal association is conducted to provide the information for decision-making toward incidence risk and mortality reduction, and action is taken by formulating public health policy to reduce risk and mortality by 10% by year 2035. Next, the epidemiologic method is used to design an intervention (education and awareness intervention on e-cigarette risk) and examine the inference and provide intervention evaluation (process, impact and outcome). Specifically, epidemiology is relevant in public policy formulation that influences public health and patient or individual health by generating the information required in decision-making for the assurance of essential public health services, optimal population health, and healthcare management (efficacy of care, compliance, quality assurance, training, planning and programming).

While the fundamental role of epidemiology in public health remains that of the assessment of the health and related-health problems and the use of the observed data to map intervention in improving population health, health and public health policies formulation require valid and reliable data. Epidemiologic findings provide such basis for practical and reliable health policies in addressing public health policies in the ever-changing human and animal populations (Figure 14.1).

The formulation of healthcare policies requires an opportunity to improve care at the patient level. Such opportunity emerges from the clinical observations of impaired, different, or unexpected outcomes that have been observed over time as well as the need to effect changes in screening, diagnostics, prognosis, and follow-up of patients. Public health policy on the other hand results from the emergence of disease or health-related events that is epidemic, endemic, and pandemic in nature. In effect, given that public health is what we do as a society to remain healthy, there is an overlap between public health and healthcare policy. However, while public health policy formulation comes from the governmental or public policy arena, healthcare policies often involve healthcare leaders and the elected officials. Consequently, the effectiveness of these policies involves knowledge of the anticipated intervention or proposed change which must be data driven, and epidemiology plays a significant role in the generation of such information for consideration by policy makers prior to health policy formulation.

What is policy, and how is public policy related to health policy? Policy had been described as the law, administrative action, regulations, or procedure utilized by government or other institutions (http://www.cdc.gov/stltpublichealth /policy/). In ensuring optimal health for all, the Centers for Disease Control and Prevention (CDC) provides guidelines and recommendations for consideration

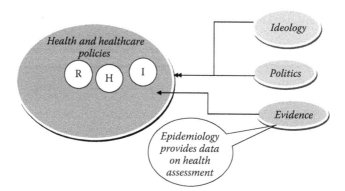

Figure 14.1 **Basis of healthcare policy.** Evidence is important in the development and implementation of health and healthcare policies. Examples of polices driven epidemiology are readmission (R), hospitalization (H), and immunization (I).

by the elected officials in health and public health policy development. Public health policies are regulations by governmental agencies toward health promotions and disease control. For example, school meal policies ensure that our children are provided with a healthy diet to reduce the obesity epidemic and its health effects. Additionally, regulations to prohibit smoking at restaurants, hospitals, health departments, schools, and public buildings are in place to enhance lung functions in reducing the incidence and mortality from lung diseases, chronic obstructive pulmonary disease, emphysema, and other related cardiopulmonary conditions. Policy remains a complex process and may involve time prior to its implementation and evaluation.

The basis of policy is ideology, value, politics, and evidence. Since the contribution of epidemiology in health policy development resides in the evidence basis of policy, epidemiologic investigation per se is insufficient in health policy formulation. However, for epidemiology to be purposive and hence consequential, policy statements in improving population health requires proactive approach. Additionally, epidemiology plays an active role in policy analysis, which is the evaluation of existing policy to determine whether or not such policies are effective in addressing a particular health problem. For example, the National Institutes of Health (NIH) in 2014 announced a proposal for policy evaluation on health disparities. Such announcement required applicants to provide a search strategy for health disparity policy analysis at the state level with respect to policies implemented in the past that has resulted in increased or decrease in health disparities.

While epidemiology plays an important investigative, analysis, and inferential role in healthcare and public health policy development and implementation, there are limits to its scientific jurisdiction. The reflection on these limits and epidemiologic accountability and scrutiny therefore serve the basis of this chapter. This chapter attempts to present a simplified notion of policy as regulatory governmental or organizational statement for actions, healthcare and public health policy as similar regulations but geared toward optimal health for individuals and the public, epidemiologic process and role in health policy development, and the future direction of epidemiology as purposive and information science in health and public health policy development in the face of limited heath resource in nation with high cost of care albeit low quality of care and preventive health services. We surmise that policies to reduce health and healthcare disparities across diverse patients and subpopulations have potentials in optimizing quality of care while lowering healthcare cost in the nation.

14.2   Health policy

While policy refers to sets of principles guiding decision-making, health policy reflects the application sets of principles in decision-making involving healthcare and population health improvement. Health policy has been described the effort taken through plans and actions to achieve specific health care goals.[1] So characterized, health policies allow for the identification of the societal health issues, set baseline for improvement, and allocate the resources for intervention and evaluation to meet the target. A broad description of health policy considers actions taken by the governmental agencies such as the CDC, Department of Health & Human Services, and Office of Minority Health to improve the health of the public. This obligation to improve the health of the population via governmental action is ensured by the US Constitution. The Affordable Care Act 2012 reflects governmental action to improve the health of all Americans by rendering healthcare value care, implying optimal quality care while lowering cost.

The decision-making by the government to advance the health of the public in a certain direction must be driven in larger part by information. Epidemiology remains an information science, and with its affiliated disciple, biostatistics is required for the investigation of the health, disease, or health-related events for an informed health policy.

14.3   Evidence-based epidemiology and "big data" practice

What is evidence-based epidemiology (EBE)? Epidemiology is an information science, implying its role to investigate, analyze, and provide inference on health and related health issues at the specific population level. Additionally, given its purposive nature, observed inference is required for the purpose of controlling disease and promoting health of the public.

The notion of EBE is derived from evidence-based medicine, which requires the guidelines of practice or care that is based on reliable and valid data including though not limited to similar studies replication, quantitative systematic review and quantitative evidence synthesis (QES). Epidemiology being an integrative science requires transdisciplinary and translational approaches in arriving at EBE.

As more "big data" concept emerges, clinical decision-making will no longer depend on assessment of one's patient or small practice data. Decision-making in clinical medicine will depend on the assessment of millions of cases across several practices, implying data sharing for "big data" clinical decision-making. Such approach will enable physicians and clinicians to assess value care, implying cost effectiveness, and value care in determining quality, outcome, and cost. The availability of big data initiative is indicative of the feasibility of comparing cost of procedure such as hip replacement surgery or spinal fusion for curve deformities correction across, cites, regions, and states. Despite the perceived gain of big data approach in clinical decision-making regarding patient care, caution must be exercised in the midst of this optimism, implying the reliance of evidence on effect size and not statistical significance since large sample data are prone to lower probability value (statistically significant finding), even when the effect size is clinically irrelevant.

14.4 Health policy formulation: Evidence, politics, and ideology

An effective policy formulation requires the logical progression involving the quantification of the burden of illness, through identifying its likely causes, to validating interventions that prevent or ameliorate it and evaluating their efficiency, to monitoring the application of these interventions and coming full circle to determine whether the burden of illness has been reduced.[2]

The policy cycle involves the assessment of population health, potential interventions, policy choices, policy implementation, and policy evaluation. An approach to policy cycle and policy subsystem describes policy process in five stages, namely, agenda setting, policy formulation, decision-making, policy implementation, and policy evaluation.[3] Policy-making is a formal struggle over ideas, values, and interests, played out by the rhetorical use of language and the enactment of social situations, much more than merely turning evidence into practice. Scientific evidence answers the question "What works?" Policy-making is about "What do we do?" Ostensibly, scientific research is about the objective establishment of facts, implying reliable and valid evidence discovery.[4]

The evidence dimension of policy development involves the assessment of population health, which reflects one of the core functions of public health: assessment, policy, and assurance. Basically, epidemiologic investigation requires the assessment of how, when, and where diseases, injuries, disabilities, and health-related events are distributed at the specific population levels (person, place, and time). By assessing the distribution of disease at the population level, epidemiology examines the trends and patterns of disease distribution and the health needs of the population while prioritizing these needs for policy formulation to address these health issues. In addition to needs assessment and patterns identification, epidemiologic investigations are utilized in assessing the risk factors, thus uncovering the determinants of the observed health needs based on the descriptive epidemiologic approach. For example, most policies regarding smoking cessation and health outcomes such as bronchial carcinoma are based on the association studies on cigarette smoking and lung cancer.[5]

Epidemiology is useful in assessing potential intervention through the analysis of the effectiveness of the current or existing health policies in addressing public health issues as well as healthcare. Basically, this function is achieved by identifying potential policy interventions, provide synthesis on existing knowledge with respect to their effectiveness, provide new data on beneficial intervention policies, and determine the potential of the proven polices in improving population within similar population dynamics context.

In terms of policy selection, epidemiology is useful in projecting or predicting the impact of potential interventions on population health, which could be achieved through computer simulation of different interventions as well as facilitating the process of consensus development (social epidemiology).

Epidemiology is beneficial in the direction of policy implementation by assisting in establishing targets for the selected policies and providing data on needs-based resource allocation for personal health services. Further, epidemiology can assist and provide guidance on the development of information systems to enhance the intervention. The evaluation of the implemented policy requires an epidemiologic investigation. This aspect is accomplished by assessing process, impact outcomes of the policy, and monitoring the direction of public health within the context and dimension of the policy.

Epidemiology has a broader role today, including, although not limited to, developing, forming, and implementing policy; addressing disease distribution (traditional role); facilitating studies on disease determinants at population level toward data generation; mapping intervention; and assessing social and economic determinants of health, health and disease risk variables modeling, healthography with geographic information system (GIS), ecologic and multilevel modeling, population dynamics, big data, transdisciplinary, translational, team, and implementation science approaches to evidence discovery.

Holmes L et al. used the data from the National Survey of Children's Health (NSCH)[6] to examine the prevalence and predisposition to the leading cause of chronic morbidity in children in the United States, namely oral health as dental disorders (DD). The NSCH is a representative sample of U.S. noninstitutionalized children, $n = 95,766$ (2011/2012). With the available data (public access use) and interactive query online (http://childhealthdata .org), the prevalence of DD (one or more than one oral health problems) was estimated at 18.7%, 95% CI, 18.1–19.4, and varied by race/ethnicity, and was highest among Hispanics (24.9, 95% CI, 23.1–26.7), and among Blacks, non-Hispanic (22.8%, 95% CI, 21.1–24.5), intermediate among other, non-Hispanic (18.9, 95% CI, and lowest among White, non-Hispanic (14.9 95% CI, 14.3–15). The data further observed geographic (state/region) variability in DD prevalence but comparable racial/ethnic patterns observed in the nationwide findings. The DD prevalence in mid-west, namely Wisconsin indicated the prevalence to be highest among Hispanics, 24.4% (95%, CI, 14.7–34.2), and other, non-Hispanic, 22.7% (95% CI, 12.2–33.2) and intermediate among Black, non-Hispanic, 20.0% (95% CI, 9.9–30.1), and lowest among White non-Hispanic, 12.7%, 95% CI, 10.1–15.3.

With the same data, the investigators examined the association between diabetes and DD, and observed a clinically and biologically relevant as well as a statistically significant association between diabetes and children dental disorders. Investigators used a "big data" reduction-based cross-sectional design termed hybrid cross-sectional as *"atypical case-noncase"* design (Figure 14.2). This design differs from traditional cross-sectional and traditional case-control. As a variant of cross-sectional, it examines both the exposure (diabetes) and outcome (dental disorder) simultaneously (snap shot) but utilizes systematic random sampling to obtain an unbiased sample from the noncase sample from the "big data" (Figure 14.3). Since the sample size for those without the outcome of interest is very large, this design sampled to reduce the "big data" to efficient sample for the noncases

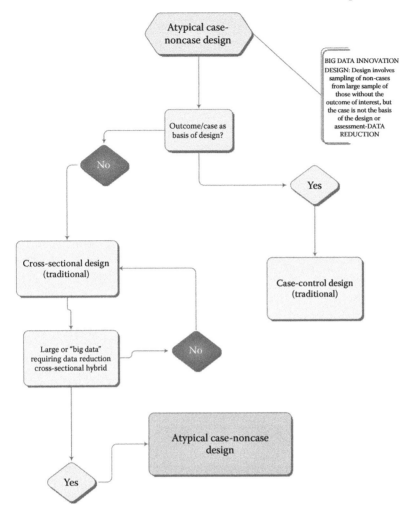

Figure 14.2 **Atypical Case–nonCase Design.** A nonexperimental design that enables efficiency of comparing events of interest in the era of "big data."

(children without diabetes) to be compared with cases (children with diabetes) with respect to the predictor or exposure of interest (dental disorders). Further, the design differs from the traditional case-control since the exposure and outcome are assessed simultaneously despite the sampling of required sample size of noncases from the large sample of noncases—"big data" reduction.

Rational policies formulation in public health requires scientific evidence based on studies replication as well as different geograpic settings and samples. Figure 14.4 is illustrative of the need for policy development and implementation in addressing dental disorders among the minorities, mainly Hispanics and non-Hispanic Blacks.

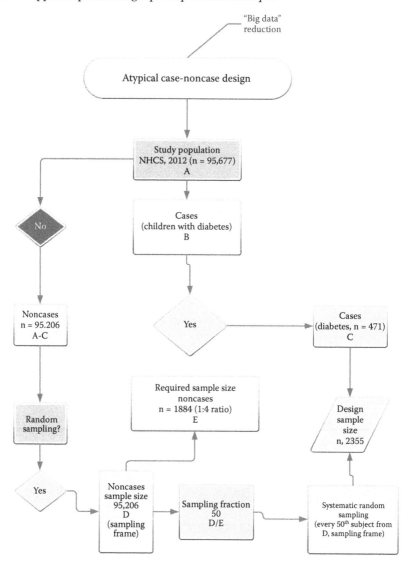

Figure 14.3 Atypical case-noncase design—sampling procedure.

Specifically compared to children without diabetes (*n* = 1884) based on systematic random sampling of 1 (cases):4 (noncases), those diagnosed with diabetes (*n* = 471) were 25% more likely to develop DD, prevalence risk ratio (PRR) = 1.25, 95% CI, 1.19–1.28, *p* < 0.001. Further racial heterogeneity was observed in this association.

The above scientific evidence presents the window of opportunity for policy formulation in addressing racial/ethnic disparities in DD among children

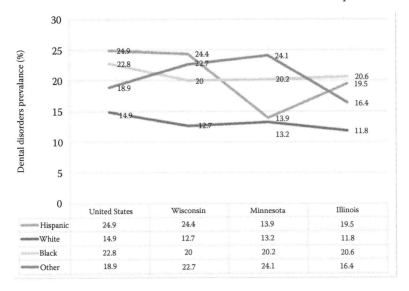

Figure 14.4 Geo-racial/ethnic prevalence of children's dental disorders. (NHCS, 2012.)

in the United States. In addition, the higher prevalence of this condition, rendering it the most prevalence chronic disease among children relative to childhood asthma, signals an urgent need for health and healthcare policy in this direction.

14.5 Decision-making (policy): Legislation, budget and resources allocation, and jurisdiction of agencies

Epidemiologic investigations are expected to be the corner stone of health, healthcare, and public health policies. This role involves the utilization of descriptive and analytic epidemiologic data in setting the agenda for policy formulation in improving individual and population level health issues.

Whereas policy development involves many dimensions, namely, ideology, politics, values, and evidence, epidemiology plays a specific role in evidence generation in guiding the basis of policy development and formulation. For epidemiology to be beneficial in policy development, it must play a fundamental role in policy analysis in the best interest of future of population health. And for policy development given its information science role, it must provide reliable and valid evidence for the legislative agenda regarding population health improvement. While a consequentialist epidemiologist would concede that epidemiology is deontological today, one argues that epidemiology not being a discipline per se but professional approach to health, healthcare, and public health improvement benefits from a mixed-model approach to health issue resolution, namely, consequentialism and deontological perspectives.

In meeting the requirements of epidemiology in health and healthcare policy formulation, there is a need to place emphasis on studies that will eventually result in causal inference. The role of epidemiology in policy development goes beyond disease exposure or risk factor association to causal inference. Policy development requires EBE and stresses the need for study replication and quantitative systematic review, including, although not limited to, meta-analysis and QES. While ecologic studies provide substantial information that may lead to hypothesis generation to address individual-level risk, for epidemiologic data to support policy developments, we need individual-level risk studies.

Cost-effectiveness analysis is necessary when it comes to budget and resource allocation. As a team science, the collaboration of epidemiologists with other disciplines, mainly economist, demographers, and statisticians, enhances evidence in budget analysis and interpretation as well as in the allocation of budget.

While there is an obvious role of epidemiology in policy formulation, this role is limited given other factors from politics, ideology, and competing values. The trends toward impaired health policy formulation stems from different backgrounds of policy-makers, different values, different time scales, and lack of credibility. While epidemiology assumes responsibility with the evidence needed for policy development and formulation, these other elements limit its pragmatic participation. But given the lack of credibility from policy makers on epidemiologic findings, data for policy formulation must be evidence based. With this scrutiny, epidemiology must be integrative and accountable toward accurate and reliable data concerning population health improvement.

14.6   Decision-making (management): Effectiveness, efficacy, training, planning, compliance, quality assurance, programming

Healthcare policies reflect the use of information in developing policies in improving the health of our patients. What role does epidemiology play in this vein? Consider the observation of a higher rate of surgical site infection (SSI) in a comprehensive pediatric tertiary hospital that resulted in increased length of stay and readmission. Is there a requirement for any form of policy to change the protocol? Consider a hypothetical study conducted to assess the determinants or risk of SSI. Using the electronic medical records, authors collected information from 246 patients, of whom 66 have SSI. The type of diagnosis, time to antibiotic administration, postoperative antibiotics received, antibiotic sensitivity, sex, body weight, age, previous SSI, type of surgery received, and duration of surgery were assessed for potential risk factors. If authors found a 65% increased risk of SSI comparing those with shorter (<30 minutes) and longer (>30 minutes) time to the administration of antibiotics, should there be a new policy if there was already one in place, and if there was no policy in this direction, should policy be developed to improve the rate of SSI?

Healthcare policy formulation involves the assessment of the effectiveness and efficacy of treatment modalities in recommending better treatment options as well as lowering cost in such recommendations. With the example from SSI, policy or protocol needs to be developed based on the epidemiologic data at the clinic setting to reduce the antibiotics administration initiation time to <30 minutes from incision. However, the implementation of this new protocol will require the planning and training of attending, residents, and the surgical team. The effectiveness of the new protocol will be assessed with reliable epidemiologic design of prospective nature as well as appropriate sampling, sample size, and statistical power estimations and appropriate statistical model such as logistic regression which is adequate predictive model if the data on SSI measure is on a binary scale. Quality assurance and compliance assessment require baseline data prior to the new protocol implementation. These assessments are conducted with rigorous epidemiologic designs and reliable data gathering techniques to ensure the accuracy quality assurance and compliance to the new protocol.

14.7   Summary

Healthcare and public health policies remain organizational and governmental actions to improve individual and population health, respectively. The formulation of these policies requires process involving significant stages, namely, agenda setting, policy formulation, implementation, and evaluation. While health policy involves evidence, implying the role of epidemiology in providing the necessary data on population health needs and risk variables, ideology, politics, and values remain major determinants of health and healthcare policies.

EBE, which is causal inference as reflected in study replication, magnitude of effect and biologic gradient (dose-response) and the analysis of analysis (meta-analysis and QES) are sources of reliable and valid data for evidence-based or data-driven policy health policy. Epidemiology plays a significant role as information, integrative, and purposive science in policy formulation. Additionally, epidemiology is concerned with policy analysis that involves the assessment of the effectiveness of health policy through its process, impact, and outcomes on population health.

Epidemiology also plays a role in healthcare policies by providing the design, analysis, and interpretation of data on effectiveness, quality assurance, planning, training, and compliance in the healthcare setting. Specifically, any change in protocol pertaining to patient care requires a quantitative assessment in providing the baseline data and the subsequent postintervention data for protocol evaluation.

Questions for discussion

1   The NIH request for proposal called for the analysis of policy that had impact on decreasing or increasing health disparities at a state level. What approach could be used in addressing this request? What are the relevant data sources that will enable such analysis?

2   Epidemiology is an information and purposive science. Discuss these notions of epidemiology with special reference to health and healthcare policy formulation. What are the obstacles to data-driven policy development?

3   Health and healthcare policy involves certain stages including formulation and evaluation. Discuss the role of epidemiology in policy evaluation.

4   Suppose you are a chair of a department within a healthcare setting and you are required to implement a new protocol for the prevention of postoperative pancreatitis following spinal fusion. Discuss the approach to achieve such initiative.

5   Differentiate among policy, healthcare, and public health policy. Does epidemiology play a role in individual-level policy formulation? Should epidemiology enhance policy formulation by influencing politics, ideology, and values?

6.   What is "big data" reduction? Describe atypical case-noncase non-experimental epidemiologic design and comment on the reliability of applying evidence from this design in developing health policies.

References

1. WHO (2015). Available at: http://www.who.int/topics/health_policy/en/ (accessed 8/5/2015).
2. P. Tugwell, K. J. Bennett, D. L. Sackett, R. B. Haynes, "The Measurement Iterative Loop: A Framework for the Critical Appraisal of Need, Benefits and Costs of Health Interventions," *J Chronic Dis* 38 (4) (1985): 339–351.
3. M. Howlett and M. Ramesh M, *Studying Public Policy: Policy Cycles and Policy Subsystems* (Toronto: Oxford University Press, 1995).
4. J. Russell, T. Greenhalgh, E. Byrne, and J. McDonnell, "Recognizing Rhetoric in Health Care Policy Analysis," *J Health Serv Res Policy* 13 (1) (2008): 40–46.
5. R. Doll and A. B. Hill, "Smoking and Carcinoma of the Lung; Preliminary Report," *Br Med J* 2 (4682) (1950): 739–748.
6. NHCS (2016). Available at: http//childhealthdata.org/ (accessed 6/1/2017).

15 Consequentialist epidemiology and translational research implication

15.1 Introduction

Epidemiology, strictly speaking, is not a discipline but a profession that evolves around information science, systems science, transdisciplinary, team science, and translational approaches. With this notion, epidemiology is purposive, accountable, and informative. The purpose of epidemiology is to assess the distribution and determinants of diseases, injuries, disabilities, and disease-related event at the population level and the application of this knowledge in mapping and implementing intervention to improve population health. Epidemiology further plays an important role in utilizing its findings that are expected to be complete and unequivocal in enhancing the understanding of complex disease etiology and process for disease prevention and treatment, this benefiting public health and clinical medicine, respectively. In this dimension, epidemiologic studies should gear toward a translational approach in assessing causal relationships between exposure and control and the utilization of that knowledge acquired from bench (molecular epidemiology), bedside (clinical epidemiology), and community (population epidemiology) in transforming human health and therapeutics through translational epidemiology that is consequential.

In meeting the extended notion of the purpose of epidemiology, improvements of population health, some epidemiologists have expressed the need to render epidemiology aw consequentialist science. While disease control and health promotion remains the goal of public health, epidemiology as the basic science of public health is challenged by providing reliable and valid evidence required in the formulation and implementation of health and public health policies in improving population health. While recognizing this amplified function of epidemiology in information provision toward policy formulation and intervention mapping, epidemiologic methods remain rigorous and robust in study design, data collection, model specification and analysis, and interpretation as well as appropriate inference.

The mixture of deontological and consequentialist approach or pathways appears to appeal to the current destiny of epidemiology. This chapter explains the traditional notion of these two philosophical theories and their applications in epidemiologic methods. Additionally, epidemiology is presented as a profession and not an exact science, implying integrative approach to addressing population health.

Clinicians and medical researchers as consumers of epidemiologic should critically appraise the methods used to arrive at the inference. Simply, accountable epidemiology requires both internal and external validity of studies prior to policy formulation and intervention mapping. Such pathways involve alternative explanation to the observed data or findings, mainly systematic error, confounding, random error, and effect measure modifier. Furthermore, in the era of evidence-based epidemiology, inconsistent findings could be addressed by appropriate designs to assess evidence accumulation through systematic review and quantitative evidence synthesis.

15.2 Consequentialist science

Is epidemiology a consequential discipline? An important role of epidemiology is to provide vital information for the development of health-related policies, as well as disease interventions and risk factors reduction. Consequently, the findings from epidemiologic studies remain relevant in health policies, clinical guidelines, and disease control at clinical and population levels. However, these significant applications do not lead to the marginalization of the primary role of epidemiology as a unique discipline concerned with the assessment of the distribution and determinants of disease, disabilities, injuries, physiologic states (pregnancy, child growth and development), and health-related event at a specific population level. Additionally, the application of these findings in developing and implementation of intervention remains extended and collaborative function or role of epidemiology.

Epidemiology had been characterized as the investigation of the various external or physical agencies and the different conditions of life that favor their development or influence their character and the sanitary and hygienic measures best fitted to check, mitigate, or prevent them.[1] This nineteenth century description of epidemiology places intervention responsivities to epidemiologist in clinical and public health settings. With this accountability, does epidemiologic investigation become consequentialist?

Consequentialism is a philosophical trend that gears scientific thinking towards the maximization of desired outcomes.[2] We can examine epidemiologic investigations at clinical and public health settings in determining whether the current trends in epidemiology warrant the label "consequentialist discipline or science." A study conducted on cerebral palsies deaths among children assessed proportionate mortality, deceased patient characteristics, and comorbidities that may be related to children discovered dead during sleep (DDDS) between 1993 and 2011.[3] The authors observed that all but 1 (18/19) had respiratory disorders, seizure, and gastrointestinal feeding tubes and were nonambulatory. With the descriptive nature of the retrospective study (case only), the authors suggested further studies in this perspective to further understanding what types of monitoring and surveillance are required to prevent such unexplained deaths and prolong survival of these patients. This example aims at understanding, although descriptively, the determinants of the DDDS phenomenon in this specific population, with the intent to utilize such knowledge in intervention to optimize survival of children with cerebral palsies in this setting. Subsequently, epidemiologic investigation without doubt as illustrated in this simple example reflects some attributes of a consequentialist discipline.

Another example involves a study performed to examine the potential contributions of comorbidities and other predisposing factors in the development of postoperative pancreatitis after spinal fusion in cerebral palsy children with curve deformities.[4] The authors retrospectively examined 355 patients, of whom 109 had postoperative pancreatitis (30.1%). Identified as predisposing factors were gastroesophageal reflux with feeding difficulties (adjusted risk ratio [ARR], 1.52; 95% confidence interval [CI], 1.01–2.29) and reactive airway diseases (ARR, 1.49; 95% CI, 1.10–2.04). Based on these findings, the authors cautioned clinicians to be aware of these comorbidities in postoperative pancreatitis predisposition in cerebral palsy patients undergoing spinal fusion. This example illustrates how epidemiologic findings could be used to develop clinical guidelines given the accumulation of evidence in the same direction.

For the medical care professionals, epidemiologic methods serve to improve the outcomes of care to benefit the patient as a member of the targeted population of care. While this obligation is an essential component of epidemiology in this unique context, rigorous methodologic approach with appropriate random sample to minimize random error, cases, and control selection to minimize selection and information biases, as well as addressing and controlling for confounding are very significant considerations in such conducts.

Because of the vital functions of epidemiology in clinical research, consequentialist epidemiology implies the transformation of the traditional function of epidemiology as merely an assessment science to the active role in intervention mapping and conduct based on epidemiologic findings. Consequentialist pathway includes, although not limited to, the following:

1 Study conceptualization in identifying the underlying risks and predisposing factors to disease, injury, disability and health-related events
2 Design and conduct of studies to assess the health and health-related events
3 Utilization of rigorous and appropriate statistical tool to obtain evidence from the collected and processed data
4 Data interpretation and intervention recommendation
5 Intervention mapping and implementation
6 Health promotion practices recommendations and disease and health-related events incidence and prevalence reduction

With these pathways or steps, consequentialist epidemiology supplements the traditional epidemiologic notion of assessing the distribution and determinants of diseases, injures, and disabilities at the population level to providing the direction on how such data should be used in planning, mapping, and conducting intervention to improve population health.

15.3   Incomplete and inconsistent clinical findings

Clinical research utilizing nonexperimental and experimental designs (clinical trial) present with conflicting findings that may be due to several factors. A classic example is the implication of sodium in hypertension. In spite of the preclinical or basic sciences consistent direct data on the direct correlation between sodium and elevated blood pressure (BP), epidemiologic studies at the community and clinical settings continue to demonstrate inconsistent findings. A significant amount of studies have implicated sodium in hypertension (references), while others have not (references).

Why are there inconsistent findings in clinical research? To address this question, suppose we sample 10 patients from the patient population of 100 with cerebral palsies for average age and systolic BP, then we replace these 10 and sample another 10, and repeat this process until we obtain five samples, how likely are we to have the same mean age or systolic BP? This simple illustration is indicative of how sampling variability and nonrepresentative sample could result in inconsistent findings, derailing public health action and well as clinical decision-making and therapeutic guidelines.

Clinical research is often conducted with small samples, which have tendency for elevated sampling error as well as measurement errors. Specifically, the degree upon which measurement errors influence results of studies is indicative of the potentials for inconsistent and conflicting findings. Consequently, consequentialist epidemiology refers in part to sampling approach that requires probability or consecutive sample prior to study conduct as well as an appropriate inference from the sample. Contrary to some consequentialists, applied and pragmatic consequentialist epidemiology requires the utilization of rigorous statistical methodology for evidence discovery. Therefore, within the clinical setting, this approach requires a team and transdisciplinary effort in which epidemiologists, biostatisticians, behavioral scientists, and other disciplines interact meaningfully to create designs and statistical models that fit the research questions and data, interpret the data appropriately, and map interventions based on the inference.

15.4   Consequentialist epidemiology: Methods

The method suggested for epidemiology of consequence involves: (a) definition or characterization of the population of interest, (b) conceptualization and development of measures of exposures and health indicators, (c) sampling with probability consideration the population at risk, (d) estimation of measures of association between exposures and health outcomes of interest, (e) rigorous evaluation of possible causal association, (f) assessment the evidence for causal web, as well as interaction (biologic/statistical), and (h) examination of the extent to which the result matters, is externally valid, to other populations.[5]

The approach by Keyes and Galea[6] in epidemiologic investigation stresses the need for appropriate design, sampling, and reliable analysis of studies.[6] There is also an implication of causal inference in a single epidemiologic investigation. While this suggestion is optimistic, it is difficult to implicate causal association based on one epidemiologic study. In effect, replication of studies with comparable samples and sampling techniques remains the hallmark of causal inference.

15.5   Addressing accountability: Sampling and confounding, adequate modeling

Epidemiology deserves scrutiny if it must exert its role of leadership in the application of clinical and population-based research in improving healthcare, health, and public health. This responsibility requires the application of reliable a valid epidemiologic findings in decision-making regarding changes in clinical and public health and services guidelines.

What is the basis of valid finding, and how could we consistently aim at internal validity? The answer to these questions reflects the extent to which clinical designs should employ designs that are relevant and efficient in providing the best yield for the research question. Often, the inferences drawn from the data are influenced by the design applied in answering the research question.

With the emphasis on internal validity, studies should examine alternative explanations for the observed data, namely, bias, potential confounding and effect measure modifier. Bias minimization is fundamental to study conduct since findings may be biased as a result of measurement errors, information bias, misclassification of exposure, etc. In effect, to enhance the internal validity of a study, epidemiologic principle requires systematic error assessment in the design and conduct phases of the study and the effort to decrease these errors prior to data collection and analysis. Several research findings remain inconclusive due to a small study size, implying random errors (external validity), mixing effect of the third variable or confounding, as well as effect measure modification. Clinical studies should attempt at measurement error reduction, potential confounding assessment, and adjustment prior to the presentation of findings. In effect, given genetic heterogeneity of humans, data must be collected of potential confounding as possible explanation of the observed relationship or effect. Specifically, authors are required to apply the guideline presented previously in this book to assess for the confounding effect and adjust for them at the analysis level with stratification or multivariable model.

Effect measure modification as previously described reflects a situation in which the result of a study, for example, odds ratio (OR), is different across stratum. Consider a study conducted to assess the effect of radiation of the development of second primary thyroid cancer (SPTC) in children. If the OR on the association between radiation therapy received and SPTC is 2.46, 95% CI, 2.00–4.35, and the stratified analysis by race/ethnicity shows, Hispanic, OR = 3.95, non-Hispanic white, OR = 1.85, and non-Hispanic Asians, OR = 2.87, then race/ethnicity remains an OR effect modifier. The accountable and responsible approach to nonmisleading results is to present these findings with race-specific stratum, adjusting for potential confounding as applicable.

Whereas the effect size assessment is fundamental to study appraisal in medicine, clinical research, and population-based research, the generalization of findings beyond the study population or the sample used to generate the data requires the quantification of random error with a probability value termed p value. The alternate to the p value is the precision as measured by the CI, which is a more informative measure of precision. As previously sustained, CI provides information on the margins of error as well as the location of the point estimate within these limits. However, p value merely reflects the arbitrary cut off point of 5% type I error in most medical and clinical research ambience.

It is worthy to note that most studies in clinical medicine do not apply probability sampling technique in the recruitment of study subjects. In such situation, it is difficult to apply a probability value of variables that were not subjected to random selection, implying equal and known probability of the subjects that generate the variables to be included in the study. The exception in the application of p value to a nonprobability sample involves the assessment of consecutive sample and disease registry. These situations reflect representative sample, hence the application of p value.

15.6 Translational epidemiology (TransEpi): Consequential or traditional

Epidemiologic designs and methods had been used to assess laboratory data (T0/T1) for evidence transfer to phases I and II clinical trials and likewise the application of such methods to phases III and IV clinical trials (T2/T4) (Figure 15.1). Clinical research largely applies epidemiologic designs to evidence discovery in enhancing patient care and improving clinical practice guidelines. Epidemiology is challenged by public health and clinical medicine to provide assessment that is adequate and clearly transferable to intervention mapping and implementation.

TransEpi is the attempt to apply epidemiologic methods and principles in enhancing studies conduct from T0 to T5, and the steps in transferring the knowledge gained in a systematic and synthesized manner in improving patient and public health. TransEpi by this characterization is the intersection of all epidemiologic initiatives in improving human health including, though not limited to, applied epidemiology, field epidemiology, occupational/environmental, nutritional, chronic disease, infectious disease, aging, neurology, social/behavioral

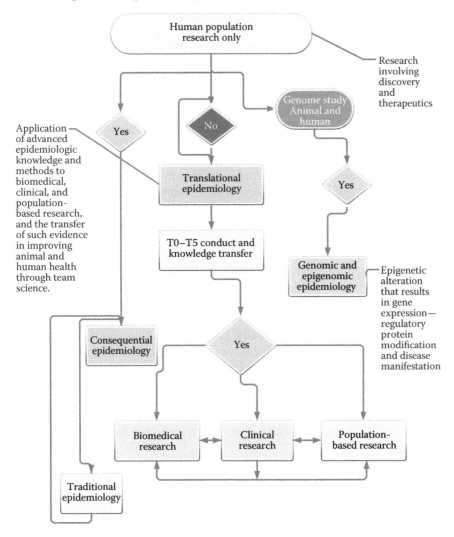

Figure 15.1 **Translational epidemiology—intersection of epidemiologic methods.**
Epidemiologic investigation is complex given environmental and genetic
factors in disease causation. As environmental influences introduce epigenetic (epigenotype) and genetic (genotype) changes in the causal pathway of diseases, translational epidemiology remains a relevant strategy
in the assessment of the role of epidemiology in genomics and epigenetic
research in disease etio-pathogenesis.

epidemiology, clinical epidemiology field epidemiology, and the recent field,
molecular and genetic epidemiology, as well as health outcomes and health
disparities epidemiology. By characterization, TransEpi is the application of
advanced and reliable epidemiologic methods and principles to advance translational research (T0–T5) and the transfer of this knowledge in the improvement

of animal and human health through collective biomedical sciences, clinical medicine, and public health effort (team science). The importance of TransEpi cannot be overemphasized given the complexities in the assessment of risk and protective factors in the pathway of therapeutics. Specifically, in the current era of gene–gene interaction, gene–environment interaction and sociogenomics in disease causations, translational epidemiology is required in assessing these risk factors with respect to incidence rates disease variation, temporal trends, risk ratios, prevalence of genetic risk factors, risk–risk interaction, sensitivity, specificity, and genetic variants' predictive values. TransEpi has a significant contribution to make in phase III randomized controlled trials where knowledge from such fields are transferred for evidence-based recommendation for professional guidelines development. For example, the recommendation of women whose family history is associated with an increased risk for deleterious mutations in BRCA1 or BRCA1 genes for genetic counseling and BRCA testing was based on the breast cancer susceptibility gene mutation testing for and breast cancer testing.[6]

TransEpi signals a departure from the traditional notion of epidemiology that restricts its application to human animals at a population level by facilitating the conduct of studies across all spectra of human health, implying bench to bedside and the populations. The growth of this field is needed more now than ever before in training of basic scientists, clinicians, and public health researchers. With such training and application, clinical medicine and public health are better strategized in transferring reliable and accurate data for advancement of knowledge in discovery and therapeutics, as well as enhancing further research in human health, changing clinical practice guidelines, and rational health and healthcare policy development (science-based policies). With enhanced responsibility of TransEpi, there remains a shared focus and pathways with consequentialist epidemiology.

15.7   Summary

Epidemiology of consequence primarily encourages epidemiologic studies to be conducted not for studies' sake but to improve population health. This approach recommends causal inference and global epidemiologic investigation in addressing health problems in the populations at greatest risk.

Philosophically, two research traditions have been applied in epidemiologic investigation, namely, deontologic and consequentialist. While the later applied the concept of the end justifying the means, deontologic tradition stresses rigorous methods implying appropriate means in arriving at the end.

The goal of epidemiology is to assess disease distribution and determinants at the population level and to apply this knowledge in intervention mapping to control disease and promote health. Epidemiology of consequence thus reaffirms the overall goal of epidemiology with more emphasis on intervention research and population health improvement.

While we support consequentialist epidemiologic approach, we caution the superficial use of this pathway in deemphasizing the need for rigorous statistical modeling in the conduct of epidemiologic studies. With this balance, epidemiology could exert its responsibility as a profession in public health indicative to improve population health.

Questions for discussion

1 Compare and contrast between deontological and consequentialist approach to evidence discovery in clinical research.
2 Suppose you are required reduce the incidence of sudden infant death syndrome in the populations at risk, outline the steps necessary to accomplish this task using epidemiology of consequence approach.
3 The director of population health at a pediatric health system requests your assistance in improving asthma readmission rate. Using the deontological approach, suggest a feasible approach in achieving this.
4 Two drugs are developed to control BP. Drug A was administered to 100 participants and illustrated a mean systolic BP reduction of 2 units ($p < 0.0001$), while drug B was administered to 25 patients and showed a mean systolic BP reduction of 10 units ($p = 0.25$). Which of these two drugs would you recommend for BP control? Should you prefer drug A or B, please provide the rationale. Additionally, if you prefer none of these agents, provide the rationale.
5 If you are required to design a course in epidemiology for medical students, please provide an outline of such course to reflect the goal of epidemiologic of consequence.

References

1. Epidemiologic Society of London, *Transactions of the Epidemiological Society of London: Sessions 1866 to 1876: Objects of the Epidemiological Society* (London, UK, 1876).
2. S. Scheffler, *Consequentialsm and Its Critiques* (New York: Oxford University Press, 1988).
3. A. F. Karatas, L. Miller, L. Holmes Jr. et al., "Cerebral Palsy Patients Discovered Dead During Sleep: Experience from a Comprehensive Tertiary Pediatric Center," *J Pediatr Rehabil Med* 6 (4) (2013): 225–231.
4. B. Borkhuu, D. Nagaraju, F. F. Miller, M. H. Moamed Ali, D. Pressel, J. Adelizzi-Delany, M. Miccolis, K. Dabney, and L. Holmes Jr., "Prevalence and Risk Factors in Postoperative Pancreatitis after Spine Fusion in Patients with Cerebral Palsy," *J Pediatr Orthop* 29 (3) (2009): 256–262. doi: 10.1097/BPO.0b013e31819bcf0a
5. K. M. Keyes and S. Galea, *Epidemiology Matters: A New Introduction to Methodological Foundations* (New York: Oxford University Press, 2014).
6. K. Keyes and S. Galea, "What Matters Most: Quantifying an Epidemiology of Consequence," *Ann Epidemiol* 25 (2015): 305–311. doi: 10.1016/j.annepidem .2015.01.016. Epub 2015 Feb 7. Review. PMID: 25749559
7. US Preventive Services Task. Genetic risk assessment and BRCA mutation testing for breast and ovarian cancer susceptibility. Washington, DC: US Preventive Service Task Force, 2005. (http://www.ahrq.gov/clinic/upstf/uspsbrgen.htm) (Accessed 6/29/2017) (pubmed—www.ncbi.nlm.nih.gov/pubmed/16144894)

Index

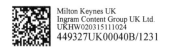
Milton Keynes UK
Ingram Content Group UK Ltd.
UKHW020315111024
449327UK00040B/1231